Measurement Concepts
in Physical Education and Exercise Science

Margaret J. Safrit, PhD
University of Wisconsin-Madison
Terry M. Wood, PhD
Oregon State University

Human Kinetics Books
Champaign, Illinois

Library of Congress Cataloging-in-Publication Data

Measurement concepts in physical education and exercise science /
   edited by Margaret J. Safrit, Terry M. Wood.
      p. cm.
   Bibliography: p.
   ISBN 0-87322-223-7
   1. Physical fitness—Testing.   2. Physical education and training-
-Evaluation.   I. Safrit, Margaret J., 1935-   . II. Wood, Terry
M., 1949-   .
   GV436.M42 1989
   613.7'1—dc19   88-39286
                                                               CIP

Developmental Editor: Joanne Fetzner
Production Director: Ernie Noa
Managing Editor: Kathy Kane
Copyeditor: Steve Otto
Assistant Editors: Valerie Hall and Holly Gilly
Typesetter: Impressions
Text Design: Keith Blomberg
Cover Design: Hunter Graphics
Printed By: R.R. Donnelley

ISBN: 0-87322-223-7

Printed in the United States of America

10 9 8 7 6 5 4 3 2 1

Human Kinetics Books
A Division of Human Kinetics Publishers, Inc.
Box 5076, Champaign, IL 61820
1-800-DIAL-HKP
1-800-334-3665 (in Illinois)

Contents

Chapter 3   Norm-Referenced Measurement: Reliability   **45**

Ted A. Baumgartner

Chapter 4   Generalizability Theory   **73**

James R. Morrow, Jr.

Chapter 5   The Use of Validity Generalization in Exercise Science   **97**

Patricia Patterson

Chapter 10   Analyzing Change   207
Robert W. Schutz

Chapter 11   New Approaches to Solving Measurement Problems   229
Judith A. Spray

Section V   Applied Measurement and Evaluation   249

Chapter 12   Measurement Methodology for Knowledge Tests   251
Dale P. Mood

Chapter 13   Measurement Methodology for Affective Tests   271
Jack K. Nelson

About the Co-Editors

 Margaret J. "Jo" Safrit is the Henry-Bascom Professor in the Department of Physical Education and Dance at the University of Wisconsin-Madison. Her areas of expertise are measurement and evaluation, in particular as they are applied to the performance of motor tasks in sport, exercise, and fundamental movement patterns. Dr. Safrit was elected a Fellow in the American Academy of Physical Education in 1980 and was the AAHPERD Alliance Scholar in 1986–87. She received the first Measurement and Evaluation Council Honor Award in 1987. In her leisure time, Jo enjoys jogging, reading, and gardening.

 Terry M. Wood is an assistant professor and the microcomputer laboratory coordinator in the College of Health and Physical Education at Oregon State University. Specializing in measurement and evaluation, computer applications, and research methods, he earned BA, BPE, and MPE degrees from the University of British Columbia and a PhD from the University of Wisconsin-Madison. Dr. Wood is a graduate fellow at both the University of British Columbia and the University of Wisconsin and is an active member of the Measurement Council and Research Consortium of the American Alliance for Health, Physical Education, Recreation and Dance; the American Educational Research Association; and the National Council on Measurement in Education. He has published manuscripts and presented scholarly papers at the state and national levels and is currently a reviewer for *Research Quarterly for Exercise and Sport* and the *Journal of Physical Education, Recreation and Dance*.

About the Authors

Ted A. Baumgartner earned a BS from Oklahoma State University, an MS from Southern Illinois University, and a PhD from the University of Iowa. He was a member of the faculty at Indiana University from 1967 to 1977; since 1977 he has been on the faculty at the University of Georgia. Dr. Baumgartner has published numerous articles on measurement issues in the *Research Quarterly for Exercise and Sport*, for which he has been a reviewer for over 15 years. He is also co-author of *Measurement for Evaluation in Physical Education and Exercise Science*. Dr. Baumgartner is a member of the American Academy of Physical Education.

James Disch is an associate professor of human performance and master of Richardson College at Rice University in Houston, Texas. A native Houstonian, Dr. Disch was a cum laude graduate of the University of Houston, majoring in physical education and mathematics. He received his MEd from the University of Houston and his PED from Indiana University in measurement and biomechanics. A member of AAHPERD since 1969, Dr. Disch has served as secretary of the Southern District Research Council and chairman of the National Measurement and Evaluation Council. He has consulted for Health and Tennis Corporation of America and the Athletic Congress and is the author of numerous articles and presentations. He has also served as a statistical advisor for the Dallas Cowboys and the Houston Astros. Dr. Disch's primary area of research is prediction in sport, particularly as related to volleyball playing capacity.

 Whitfield B. "Chip" East earned his BA and MA from the University of North Carolina, Chapel Hill, and his EdD from the University of Georgia. Dr. East is currently an associate professor and the chairperson of the Department of Physical Education and Recreation at East Tennessee State University and is serving as chairperson of the Measurement and Evaluation Council of ARAPCS. Dr. East teaches measurement and evaluation, research design, and statistics and has conducted research in grading and evaluation, including estimating skill improvement from measures of pre- and postinstructional scores.

 Larry D. Hensley, a native of Texas, received his master's degree from Indiana University and his doctorate from the University of Georgia. He is currently an associate professor and coordinator of the graduate programs in health and physical education at the University of Northern Iowa. Primarily interested in applied research in measurement and evaluation, Dr. Hensley has been involved with the development of a number of sports skills tests and has recently focused his research activities on grading practices in physical education. He has published a number of articles and made numerous presentations at professional conferences; recently he served as president of the Iowa AHPERD. Formerly a ranked badminton player, he now enjoys racquetball and golf as well.

 Andrew S. "Tony" Jackson received his doctorate from Indiana University in 1969 and is a professor in the Department of Health and Human Performance at the University of Houston. He also holds a full (adjunct) professorship in the Department of Medicine at Baylor College of Medicine. He is a fellow of the American College of Sports Medicine and the American Academy of Physical Education. Dr. Jackson has published extensively in the areas of exercise physiology, cardiology, and human factors and is best known for his research on the measurement of body composition. He is a research consultant to the Cardio-Pulmonary Laboratory at NASA/Johnson Space Center, the Section of Cardiology of the Kelsey-Sybold Clinic, Shell Oil Company, and the Diet Modification Clinic of Baylor College of Medicine. A computer enthusiast, he is a member of the "Macintosh cult."

 Harry A. King received the BSc degree in pure mathematics/physics from the University of Wales (where he was a universities international soccer player), an MSc in kinesiology from Simon Fraser University (Canada), and a PhD from the University of Iowa. He spent 5 years working in English schools, teaching the sciences and coaching soccer, rugby, sailing, swimming, and other activities. In 1978 he joined the physical education department at San Diego State University. His research has concerned the application of quantitative and computer methods to physical education, though his current interests favor a humanistic perspective toward these measurement technologies. In heaven he intends to spend the first million years perfecting his tennis game.

Marilyn A. Looney earned her doctorate in physical education from Indiana University. Her research interests concern reliability and validity issues of criterion-referenced measurement and the application of generalizability theory. Dr. Looney is a fellow of the American Alliance for Health, Physical Education, Recreation and Dance Research Consortium and has been a member of the Measurement and Evaluation Advisory Committee. She currently teaches at Northern Illinois University. Racquet sports, whitewater rafting, and golf are her favorite recreational activities.

Rosemary McGee, whose work focuses on the practical application of measurement in school settings, is a well-known contributor to the field of measurement and evaluation. She has coauthored several books and articles that encourage the testing of both skills and knowledge, as well as the increased use of affective measures, in physical education. Dr. McGee earned her PhD from the University of Iowa and is professor emeritus of physical education at the University of North Carolina at Greensboro, where she taught from 1954 to 1988. She also serves as an evaluation and curriculum consultant.

In 1970, **Dale P. Mood** received his PhD in physical education with an emphasis in measurement and statistics from the University of Iowa. Since then he has been a member of the faculty of the University of Colorado in Boulder, serving as chair of the Boulder Faculty Assembly from 1983 to 1985 and as chair of the Department of Kinesiology since 1982. He has been active in many aspects of the American Alliance for Health, Physical Education, Recreation and Dance at both state and national levels, holding numerous offices including president of the Association for Research, Administration, Professional Councils and Societies. His research interests include developing tests for use in predicting sports performance, measuring physical fitness parameters, and applying statistical techniques to measurement in the cognitive domain. Dr. Mood has made over 20 national or international presentations, published over 40 articles, and authored two college-level textbooks. He lives with his wife and five children in Boulder, where he enjoys running and hiking.

James R. Morrow, Jr. earned his doctorate in education research and evaluation methodology from the University of Colorado. He has taught since 1976 at the University of Houston, where he serves as the associate department chair and the graduate coordinator of physical education. His research interests are measurement and research in exercise science. He has published packages related to assessment in exercise science and youth fitness. He is a fellow in both the American College of Sports Medicine and the Research Consortium of the American Alliance for Health, Physical Education, Recreation and Dance.

Jack K. Nelson is a professor of physical education at Louisiana State University. He received his doctorate from the University of Oregon, where he studied under H. Harrison Clarke. His research interests are in the measurement of physical fitness and sport skills, primarily as they apply to field tests. Dr. Nelson has coauthored four books in the areas of measurement, fitness, and research and has written numerous articles in professional journals. He enjoys tennis, running, golf, and other outdoor activities.

Patricia Patterson received her doctorate in assessment from the University of Wisconsin-Madison in 1985 and teaches at San Diego State University. Her research interests include sequential testing, item response theory, and validity generalization, with a particular emphasis on the application of these approaches to exercise science. Dr. Patterson is also a consultant in dance exercise. Her recreational pursuits include distance running, aerobic dance, and weight training.

Robert W. Schutz received an MSc Degree from the University of Alberta and a PhD from the University of Wisconsin. Since 1970 he has been on the faculty of the University of British Columbia (School of Physical Education and Recreation, Department of Sport Science). Dr. Schutz's research activities fall into three general areas: applied statistics (focusing on multivariate procedures and repeated measures analyses), mathematical analyses of sport, and the measurement of attitudes. He has published methodological papers in a variety of disciplines and is on the editorial board of a number of journals. He is a member of the American Statistical Association, a Fellow of the American Academy of Physical Education, and active in numerous national and international scholarly organizations.

Judy Spray is a research psychologist at the American College Testing Program in Iowa City, Iowa. She earned her doctorate in measurement and assessment at the University of Wisconsin-Madison and taught measurement and research technique courses at the University of Iowa and San Diego State University before assuming her research position with ACT. Dr. Spray has also taught and coached in the state of Arizona and is an avid golfer.

Preface

Although many textbooks have been written on the practical applications of measurement in physical education, never before has a book been devoted primarily to concepts of measurement in physical education and exercise science. The knowledge base has been growing for many years, but this knowledge has been accessible only through original journal articles and, to a lesser extent, chapters in books dealing with measurement theory. The idea for this book was conceived out of a felt need for a concise reference that could be used by students in graduate measurement courses in physical education and exercise science as well as by scholars in the field. The book is intended for the non-specialist in measurement; therefore, the coverage of measurement theory will be basic and limited to theories most directly relevant in physical education and exercise science.

One of the strengths of the book is the authors' high level of expertise. All are prominent measurement specialists in physical education and exercise science. Many authors have themselves written textbooks in measurement at the undergraduate level. A vast amount of knowledge, insight, and experience has been brought together in this treatise.

The first section of the book provides an overview of the scope of measurement as it applies to exercise, sport, and other forms of physical activity. A distinction is made between applied and theoretical research in measurement, although most of the research that has been conducted has direct application to measurement problems in our field. In the second section, one of the long-standing approaches to measurement—norm-referenced measurement—is covered. This approach is discussed within the context of classical test theory (CTT) and an extension of CTT known as generalizability theory. Applications to physical education and exercise science are included throughout these four chapters, along with step-by-step procedures for carrying out validity and reliability studies.

Criterion-referenced measurement, a more recently emphasized approach to measurement in our field, is the topic of the third section. Although research on mastery testing of motor tasks has not been extensive, the practical use of this form of testing is prevalent in school settings. Once again, examples and explicit procedures are set forth.

The fourth section deals with advanced measurement and statistics. Each of the four chapters in this section were included because past experience has demonstrated the versatility of several statistical methods in the physical education and exercise setting. The first chapter deals with multivariate statistical techniques, particularly those that can be used to establish construct validity. Applications of regression analysis to exercise science, primarily in the context of predictive validity, are explored in the second chapter. This is followed by an examination of one of the long-standing problems in measurement—the analysis of change. The section ends with a discussion of new approaches to solving measurement problems in our field, such as item response theory and sequential testing.

In the fifth and final section, selected applied measurement and evaluation methods are examined. The traditional areas of human behavior—cognitive, affective, and psychomotor—form the basis of the first three chapters. The focus of the section then shifts to an evaluation topic of great interest in our field—program evaluation. Various program evaluation models are described and compared. The final chapter is devoted to the use of computers in measurement.

To facilitate reading this book, an explanation of the use of boldface type and italics follows. Words in boldface type are key words which are defined in the glossary at the end of the book. Italics are used in a more general way. Words are italicized for emphasis, but are not necessarily defined in the glossary.

Grateful appreciation is expressed to all authors for their outstanding contributions to this book. In addition to the editors, who are also authors, the group of contributors consists of Ted A. Baumgartner, University of Georgia; James R. Morrow, Jr., University of Houston; Patricia Patterson, San Diego State University; Marilyn A. Looney, Northern Illinois University; James Disch, Rice University; Andrew S. Jackson, University of Houston; Robert W. Schutz, University of British Columbia; Judith A. Spray, American College Testing; Dale P. Mood, University of Colorado; Jack K. Nelson, Louisiana State University; Whitfield B. East, East Tennessee State University; Larry D. Hensley, Northern Iowa University; Rosemary McGee, University of North Carolina at Greensboro; and Harry A. King, San Diego State University.

Gratitude is also extended to the staff at Human Kinetics Publishers, Inc. for their assistance in developing and producing this book. Special thanks go to Rainer Martens for his encouragement of the editors and to Joanne Fetzner for her competent work as developmental editor. Special thanks also go to the reviewers of the book for their careful analyses and helpful input.

Margaret J. Safrit
Terry M. Wood

The Scope of Measurement in Physical Education and the Exercise Sciences

Measurement plays an important role in both physical education and research dealing with human movement studies and the exercise sciences. This role is delineated in chapter 1 of the book by Margaret J. Safrit, a co-editor of the book. Safrit provides a rationale for the study of advanced topics in measurement and properly identifies measurement as a subdisciplinary area of study in physical education and exercise science. It is an area possessing a broad theoretical base. A brief overview of a few measurement theories is presented by Safrit, followed by a description of applied and theoretical research in the measurement of motor behavior. Several terms basic to the study of measurement are also defined. This introductory material sets the stage for the remainder of the book.

CHAPTER 1

An Overview of Measurement

Margaret J. Safrit
University of Wisconsin, Madison

Most of the activities undertaken in physical education and exercise science involve measurement. Data are collected from subjects in an experiment, test scores are obtained from students in a physical education class, measures of fitness are administered to members of a fitness club, and so forth. The goal is the same in all of these instances: to measure as accurately and precisely as possible the underlying attribute of interest. In certain areas of specialization, such as exercise physiology, it is often possible to measure the attribute directly; in other areas, such as sport psychology, many attributes must be measured indirectly. Yet the basic concepts of measurement apply to all areas. In designing a study, measurement principles are as important as the research design, experimental protocol, and statistical analyses. Indeed, paying careful attention only to the latter three components may be worthless if measurement principles are ignored. In the absence of valid and reliable measures, the results of a study are meaningless. The importance of measurement is equally relevant in other career options in physical education and exercise science. For example, it would be hazardous to prescribe an exercise program for a person based on inappropriate or improperly administered measures. Measurement pervades every corner of our field.

This chapter is divided into two major subsections. The first subsection is an introductory overview of the field of measurement, from both an applied and a theoretical perspective. The second subsection contains basic measurement definitions and concepts that should be mastered before reading the remainder of the book.

Overview of the Measurement Area

Measurement as a formal area of study has never been clearly defined in physical education and exercise science. There is no label to represent the study of measurement of motor behavior. Measurement can be considered in a generic sense, and basic concepts such as validity and reliability within various measurement theories can be described. However, many measurement specialists in other disciplines are affiliated with a field of study in addition to measurement. While they may undertake basic work in measurement, it is often pursued to solve a measurement problem in their field. Thus, measurement may be subsumed under a field and renamed (e.g, psychology, psychometrics, economics, econometrics). Although efforts have been made to propose a comparable name for measurement in physical education and exercise science, these labels have never been well received. Two examples proposed in the past are physical edumetrics and psychomotormetrics.

Aside from not having a widely accepted label to identify the measurement of motor behavior as an area of study, measurement frequently is perceived as an atheoretical area of specialization. There are probably several reasons for this perception. First, many scholars have viewed measurement merely as a tool to be used in answering questions in other areas of specialization. This view still persists to some extent in our field. Second—and this is tied to the first reason—few scholars understand theoretical work in measurement. At best there may be a vague awareness of one or two measurement models, but the idea of developing and refining these models under experimental conditions is almost unheard of in physical education and exercise science. Third, scholars identified as measurement specialists in our field have, in the past, dealt primarily with applied measurement research rather than theoretical research. Furthermore, until the late 1950s, the most prominent scholars in physical education could be classified as "renaissance" people, who were at the forefront of what would now be considered several areas of specialization. This was possible in those days because the knowledge base in each of the areas was much smaller than it is today. Even today few people in physical education and exercise science identify measurement as their primary area of specialization, and much of their work can be categorized as applied. Applied research is badly needed in measurement, and no negative connotation is intended in referring to this type of work. The distinction between applied and theoretical work is emphasized here to reinforce the fact that measurement models are theoretically based, and applied work is an outgrowth of theory.

Because this chapter serves as an introduction to the book as a whole, it is designed to provide a unifying view of measurement. Although an overall rationale exists for selecting the topics of the remaining chapters, these chapters—taken as a whole—do not necessarily form a complete picture of measurement in physical education and exercise science. No book can do this.

However, it is important for the reader to have a general understanding of the entire area. For example, some very interesting work is being done with measurement models and their appropriateness for measures of motor behavior. Because some of these models are not yet being applied in physical education and exercise science, detailed information on them is not included in this book. But if the reader is to have an accurate perception of the field of measurement, at least a minimal reference to these theoretical approaches must be included. One of the purposes of this chapter is to describe, however briefly, aspects of measurement that may not be dealt with in detail in subsequent chapters.

The next section of this chapter discusses the role of measurement research in physical education and exercise science, and how it has changed over the years. Two categories of research—applied and theoretical—are described. Applied measurement research is presented in a historical context to provide a perspective of (a) the evolution of measurement as a field of study and (b) the breadth of the applied work in the field. Theoretical measurement research is presented in a topical context, although there are historical overtones to this section as well.

Applied Measurement

Early physical educators were interested in measurement, mostly of the physical type. Edward Hitchcock, often called the father of measurement in physical education, used anthropometric measures in his work during the late 1800s. Hitchcock, a medical doctor, was primarily interested in body symmetry and proportion, and prescribed exercise to modify body size. In 1861, he developed standards of age, height, and weight and of chest, arm, and forearm girths. His interests also extended to strength measurement, especially strength of the upper arm. Hitchcock was considered the leading authority in anthropometry during this era. Around the same period, Dudley Sargent developed similar tables of standards at Harvard University. Sargent developed the Intercollegiate Strength Test in the 1870s.

Widespread usage of both strength and anthropometric measurement lagged in the early 1900s. Although interest in the measurement of strength subsequently resumed, anthropometric measures never regained their early prominence. Nonetheless, this type of measure still holds an important place in measuring growth, body composition, and body type.

At the turn of the century, there was considerable interest in measuring cardiorespiratory function. This was made possible by the development of endurance measures and heart and lung tests. At the time there was a general perception that strength development was overemphasized. Athletes were thought to become muscle bound—a condition that hindered athletic performance—as a result of strength exercises. The first test of cardiac function, the Blood Ptosis Test, was developed by C. Ward Crampton in 1905. Crampton noted changes in cardiac rate and arterial pressure on assuming the erect position from a supine position. In the 1920s more sophisticated work was published on the measurement of physical efficiency. E.C. Schneider designed a test used in aviation in World War I to determine fatigue and physical condition for flying. The relationship between pulse rate and blood pressure in the reclining position and the standing position was determined, along with the ability to recover to normal standing values after a measured bout of exercise. In 1931 W.W. Tuttle modified a block-stepping test, similar to a step test, that measured endurance and the general state of training. This was known as the Tuttle Pulse-Ratio Test—a forerunner of the Harvard Step Test, which was developed in 1943. The efficiency of the circulatory system was indicated by the increase in heart rate during exercise and the speed with which the heart rate returned to a normal rate after exercise. Work in this area became increasingly sophisticated with the development of the Balke Treadmill Test in 1954 and other similar measures. Maximal stress tests on a treadmill still represent the standard for measuring cardiorespiratory function in a laboratory setting.

Turning to the development of tests of sports skills, the earliest versions of these tests were developed as part of athletic performance batteries. For example, in 1913 the Athletic Badge Tests were published by the Playground and Recreation Association of America. David Brace, who spent most of his career at the University of Texas, made one of the first systematic attempts to measure a group of fundamental skills for a specific sport (basketball) in 1924. He also worked on the development of tests for indoor baseball and soccer. In their 1930 measurement textbook, Bovard and Cozens noted that the area of skills testing was relatively untouched. They identified 1916 as the approximate year in which the physical education curriculum was broadened to include games and sports. Because of this curricular expansion, they noted, physical educators needed to be prepared to measure sports skills and other aspects of physical activity. Although some tests were developed during this time, many were not published. Skills test development was emphasized at the University of Wisconsin during those years; Ruth Glassow and Marion Broer published a measurement book in 1938 that was devoted almost entirely to skills tests and batteries. Charles McCloy at the University of Iowa strongly criticized the subjective measurement of skill in his 1939 textbook, as did Harrison Clarke (University of Oregon) in his 1945 textbook. Subsequently, Gladys Scott and her students at the University of Iowa made many contributions to the development of skills tests in the field of physical education. A number of these tests were described in the 1959 textbook by Scott and French.

Unfortunately, the development of sports skills tests has never been systematically undertaken by physical educators, with the exception of the AAHPERD Measurement and Evaluation Council. As a result, most skills tests have been developed by graduate students, experts in a sport with a special interest in testing, and interest groups usually sponsored by the American Alliance for Health, Physical Education, Recreation and Dance. Thus, test development has been sporadic and has not been based on a standard set of criteria. The Alliance has made an effort to fill the void in the skills-testing area by publishing a series of skills test batteries in a variety of sports. However, most of these manuals now need to be revised and updated. One of the best sources of sports skills tests is a book by Collins and Hodges (1978). They have attempted to pull together all of the existing tests of sports skills.

After a temporary lag in the use of strength tests, interest was restored with the development of new tests in the area, such as the Strength Index and Physical Fitness Index developed by Frederick Rand Rogers around 1925. This type of measurement became much more precise with the development of cable tensiometer tests by Harrison Clarke. Clarke's innovative thinking led to the design of equipment allowing an investigator to measure the strength of many different body parts. As more sophisticated equipment (e.g., dynamometers and weight training machines) was made available to the physical educator, other approaches to testing strength became feasible.

Physical fitness testing has received the greatest emphasis of any type of test used in practical settings in physical education and exercise science. Historically, national interest in physical fitness has peaked during times of war, when many men have been unable to meet the physical requirements of the draft. This inability has focused the attention of government officials on the level of physical fitness of American citizens. After World War II, President Eisenhower strongly advocated the development of physical fitness throughout the United States. His support was partly a reaction to the results of the Kraus-Weber Test, which when administered to elementary school children in the United States and Europe resulted in the superior performance of European children. Interestingly, the Kraus-Weber Test was not designed as a measure of overall physical fitness, but rather as a measure of minimal functioning of the low back area. More valid tests of physical fitness have been developed since. In the 1970s interest in fitness surged throughout the United States, although the emphasis was tied more closely to personal health and well-being than fitness for fighting wars.

Recently many changes have taken place in the development and promotion of physical fitness tests for children and youth. Two familiar tests no longer exist in their original form. The Youth Fitness Test (AAHPERD, 1976) was designed to measure both performance and health-related physical fitness. This test was sponsored by the Alliance and by the President's Council on Physical Fitness and Sports. The Health-Related Physical Fitness Test (AAHPERD, 1980) was sponsored by the Alliance and by the Institute for Aerobics Research. Efforts in 1987 and 1988 to promote a national youth fitness test were unsuccessful. As a result, five tests have now been published by various agencies. The Alliance proposed the AAHPERD Physical Best Program (AAHPERD, 1988), which includes a health-related physical fitness test. This test is similar to the FITNESSGRAM test (Institute for Aerobics Research, 1987) and the Fit Youth Today test (American Health and Fitness Foundation, 1986). The President's Council (1987) and Chrysler/AAU (1987) also published revised versions of fitness tests. In general, the test batteries are more alike than different with regard to the components of physical fitness they measure. A much greater emphasis is now placed on fitness education rather than stressing only the tests used to measure fitness. Although advances in the development and use of physical fitness tests in the United States have been impressive, much remains to be done.

One other type of testing in physical education has not yet been mentioned: the measurement of general motor ability. Motor ability is an expression that was familiar to physical educators in the early 1900s. As early as 1894 the Normal School of Gymnastics in Milwaukee and the Gymnastics Societies in Cleveland administered batteries of tests that measured ability in jumping, climbing, shot-putting, lifting, and so forth.

As time passed, many schools began to institute testing programs, including basic events in track and field. Most of the test batteries developed then had many similarities, and none of the original batteries was based on sound test development as we know it today. However, the test technology used in those days represented the best scientific thinking at the time. In the 1930s, test batteries purporting to measure basic motor ability were published, based on a more substantial scientific rationale. Although the overall validity of these batteries was never firmly established, the popularity of the concept of motor ability continued into the late 1950s. At that time emerging research evidence called the concept into question. The idea of general motor ability, while intuitively appealing, has never been verified scientifically.

In summary, most of the applied work in measurement has revolved around the development of tests, including the determination of test validity and reliability. A few studies have been published on test objectivity, especially when the use of judges or observers is part of the measurement process. In the exercise sciences, considerable work has been published on the development and improvement of instrumentation used to measure physical and physiological parameters. Little work has been devoted to knowledge test development, although a book published by McGee and Farrow (1987) reproduces many knowledge tests in physical education and is a useful contribution to the field. Finally, research has been conducted on the application of various measurement theories to measures of motor performance. This type of research is described in the next section.

Theoretical Measurement

An overview of measurement models. Any well-developed test is based on a measurement model. If test validity and reliability have been obtained, the procedures for estimating these characteristics are dictated by the model. This fact is often not recognized by test users and even by some test developers. Many physical educators and exercise scientists do not realize that most of the tests developed in their respective areas are based on classical test theory. Each model has a unique set of assumptions and is based on a mathematical model.

The most widely used models in our field have been those derived from classical test theory. They have been the basis of psychometrics for over 75 years. Classical test theory is built around the concept of a true score and an error score. The obtained score, the score an examinee actually obtains on a test, consists of a true score component and an error score component. The true score is the score the examinee would have made if no measurement error existed. The error score is attributed to measurement error.

Three basic assumptions underlie classical test theory: (a) The true score is independent of the error score; (b) the mean of error scores is zero; and (c) error scores from different distributions of the same test are independent of one another. The development of this test technology was initiated by Charles Spearman in the early 1900s. Conceptually, the individual differences approach to testing was developed by Alfred Binet. This theory, which has appealed to psychologists for many decades, is based on the notion that because individuals differ on various traits, a good test should reflect these differences. Procedurally this is accomplished by examining an individual's observed score relative to the score of others in a group of examinees. The popular term *norm-referenced measurement* describes an implementation of classical test theory.

Measurement models can be classified into two categories: weak true-score models and strong true-score models. The terms *weak* and *strong* refer to the assumptions underlying the model. The assumptions of a weak model are not rigorous and can be met by many data sets; the assumptions of a strong model are satisified only under limited conditions.

Of the strong true-score models, the binomial error model has been used to develop criterion-referenced tests. Although some research has been done on criterion-referenced measurement (CRM) in physical education and exercise science, very few tests of this type have been published. Yet physical educators seem to find this approach to testing intuitively appealing.

A powerful measurement theory that has been studied extensively in education and psychology in recent years, with very little attention from physical education and the exercise sciences, is item response theory (IRT), also known as latent trait theory. It is an appealing approach to measurement in our field, because it specifies a relationship between an observable examinee test performance and the unobservable trait or ability assumed to underlie performance on the test. This relationship is described by a mathematical function; thus, IRT is a mathematical model, based on specific assumptions about the test data. A large number of choices are available for the mathematical form of the relationship; thus, a family of IRT models exists. Because an examinee's ability level on a trait can be estimated from a test score, this provides a sophisticated means of testing motor behavior that has not been available previously.

Theoretical measurement research. Modest amounts of theoretical work in measurement have been undertaken in physical education and exercise science from the 1940s to the present. In 1947 Brosek and Alexander published an article describing the use of analysis of variance to estimate the reliability of repeated measures. The application of this approach to measures of motor behavior was described in 1958 by Feldt and McKee. This work was extended to include the use of trend analysis to obtain a more complete picture of repeated measures data (Alexander, 1947; Baumgartner & Jackson, 1970; Liba, 1962). Kroll (1967) also described this procedure in several articles. Eventually a monograph was published describing several models that could be used to estimate reliability (Safrit, Atwater, Baumgartner, & West, 1976). An overview of generalizability theory, an extension of the analysis of variance approach, was also included in this monograph. Although generalizability theory was not developed by these measurement specialists, the first discussion of this theory directed to physical educators was presented in the monograph. More recently, theoretical work has been done on generalizability theory. This includes a description of various models of generalizability theory (Godbout & Schutz, 1983) and an empirical study comparing two indices of dependability from criterion-referenced generalizability theory (Patterson & Safrit, 1987a, 1987b). Several applied studies using generalizability theory have also been published in our field (Morrow, Fridye, & Monaghen, 1986; Mosher & Schutz, 1983; Oppliger & Spray, 1987; Stamm & Moore, 1980; Stamm & Kelso, 1978; Taylor, 1979). A multivariate approach for estimating the reliability of batteries of psychomotor tests was explicated, tested, and applied in a practical setting (Safrit & Wood, 1987; Wood & Safrit, 1984; Wood & Safrit, 1987).

Construct validity has been explored, often with the use of multivariate techniques (Korell & Safrit, 1977; Safrit, Korell, McDonald, & Yeates, 1977; Safrit, Stamm, Russell, & Sloan, 1977). A number of factor analytic studies have been published, some of which are exemplary in nature (Disch, Frankiewicz, & Jackson, 1975; Jackson & Coleman, 1976; Safrit, Wood, & Dishman, 1985). More recently, studies of predictive validity have been undertaken in employment settings (Laughery & Jackson, 1984; Jackson, 1986).

As criterion-referenced measurement (CRM) became a heavily researched topic in other areas, the use of this model was explored in a physical education setting (Safrit, 1977). CRM reliability estimates, P and k, were compared (Safrit & Stamm, 1980; Safrit, Stamm, & Douglass, 1982) and modifications of these estimates were examined (Looney, 1987). Validity studies were also undertaken (Douglass & Safrit, 1983; Washburn & Safrit, 1982).

Item response theory, also known as latent trait theory, is becoming a topic of great interest in our field. Work on this theory in physical education has been virtually nonexistent, with the exception of two recent studies (Costa, Safrit, & Cohen, 1988; Hooper, 1987).

An introductory article on item response theory by Spray (1987) along with a series of responses to her article (Disch, 1987; Safrit, 1987; Wood, 1987) provided the first overview of this theory and its potential application to measures of motor behavior. A tutorial (Safrit, Costa, & Cohen, in press), describing in more detail the application of item response theory in psychomotor testing, included a step-by-step approach to using one of the models.

Other areas of research include measures of error in motor control (Gessaroli & Schutz, 1984; Safrit, Spray, & Diewert, 1980; Schutz, 1974; Spray, 1987) and several spin-offs of criterion-referenced measurement. One is sequential testing, which is a general approach to making classification decisions when repeated measures are obtained. Two sequential testing models have been studied: the sequential probability ratio test (Safrit, Wood, Patterson, Ehlert, & Hooper, 1985); and inverse sampling, also known as the trials-to-criterion testing (Spray, Sorenson, & Hooper, 1986; Shifflett, 1985). Very little has been done in physical education and exercise science to develop and promote new measurement models especially designed for motor performance data. The one prominent exception is the work of Spray (e.g., 1982, 1987).

The interest in meta-analytic techniques for analyzing a group of research studies spawned an interest in examining the validity of all studies of a specific test. This process is known as the validity generalization model. A tutorial-type paper directed to the exercise scientist has recently been published (Safrit, Costa, & Hooper, 1986), and a large-scale study of the generalizability of distance run tests has been conducted (Safrit, Costa, Hooper, Patterson, & Ehlert, 1988). The measurement of change has also been a research topic of interest in our field. Two theoretical models for measuring change have been proposed (Hale & Hale, 1972; East, 1985), and one of these models has been examined in an applied setting (Wells & Baumgartner, 1974).

Although many measurement topics have received theoretical consideration in our field, none of this work has been extensive. There is a great need for systematic research on a variety of topics of this nature. Furthermore, the exploration of new or little-known measurement theories that might be more appropriate for the measurement of motor behavior should be stressed, as Spray (1987) has advocated repeatedly. On the positive side, some interesting new exploratory work in measurement could have a major impact on the field in future years.

Measurement Definitions and Concepts

Now that an overview of measurement as a disciplinary area has been presented, a few basic terms will be defined and exemplified. Measurement is typically defined as the process of assigning numbers to properties of objects, organisms, or events according to some rule. It must be possible to define the attribute in quantifiable terms, so that a meaningful interpretation can be given to a comparison of the magnitude of any two scores on the attribute. This definition also calls for the use of a defined unit of measurement.

Nunnally (1978) presents a useful summary of the advantages of measurement. They include objectivity, quantification, communication, economy, and scientific generalization. Measurement leads to *objectivity* by allowing educators and scientists to make statements that can be verified independently by their colleagues.

Another advantage of measurement is that the process of *quantification* permits educators and scientists to report results with greater precision. Of greater significance is the fact that powerful methods of mathematical analysis can be used with the data when results are quantified. A third advantage, *communication*, refers to the usefulness of standardized measures in permitting an accurate comparison of results. When means and standard deviations of the same measure can be compared across studies (rather than subjective observations of the attribute), this leads to precise rather than general communication. A fourth advantage is that measurement is more *economical* of time and money than subjective evaluation.

A final advantage is *scientific generalization*. A scientist cannot develop a network of principles and laws without standardized measurement methods based on precise operational definitions. Appropriate measurement methodology is basic to the development of theory. For example, a sport psychologist may formulate hypotheses about the validity of arousal theory in a sport setting. To test these hypotheses, a satisfactory measure of arousal must be developed for the sport-specific setting. In the absence of appropriate measures, theories cannot be developed and expanded.

Two additional terms are important for understanding the next section: evaluation and statistics. *Evaluation* is the process of making judgments about the results of measurement in terms of the purpose of measuring. *Statistics* is a method of summarizing and analyzing data for purposes of interpretation. Statistics used to describe a set of test scores are referred to as descriptive statistics. If test scores are used to make inferences about a population based on the information derived from a sample of examinees, the use of inferential statistics is appropriate.

Measurement Scales

Whenever a measurement instrument is used, a score of some sort is obtained. To interpret a set of scores, one must understand what the score represents. An accurate interpretation depends in part on the type of scale the score reflects. According to the definition of measurement, numbers are assigned according to some rule. The rule for assigning numbers identifies the scale. The rule is determined primarily by the features of the real number series.

Real number series. When numbers are assigned to properties (of objects, people, etc.) so that the relations between the numbers reflect the relations between the properties, the property has been measured. The classification of types of scales is determined by whether the numbers (scores) reflect none, one, two, or all three of the features of the real number system.

The real number system consists of three features: order, distance, and origin.

Order: Numbers are ordered. Higher numbers represent greater amounts of the attribute being measured.

Distance: Differences between pairs of numbers are ordered. That is, the numbers describe the magnitude of the differences among the observational units (Hopkins & Glass, 1978, p. 11).

Origin: The series has a unique origin indicated by the number zero. The zero value represents total absence of the attribute being measured.

Types of scales. Although the possibility of an unlimited number of different types of scales exists, traditionally four types are described. These are nominal, ordinal, interval, and ratio. These scales can be characterized by features of the real number system but also by the range of invariance. Invariance is defined as the kinds of transformations that leave the structure of the scale undistorted.

A **nominal scale** contains none of the three features of the real number system. When objects that have attributes in common are grouped into classes, a nominal scale is formed. The classes are mutually exclusive, meaning that no object can fall into more than one class.

Classifying football players by numbers is an example of nominal scaling. A player who is assigned number 42 is not necessarily better than a player who is assigned number 12. Order is not a feature of the nominal scale, because membership in any one category does not represent greater or lesser magnitude than membership in any other category. As another example, microcomputers in an instructional laboratory might be classified according to whether they have a single disk drive, a dual disk drive, or a single disk drive/hard disk combination. Because order is not a meaningful factor, neither distance nor origin can be features of the nominal scale.

The invariance range of the nominal scale is one of general substitution. Any one-to-one substitution is legitimate and does not change the structure of the scale. One might label the defensive and offensive units of a football team in some other way, but the new labels would not change the common properties associated with the persons belonging to each unit.

Because any number used in nominal scaling is not important in terms of magnitude, the nominal scale should not be subsumed under the label *measurement*, according to some statisticians (e.g., Glass & Stanley, 1970). But because it is impossible to measure human beings in the precise manner of the physical sciences, nominal scales are sometimes useful to educators.

Sometimes nominal scales have an underlying order in a gross sense. For example, students might be classified at a high, medium, or low level of physical fitness. The categories are mutually exclusive, but membership in the high category represents a higher level of fitness than does membership in the low category. This type of scale can be referred to as *quasi-ordinal* or *summated* (Gardner, 1975), falling somewhere between nominal and ordinal.

An **ordinal scale** reflects one feature of the real number series: order. The simplest form of ranking is to order the properties of objects of concern and to assign ranks to these properties. A basketball coach might be asked to rank the basketball teams in a league on the basis of predicted success at the end of the season. If there are ten teams in the league, a rank of one would be assigned to the team that is predicted to win the league title, and a rank of ten to the team predicted to place last. Because a rank of one is better than a rank of two, order is important. However, the first-ranked team may be considerably better than the teams ranked two, three, and four, while the latter three teams might be considered similar in ability. These differences are not reflected in the differences between ranks. Thus distance, the second feature of the real number series, is not a characteristic of ordinal scales.

Ordinal scales are also represented when an attribute is scored rather than ranked, but the differences between the scores have no meaning. When a national press selects all-star teams, each sportswriter votes for a chosen player. Suppose player F receives 232 votes; player R, 190 votes; and player N, 93 votes. Clearly player F is considered outstanding by the largest number of sportswriters, but the number of votes does not disclose how much better player F is than player R. Because the distance between numbers is not meaningful, these scores are ordinal data. Although the actual number of votes may be published by the press, future reference to the all-star players generally centers on the ranks of the players.

Any order-preserving transformation will leave the ordinal scale invariant. The number of votes for our all-star players can be altered in any way we wish as long as the ranking of players remains unchanged. Even though the actual number of votes may be of interest to some people, a player is ranked number one whether he won by 2 votes or 200 votes. Many players will not receive any votes; however, a zero vote does not reflect an absence of ability in football. Thus the third feature of the real number series, origin, is also not a characteristic of ordinal scales, except in special cases where the existence of an absolute origin is indicated.

An **interval scale** has two features of the real number series: order and distance. If a zero point exists, it is a matter of convention or convenience. A child who scores a zero on a test of ball-throwing accuracy probably does not totally lack throwing ability. Thus, origin is not a characteristic of the interval scale.

In addition to having a meaningful order, interval scores have equal distances between scores. That is, the difference between 80° and 70° is the same as the difference between 40° and 30°. The difference between 93 and 90 points on a motor performance test is the same as the distance between 53 and 50. (In reality, the latter statement may not always be true. It may be more difficult to gain 3 points when one's score is 90 than when one's score is 50.)

Any linear transformation of the scale is possible without altering the invariance of the scale. Multiplication or division of each value by a specified number merely changes the unit of measurement. Addition or subtraction of a specified number from each value shifts the origin of the number. We cannot take the ratio of any two values on the scale, because this would change the property of the scale. Because there is an arbitrary origin rather than an absolute origin, one value cannot be described as twice or one-third as much as another. These kinds of comparisons are possible only when a meaningful zero point exists, that is, when zero represents absence of the attribute being measured.

A **ratio scale** has all three features of the real number series. Ratio data are invariant under somewhat more restricted conditions than are interval data. Because an absolute origin (zero equals absence of the attribute measured) is determined, only the unit of measurement is free to vary. Therefore, we cannot add or subtract a given number to each value of the variable without changing the origin, and thus losing one of the properties of the ratio scale. Multiplication and division leave the scale invariant.

Ratio data include measures of length, weight, and time, which frequently are used in measuring motor behavior. There are problems associated with some of the underlying assumptions of ratio data when athletic performance is measured. Consider a field event, the pole vault. Is the difference between an 18 ft, 1 in. and 18 ft, 5 in. pole vault the same as the difference between a 12 ft, 1 in. and 12 ft, 5 in. vault? In terms of distance as a pure measure, they are the same. In terms of performance, the difference at 18 ft is much more significant than the difference at 12 ft. Is a vault of 18 ft twice as good as a vault of 9 ft? In reality, an 18-ft vault is much more than twice as good as a 9-ft vault. In practice these types of scores often are treated as interval data, even though the assumption of equal distance may be violated.

Clearly an attempt to fit all existing data into these four categories is restrictive. This point is reinforced by a number of statisticians (e.g., Glass & Stanley, 1970; Gardner, 1975; Hays, 1981). They stress the importance of judgment in categorizing the scale of measurement used. Gardner used the term *summated scale* to refer to scales that fall between the categories of nominal, ordinal, interval, and ratio. For example, members of a corporate fitness center might be placed into high, medium, and low levels of physical fitness. Although the use of categories points to a nominal scale, in this case there is a meaningful order to the category labels. The data represent a summated scale, which would fall somewhere between the nominal and ordinal scales.

The main point to remember about measurement scales is that the scale should accurately reflect the underlying attribute being measured. If two people receive markedly different scores on a measure of sport competition anxiety, it usually is assumed that they possess different levels of anxiety. If the test is not valid, however, the score differences may be meaningless. In reality, the examinees may be quite similar in their anxiety levels and the scale represented by the test scores not accurately reflective of their real status.

For many years, there was considerable disagreement among statisticians about the appropriate statistics to be used with various scales. One view held that parametric statistics should be used to analyze interval and ratio data, and nonparametric statistics for ordinal data. The other view, now widely accepted, noted that any data set could be analyzed using parametric statistics as long as the underlying assumptions of the statistic were met. This point has been reinforced by many statisticians and was summarized clearly by Gaito (1960). Gaito also reviewed a number of studies demonstrating the conditions under which these assumptions could be violated safely. A more recent overview of the controversy over the limitations that scales of measurement impose on statistical procedures was published by Marcus-Roberts and Roberts (1987).

Discrete and
Continuous Variables

In addition to understanding the properties of the scale used to measure a variable, it is important to identify the variable as continuous or discrete. A **continuous variable** is one that, in theory, can be measured to finer and finer degrees. Many physical measures, such as distance, time, and weight or mass, are examples of continuous variables. The long jump, for example, can be measured to the nearest foot, the nearest inch, the nearest half-inch, and so on.

Discrete variables can assume values only at distinct or discrete points on a scale. A baseball team might get 16 hits during a game but never 16.5 or 16.25 hits. Other examples of discrete variables are the number of students in a class, the number of teams in a league, and the number of books in a library.

It is important to remember that although a *variable* may be either continuous or discrete, the *scores* or measures collected on that variable are always discrete in nature. If times are recorded in some event, such as the 50-yd dash or the 100-m freestyle, the record will consist of discrete times measured to the accuracy permitted by the timing device.

Most of the statistical procedures described in this book deal with test scores that are assumed to come from continuous variables. This assumption is not an unreasonable one and can even be made for some variables that are intuitively discrete. For example, the number of pull-ups or sit-ups an individual can perform in 60 seconds can be considered a continuous variable, even though some fractional part of a pull-up or sit-up has little practical significance.

Conclusion

This chapter was designed to provide an overview of measurement in physical education and exercise science. The initial focus was on applied and theoretical research dealing with the measurement of motor behavior. The applied work was reviewed in a historical context, while the theoretical work was essentially summarized on a topical basis. The need for more research, particularly at the theoretical level, was emphasized. Finally, the framework was laid for a discussion of measurement by defining measurement, describing measurement scales, and differentiating between continuous and discrete measures.

References

Alexander, H.W. (1947). The estimation of reliability when several trials are available. *Psychometrika, 12,* 79–100.

American Alliance for Health, Physical Education, Recreation and Dance (1976). *Youth Fitness Test Manual.* Reston, VA: Author.

American Alliance for Health, Physical Education, Recreation and Dance (1980). *Health-Related Physical Fitness Test Manual.* Reston, VA: Author.

American Alliance for Health, Physical Education, Recreation and Dance (1988). *The AAHPERD Physical Best Program.* Reston, VA: Author.

American Health and Fitness Foundation (1986). *Fit Youth Today.* Austin, TX: Author.

Baumgartner, T.A., & Jackson, A.S. (1970). Measurement schedules for tests of motor performance. *Research Quarterly, 41,* 10–14.

Brosek, J., & Alexander, H. (1947). Components of variation and consistency of repeated measurements. *Research Quarterly, 18,* 152–166.

Chrysler Fund-Amateur Athletic Union (1987). *Physical fitness program.* Bloomington, IN: Author.

Collins, D.R., & Hodges, P.B. (1978). *A comprehensive guide to sports skills tests and measurement.* Springfield, IL: Charles C. Thomas.

Costa, M.G., Safrit, M.J., & Cohen, A.S. (1988). *A comparison of two IRT models used with a measure of motor behavior.* Manuscript submitted for publication.

Disch, J. (1987). Recent developments in measurement and possible applications to the measurement of psychomotor behavior: A response. *Research Quarterly for Exercise and Sport, 58,* 210–212.

Disch, J., Frankiewicz, R., & Jackson, A. (1975). Construct validation of distance run tests. *Research Quarterly, 46*(2), 169–176.

Douglass, J.A., & Safrit, M.J. (1983). An empirical approach to the validation of a criterion-referenced measure of motor performance. *Journal of Human Movement Studies, 9,* 57–69.

East, W. (1985). *Program change.* Johnson City, TN: East Tennessee State University.

Feldt, L.S., & McKee, M.E. (1958). Estimation of the reliability of skills tests. *Research Quarterly, 29*, 279–293.

Gaito, J. (1960). Scale classification and statistics. *Psychological Review, 67*, 277–278.

Gardner, P.L. (1975). Scales and statistics. *Review of Educational Research, 45*, 43–57.

Gessaroli, M., & Schutz, R. (1984). Variable error: A blessing in disguise. In L. Wankel & R. Wilberg (Eds.) *Psychology of sport and motor behavior: Research and practice,* pp. 365–372. Champaign, IL: Human Kinetics.

Glass, G.V., & Stanley, J.C. (1970). *Statistical methods in education and psychology.* Englewood Cliffs, NJ: Prentice-Hall.

Godbout, P., & Schutz, R.W. (1983). Generalizability of ratings of motor performance to various observational designs. *Research Quarterly for Exercise and Sport, 54*, 20–27.

Hale, P.W., & Hale, R.M. (1972). Comparison of student improvement by exponential modification of test-retest scores. *Research Quarterly, 43*, 113–120.

Hays, W.L. (1981). *Statistics* (3rd ed.). Chicago: Holt, Rinehart, and Winston.

Hooper, L.M. (1987). *The sensitivity of two goodness of fit statistics when the local independence assumption is violated.* Unpublished doctoral dissertation, University of Wisconsin, Madison.

Hopkins, K.D., & Glass, G.V. (1978). *Basic statistics for the behavioral sciences.* Englewood Cliffs, NJ: Prentice-Hall.

Institute for Aerobics Research. (1987). *FITNESSGRAM user's manual.* Dallas, TX: Author.

Jackson, A.S. (1986). *Validity of isometric strength tests for predicting work performance in offshore drilling and producing environments.* Houston: Shell Oil Company Technical Report.

Jackson, A.S., & Coleman, A.E. (1976). Validity of distance run tests for children. *Research Quarterly, 47*, 86–94.

Korell, D.M., & Safrit, M.J. (1977). A comparison of seriation and multi-dimensional scaling: Two techniques for validating constructs in physical education. *Research Quarterly, 48*, 333–340.

Kroll, W. (1967). Reliability theory and research decision in selection of a criterion score. *Research Quarterly, 38*, 412–419.

Laughery, K.R., & Jackson, A.S. (1984). *Preemployment physical test development for roustabout jobs on offshore production facilities.* Lafayette, LA: Kerr McGee Corporation Technical Report.

Liba, M. (1962). A trend test as a preliminary to reliability estimation. *Research Quarterly, 33*, 245–248.

Looney, M.A. (1987). Coefficients of agreement: Interpretation differences for reliability applications. *Research Quarterly for Exercise and Sport, 58*, 360–368.

Marcus-Roberts, H.M., & Roberts, F.S. (1987). Meaningless statistics. *Journal of Educational Statistics, 12*, 383–394.

McGee, R., & Farrow, A. (1987). *Test questions for physical education activities.* Champaign, IL: Human Kinetics.

Morrow, J.R., Jr., Fridye, T., & Monaghen, S.D. (1986). Generalizability of the AAHPERD health related skinfold test. *Research Quarterly for Exercise and Sport, 57*, 187–195.

Mosher, R.E., & Schutz, R.W. (1983). The development of a test of overarm throwing: An application of generalizability theory. *Canadian Journal of Applied Sport Sciences*, *8*, 1–8.

Nunnally, J.C. (1978). *Psychometric theory* (2nd ed.). St. Louis: McGraw-Hill.

Patterson, P., & Safrit, M.J. (1987). *The dependability of criterion-referenced test scores in the psychomotor domain using criterion-referenced generalizability theory.* Manuscript submitted for publication.

Patterson, P., & Safrit, M.J. (1987). *A theoretical study of dependability indices using criterion-referenced generalizability theory.* Manuscript submitted for publication.

Oppliger, R.A., & Spray, J.A. (1987). Skinfold measurement variability in body density prediction. *Research Quarterly for Exercise and Sport*, *58*, 178–183.

President's Council on Physical Fitness and Sports. (1987). *The Presidential Physical Fitness Award Program.* Washington, DC: Author.

Safrit, M.J. (1977). Criterion-referenced measurement: Applications in physical education. *Motor Skills: Theory into Practice*, *2*, 17–25.

Safrit, M.J. (1987). The applicability of item response theory to tests of motor behavior. *Research Quarterly for Exercise and Sport*, *58*, 213–215.

Safrit, M.J., Atwater, A.E., Baumgartner, T.A., & West, C. (1976). *Reliability theory.* Washington, DC: American Alliance for Health, Physical Education, and Recreation.

Safrit, M.J., Costa, M.G., & Cohen, A.S. (in press). Item response theory and the measurement of motor behavior. *Research Quarterly for Exercise and Sport*.

Safrit, M.J., Costa, M.G., & Hooper, L.M. (1986). The validity generalization model: An approach to the analysis of validity studies in physical education. *Research Quarterly for Exercise and Sport*, *57*, 288–297.

Safrit, M.J., Costa, M.G., Hooper, L.M., Patterson, P., & Ehlert, S.A. (in press). The validity generalization of distance run tests. *Canadian Journal of Sports Sciences*.

Safrit, M.J., Korell, D.M., McDonald, E.D., & Yeates, M.E. (1977). The participant-observer: A source of invalidity in measuring motor skills. *Perceptual and Motor Skills*, *45*, 75–80.

Safrit, M.J., Spray, J.A., & Diewert, G.L. (1980). Methodological issues in short-term motor memory research. *Journal of Motor Behavior*, *12*, 13–28.

Safrit, M.J., & Stamm, C.L. (1980). Reliability estimates for criterion referenced measures in the psychomotor domain. *Research Quarterly for Exercise and Sport*, *51*, 359–368.

Safrit, M.J., Stamm, C.L., & Douglass, J.A. (1982). The consistency of mastery classifications for a criterion-referenced test of motor behavior: The effect of varying sample size. *Journal of Human Movement Studies*, *7*, 131–143.

Safrit, M.J., Stamm, C.L., Russell, K.R.E., & Sloan, M.R. (1977). Measurement artifacts: The effect of environment and order of testing on the measurement of a gross motor skill. *Research Quarterly*, *48*, 376–381.

Safrit, M.J., & Wood, T.M. (1987). The test battery reliability of the Health-Related Physical Fitness Test. *Research Quarterly for Exercise and Sport*, *58*, 160–167.

Safrit, M.J., Wood, T.M., Patterson, P., Ehlert, S.A., & Hooper, L.M. (1985). The application of sequential probability ratio testing to a test of motor skill. *Research Quarterly for Exercise and Sport*, *56*(1), 58–65.

Safrit, M.J., Wood, T.M., & Dishman, R.K. (1985). The factorial validity of the Physical Estimation and Attraction Scale. *Journal of Sport Psychology, 7*, 166–190.

Schutz, R.W. (1974). Absolute error. *Journal of Motor Behavior, 6*, 295–301.

Shifflett, B. (1985). Reliability estimation for trials-to-criterion testing. *Research Quarterly for Exercise and Sport, 5*, 266–274.

Spray, J.A. (1982). Effects of autocorrelated errors on intraclass reliability estimation. *Research Quarterly for Exercise and Sport, 53*, 226–231.

Spray, J.A. (1987). Recent developments in measurement and possible applications to the measurement of psychomotor behavior. *Research Quarterly for Exercise and Sport, 58*, 203–207.

Spray, J.A., Sorenson, C., & Hooper, L. (1986). The applicability of inverse sampling procedures for criterion-referenced testing in the elementary school. *Motor Skills: Theory into Practice, 8*, 103–112.

Stamm, C.L., & Kelso, J.A.S. (1978). Reliability and motor memory. *Journal of Motor Behavior, 10*, 15–23.

Stamm, C.L., & Moore, J.E. (1980). Application of generalizability theory in estimating the reliability of a motor performance test. *Research Quarterly for Exercise and Sport, 51*, 382–388.

Taylor, J.L. (1979). Development of the physical education observation instrument using generalizability study theory. *Research Quarterly, 50*, 468–481.

Washburn, R.A., & Safrit, M.J. (1982). Physical performance tests in job selection: A model for empirical validation. *Research Quarterly for Exercise and Sport, 53*, 267–270.

Wells, W.T., & Baumgartner, T.A. (1974). An investigation into the practicability of using the Hales' exponential method of evaluating improvement. *Research Quarterly, 45*, 460–464.

Wood, T.M. (1987). Putting item response theory in perspective. *Research Quarterly for Exercise and Sport, 58*, 216–220.

Wood, T.M., & Safrit, M.J. (1984). A model for estimating the reliability of psychomotor test batteries. *Research Quarterly for Exercise and Sport, 55*, 53–63.

Wood, T.M., & Safrit, M.J. (1987). A comparison of three multivariate models for estimating test battery reliability. *Research Quarterly for Exercise and Sport, 58*, 150–159.

Supplementary Readings

Barrow, H.M., & McGee, R. (1979). *A practical approach to measurement in physical education* (3rd ed.). Philadelphia: Lea & Febiger.

Baumgartner, T.A., & Jackson, A.S. (1987). *Measurement for evaluation in physical education and exercise science* (3rd ed.). Dubuque, IA: Brown.

Bosco, J.S., & Gustafson, W.F. (1983). *Measurement and evaluation in physical education, fitness, and sport.* Englewood Cliffs, NJ: Prentice-Hall.

Clarke, H.H., & Clarke, D.H. (1987). *Application of measurement to physical education* (6th ed.). Englewood Cliffs, NJ: Prentice-Hall.

Crocker, L., & Algina, J. (1986). *Introduction to classical and modern test theory.* New York: Holt, Rinehart, and Winston.

Jensen, C.R., & Hirst, C.C. (1980). *Measurement in physical education and athletics.* New York: Macmillan.

Johnson, B.L., & Nelson, J.K. (1986). *Practical measurements for evaluation in physical education* (2nd ed.). Edina, MN: Burgess.

Nunnally, J.C. (1978). *Psychometric theory.* St. Louis: McGraw-Hill.

Thorndike, R.L. (1982). *Applied psychometrics.* Boston: Houghton Mifflin.

Norm-Referenced Measurement

Norm-referenced measurement is an approach to measurement typically subsumed under classical test theory. Section II describes the theory associated with test characterics used in the norm-referenced measurement approach. These test characteristics—validity and reliability—have been used extensively in the development of tests of exercise, sport, and basic movement. Terry M. Wood, co-editor of this book, has prepared chapter 2, which deals with validity concepts associated with norm-referenced measurement. Nowhere in the field of physical education and exercise science has this topic been treated so extensively and thoroughly. Teachers, researchers, and graduate students will benefit from Wood's treatise. Chapter 3, written by Ted A. Baumgartner, covers reliability concepts associated with norm-referenced measurement. Baumgartner, long acknowledged as an expert on this topic, began studying reliability theory as a doctoral student in physical education. The step-by-step procedures for calculating reliability estimates should be an invaluable aid to researchers and test developers.

Chapter 4, by James R. Morrow, Jr., deals with generalizability theory, which is an extension of reliability theory as covered in the Baumgartner chapter. Morrow's explication of this complex topic makes it readily understandable to non-specialists in measurement. He demonstrates how the theory can be understood more easily by breaking it down into manageable elements. The last chapter in this section, chapter 5, was written by Patricia Patterson. Patterson's lucid treatment of validity generalization relfects her expertise in the area. Both the strengths and weaknesses of the validity generalization model are described, and an example using a small data set makes this approach accessible to the reader.

CHAPTER 2

The Changing Nature of Norm-Referenced Validity

Terry M. Wood
Oregon State University

Judged by many measurement specialists to be the single most important concept in measurement (American Psychological Association, 1985; Safrit, 1986), test validity continues to play a central role in test construction and in the evolution of measurement theory and practice. Questions concerning test validity affect the test constructor, the test user, and the test taker, necessitating a firm understanding of test validity by all individuals involved in the measurement process.

The concepts of test validity for norm-referenced and criterion-referenced measurement are similar; however, the methodologies for determining validity under these measurement models can vary substantially. This chapter focuses on test validity in the norm-referenced model; chapter 6 discusses test validity under the criterion-referenced model.

Test Validity: An Overview

The term *validity* takes on various meanings in research literature. It is not uncommon in a single research paper to find reference to validity of an experiment (e.g., internal validity, external validity, statistical conclusion validity, ecological validity) along with reference to validity of a test (e.g., content validity, criterion-related validity, construct validity). In the former case, validity refers to the appropriateness of interpreting the results of an experiment; in the latter case, validity is concerned with the appropriateness of interpreting the scores of a test. The discussion that follows concerns the validity of test scores.

Conceptually, validity can be defined along two separate yet related dimensions—relevancy and reliability (Safrit, 1981). Test *reliability* refers to freedom from measurement error (American Psychological Association, 1985) or to the degree of consistency of scores over repeated testing (e.g., stability of scores over time, consistency of scores across parallel tests, consistency over repeated trials of the same test). *Relevancy* refers to the ability of test scores to measure accurately, under specified conditions, what they are supposed to measure. To claim evidence for validity a test must exhibit both relevancy and reliability; however, a test can be reliable without being relevant. For example, height can be measured reliably, but it is not a relevant measure of one's basketball playing ability. A quantitative description of the relationship between relevancy and reliability is given as

$$|r_{xy}| \le \sqrt{r_{xx'}} \tag{2.1}$$

where r_{xy} is the validity coefficient of test x with test y and $r_{xx'}$ is the reliability coefficient for test x. Equation 2.1 shows that the square root of a test's reliability coefficient provides an upper limit to the extent that a test will correlate with another test. In other words, a test will not correlate more highly with another test than it correlates with itself. From a practical standpoint Equation 2.1 shows the importance of test reliability in the test construction process.

There appears to be little disagreement concerning a definition of **test validity**. The 1985 *Standards for Educational and Psychological Testing* refers to validity as "the appropriateness, meaningfulness, and usefulness of the specific inferences made from test scores. Test validation is the process of accumulating evidence to support such inferences" (American Psychological Association, 1985, p. 9). Similarly, Cronbach (1971) provided a broad interpretation of validity as "the soundness of all interpretations of a test" (p. 443), while Messick (1980) interjected ethical considerations into the definition, describing validity as "the overall evaluative judgement of the adequacy and appropriateness of inferences drawn from test scores" (p. 1023). Several facets of the validity concept are evident from the preceding definitions. First, test validation concerns the accuracy of test scores (Cronbach, 1971). More specifically, it is the accuracy of interpretations of test scores and not tests that are validated. Test scores can be employed for many purposes, with varied populations, under changing conditions. For example, test scores reflecting volleyball spiking ability might be used to classify individuals into ability levels for class instruction, to contribute to the final grade in a

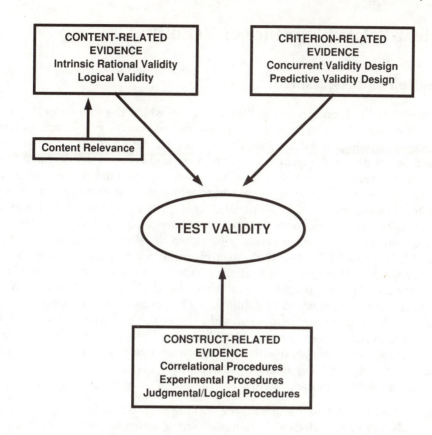

Figure 2.1 Classification of test validity evidence.

volleyball unit of instruction, or to diagnose student weaknesses in volleyball spiking ability. Such a test must be validated for each purpose. Because it is the interpretations of test scores that are validated, it follows that there is no such thing as "the validity" of a test. Validation of a test is an ongoing evaluative process that involves marshalling a body of evidence and employing a variety of methods aimed at determining the degree of accuracy in using test scores for making specific inferences.

Although test validity is a unitary concept, it has been customary to delineate several types of test validity evidence based on various types and uses of tests. Figure 2.1 presents the triad classification of validity types featured in the 1985 *Standards for Educational and Psychological Tests* (American Psychological Association, 1985)—content-related evidence of validity, criterion-related evidence of validity (concurrent validity and predictive validity), and construct-related evidence of validity. Brief descriptions of these classifications and methods used to provide evidence for each are discussed below.

Content-Related Evidence of Validity

Definition and Assessment

Content-related evidence refers to "the degree to which the sample of items, tasks, or questions on a test are representative of some defined universe or domain of content" (American Psychological Association, 1985, p. 10). Gathering content-related evidence typically occurs during the test construction phase and involves defining a universe of content and behaviors to be reflected by a test, writing test items or defining tasks that reflect the universe, and judging the extent to which the test items or tasks accurately reflect the defined universe. In written test construction, a table of specifications or blueprint is commonly employed to gather content-related evidence. An adaptation of the procedure known as *logical validity* has been developed for tests of motor skill (Safrit, 1981). Figure 2.2 presents the test blueprint for a written test of badminton rules for college-aged players in a beginning badminton class. The universe of content and behaviors is defined by the content areas, listed along the left side, and by the levels of cognitive behaviors to be exhibited by respondents, listed along the top. The percentages listed along the bottom and right side of the blueprint give the weightings or relative importance of each content and behavioral category. Numbers within each cell of the blueprint correspond with test items written to reflect the content/behavior characteristic of the cell. For example, item number 29 was written to examine a respondent's knowledge in the content area "rules for service reception in doubles play":

Player X serves to player Y and wins the ensuing rally. Before the next serve player Y and his/her partner decide to change receiving courts so that player Y is again the receiver for player X's serve.

The receiving team wins the next rally before the error is discovered. What is the correct ruling?
a) A let is awarded for the last point only.
b) The serving team is awarded the point.
c) The receiving team's victory in the rally is upheld.
d) The receiving team is given a warning.

Assessing content-related evidence of such a test involves comparing the test blueprint with a copy of the test items to ensure that test items accurately sample the defined universe. Safrit and Wood (1983) give an example of assessing content-related evidence for the Health-Related Physical Fitness Test Opinionnaire. Assessment typically is made by a number of qualified judges. To enhance the assessment, quantitative analysis of agreement among judges' ratings can be made using one of several indices, including the content validity ratio developed by Lawshe (1975) or the *V* index offered by Aiken (1985). As an alternative approach, Cronbach (1971) suggested that content-related evidence could be quantified by comparing respondents' scores on two versions of a test constructed independently by test developers using the same detailed description of the content/behavior universe.

BEHAVIORS

CONTENT	KNOWLEDGE	COMPREHENSION	APPLICATION	
Playing Surface	1, 2, 3			7.5%
Equipment	8			2.5%
General Rules				
Scoring	4		6	5.0%
Serving	12	22, 19	10	10.0%
Receiving	13	15	16	7.5%
Playing	20, 23, 39, 37	18, 17	21	17.5%
Singles Rules				
Scoring	9, 11			5.0%
Serving			14	2.5%
Doubles Rules				
Scoring	25, 27, 36	34		10.0%
Serving	32, 36	24		7.5%
Receiving	30, 29, 31	28	33	12.5%
Playing	35		38, 40	7.5%
Etiquette	5, 7			5.0%
	60.0%	20.0%	20.0%	

Figure 2.2   Test blueprint for a classroom test of badminton rules.

Discussion

The meaning of content validity.   Assessment of content-related evidence is a necessary but not sufficient step in test score validation, because the procedure refers to proper test construction but does not involve administration of the test to a sample of respondents and the analysis of test score interpretation (Guion, 1978b). This feature conflicts with the definition of test validity and has generated controversy among measurement specialists (e.g., Benson, 1981; Fitzpatrick, 1983; Guion, 1978a, 1978b; Messick, 1975, 1980; Tenopyr, 1977). Messick (1975) succinctly summed up the issue:

> The major problem here is that content validity . . . is focused upon test *forms* rather than test *scores*, upon *instruments* rather than measurements. Inferences in educational and psychological measurement are made from scores and scores are

a function of subject responses. Any concept of validity of measurement must include inference to empirical consistency. Content coverage is an important consideration in test construction and interpretation, to be sure, but in itself does not provide validity. (p. 960)

In an insightful exploration into the meaning of content validity, Fitzpatrick (1983) showed that the term has been employed to reflect various meanings, such as the sampling adequacy of content and behaviors, the relevance of content and behaviors, the clarity with which content and behavioral domains are defined, and the technical quality of test tasks and items. Fitzpatrick suggested that because the assessment of sampling adequacy of content, relevance of content, and clarity of domain definition involve judgments rather than analysis of test scores, these concepts would be more appropriately labeled *content representativeness*, *content relevance*, and *domain clarity*, respectively. Furthermore, sampling adequacy of behaviors and relevance of behaviors question the underlying meaning of scores and are thus matters of construct validity, while technical quality of tasks and items is an important test attribute but does not reflect validity. Therefore, "no adequate means of defining content validity was found. In light of this, it seems reasonable to conclude that content validity is not a useful term for test specialists to retain in their vocabulary" (Fitzpatrick, 1983, p. 11). In line with such reasoning, the latest *Standards for Educational and Psychological Testing* (American Psychological Association, 1985) refers to "content-related evidence" rather than to content validity.

Content relevance. By definition, assessment of content-related evidence does not include questions directed at the appropriateness of the defined universe. Questions concerning the appropriateness of the universe definition are categorized as **content relevance** (Fitzpatrick, 1983; Messick, 1980) and include inquiry into the omission of important content or behaviors from the defined universe, inclusion of unimportant content or behaviors, and inappropriate weighting (underemphasis or overemphasis) of content or behaviors (Safrit, 1981). Analysis of content relevance should accompany assessment of content-related evidence of validity.

Intrinsic rational validity and logical validity. For some types of tests the universe of content is not so clear-cut, and a table of specifications is difficult to develop (e.g., tests employed for assessing specific abilities such as those measured by teacher-made classroom tests and tests of motor skill). For such tests Ebel (1983) suggested a method he termed **intrinsic rational validity**, which involves developing "a written document that (a) defines the ability to be measured, (b) describes the tasks to be included in the test, and (c) explains the reasons for using such tasks to measure such an ability" (p. 8). A concept similar to intrinsic validity has been adapted for use in providing content-related evidence for tests of motor skill (e.g., Chapman, 1982; Safrit, Wood, Ehlert, Hooper, & Patterson, 1985). Termed **logical validity**, the procedure entails defining the components of good performance, developing a test that measures the defined components, and scoring the test so that better scores reflect successful performance (Safrit, 1981). As in assessing other types of content-related evidence, it is important to consider content relevance of the universe when examining logical validity.

Face validity. Few concepts in measurement have generated such heated debate as the concept of *face validity*. More than three decades ago, Mosier (1947) remarked that "beautiful friendships have been jeopardized when a chance remark about face validity has classed the speaker among the infidels" (p. 191), while Safrit (1981) described the term as "not only obsolete but also inaccurate" (p. 83). Similarly, the 1974 *Standards for Educational and Psychological Tests* (American Psychological Association, 1974) concluded that face validity was unacceptable as a basis for interpreting scores. Few concepts could weather such attacks, yet debate over face validity continues to rage (Nevo, 1985; Nichols, Licht, & Pearl, 1982, 1983; Secolsky, 1987). The object of such attention is a term with several meanings. Mosier (1947) attributed four meanings to the term face validity, none of which provides direct evidence regarding the proper interpretation of test scores:

- *validity by assumption* or evidence for validity of a test based on a commonsense relationship between the items on a test and the objectives of the test;
- *validity by definition* or the fact that a test represents a sample from a population of items that are assumed to represent a universe of responses;
- *appearance of validity* or the degree to which a test looks like an appropriate measure of a characteristic; and
- *validity by hypothesis* or evidence for validity based on the similarity between the test and other tests of known validity.

It can be readily seen that none of the definitions listed above is concerned with actual test scores, and none provides much evidence regarding the underlying meaning of test scores. Furthermore, the use of such methods has a tendency to draw attention away from meaningful sources of evidence for validity. While it could be argued that all four interpretations are attributes of valid tests, none of the interpretations by itself or in combination with the others constitutes sufficient evidence for test validity. Therefore, use of the term *face validity* is not recommended.

Criterion-Related Evidence of Validity

Definition and Assessment

From a logical perspective, test scores are expected to relate well to scores on another test measuring the same characteristic. For example, individuals who score well on the 12-min run test of aerobic endurance are expected to score well on a treadmill test measuring $\dot{V}O_2max$, and those who perform poorly on the 12-min run test are expected to exhibit low $\dot{V}O_2max$ scores on the treadmill. **Criterion-related evidence** quantifies such a relationship between test scores (e.g., 12-min run scores) and scores from one or more criterion tests (e.g., treadmill test) which are presumed to be a more accurate measure of the characteristic of interest. Criterion-related evidence can take several forms using various methodologies. The two most common forms are evidence of concurrent validity and evidence of predictive validity. Correlational methods are used primarily in concurrent validity designs, whereas both regression and correlation are used in predictive validity designs. Validity generalization and differential validation (Katzell & Dyer, 1977; Linn, 1978) are more recent contributions to the methodology of criterion-related evidence.

Concurrent validity designs. Depending on the use of test scores, two types of designs for obtaining criterion-related evidence can be delineated—**concurrent validity designs** and **predictive validity designs** (American Psychological Association, 1985). In concurrent validity studies, scores from the test and the criterion test(s) are collected at the same time with the aim "to appraise the diagnostic effectiveness of the test in detecting current behavioral patterns or to assess the suitability of substituting the test for a longer, more cumbersome, or more expensive criterion measure" (Messick, 1980, p. 1017). Examples of concurrent validity studies abound in the physical education literature. In the area of physical fitness appraisal, researchers have explored the concurrent validation of distance run tests as substitutes for more expensive and time-consuming criterion aerobic measures, such as estimating $\dot{V}o_2max$ from a treadmill test (e.g., Getchell, Kirkendall, & Robbins, 1977), or the validity of sit-and-reach flexibility test scores as a measure of low-back musculoskeletal function (Jackson & Baker, 1986). Validation of motor skill tests has depended largely on concurrent validity studies. Questioning the validity evidence provided by previously published golf skill tests, Green, East, and Hensley (1987) recently provided concurrent validity evidence for the Green Golf Test by examining the multiple correlation between the four skills in the golf test and a criterion measure of total score on 36 holes of golf ($R = .77$ for a four-task battery). Assessing concurrent validity involves developing the field test and assessing the content (logical) related evidence for the test, choosing an appropriate criterion measure(s), administering both tests to a large sample from the population of interest, computing the validity coefficient (r_{xy}) by correlating the scores on the field test and the criterion measure, and examining the stability of r_{xy} by cross-validating the results. **Cross-validation** provides evidence for the sampling variability of r_{xy} through random division of the sample into two groups, followed by computation and statistical comparison of r_{xy} for each group. Jackson and Baker (1986) give an example of cross-validation used in a concurrent validity design examining low back and hamstring flexibility. Evidence for stability of r_{xy} is given by coefficients that are not statistically different.

Predictive validity designs. Evidence for predictive validity is necessary for test scores that will be used either to predict directly, through regression equations, criterion scores, or to make decisions about future behavior. In anthropometry, for example, skinfold measures have been used in prediction equations to estimate body density scores (e.g., Durnin & Womersly, 1974; Lohman, 1981), whereas in sport psychology, personality characteristics have been utilized to predict future success in rowing (Morgan & Johnson, 1978). Predictive validity studies are employed to validate such uses of scores. Based on the time period between administration of the **predictor test** and administration of the **criterion test**, two predictive validity designs can be identified: prediction of present performance and prediction of future performance (Safrit, 1981). In the former design, the predictor and criterion tests are administered at the same time, followed by development and analysis of prediction equations. The aim of such designs is to develop prediction equations that will accurately predict present performance on the criterion variable from knowledge of the predictor variable(s). Examples of test scores used for this purpose include the use in anthropometry of skinfold measures to estimate body density, and the use in exercise physiology of performance time during graded exercise on a treadmill to predict $\dot{V}O_2$max (Alexander, Liang, Stull, Serface, Wolfe, & Ewing, 1984). Safrit (1981) outlined five steps commonly employed in presenting evidence of the accuracy of test scores in predicting present behavior of a criterion measure:

1. Assuming that evidence for the content-relatedness of both the predictor test(s) and the criterion measure(s) has been examined, randomly sample approximately 200 subjects from the population of interest (more subjects will be required if more than one predictor is employed).
2. Administer the predictor test(s) and criterion measure(s) to all subjects.
3. Compute and interpret the validity coefficient. If the validity coefficient is large enough for the purposes of the test, continue with the predictive validity study; otherwise abandon the study.
4. Cross-validate the prediction equation. Randomly divide the group in half (100 respondents per group) and compute the prediction equation for group 1 respondents (the derivation sample). Using the group 1 prediction equation, estimate the criterion score for group 2 respondents (the validation sample) by substituting group 2 predictor scores into the prediction equation.
5. Determine the accuracy of prediction by computing the *standard error of estimate* (*SEE*). The *SEE* provides an estimate of the average error associated with estimating criterion scores from the prediction equation and is given in the following definitional formula:

$$SEE = \sqrt{\frac{\Sigma(y_i - y'_i)^2}{n-1}} \qquad (2.2)$$

where y_i is the known score on the criterion for the ith respondent in group 2, y'_i is the predicted criterion score for the ith respondent in group 2, and n is the number of respondents in group 2. If the *SEE* is sufficiently small for the purposes of the test, predictive validity can be claimed. An index of the prediction's stability is given by the cross-validation coefficient (R_{cv}), defined as "the simple correlation between predicted and actual criterion scores where the predictions are obtained by applying the derivation sample weights to validation sample observed scores" (Dorans & Drasgow, 1980, p. 728).

When test scores are used to predict future performance, the aim of prediction is often to garner evidence for selection decisions. For example, the accuracy of the Scholastic Aptitude Test (SAT) as a predictor of success in college has received much attention in the educational literature, because SAT scores are often used as criteria for admission into colleges and universities. A number of researchers in exercise science have employed predictive validity methods to explore the accuracy of predicting team membership from knowledge of antecedent variables (Morgan & Johnson, 1978; Nagle, Morgan, Hellickson, Serfass, & Alexander, 1975). Designs for predicting future performance involve administering the predictor test to a sample of interest, waiting for a period of time, administering the criterion test(s), computing the most accurate prediction equations, and determining through one of several indices of agreement the decision accuracy of the predictor test scores.

Discussion

The criterion measure. Several factors concerning criterion-related evidence deserve emphasis. Of primary concern is the dependence of the method on the criterion test scores as an accurate measure of the characteristic being investigated. A low validity coefficient can be interpreted in one of three ways: (a) the predictor test lacks validity, (b) the predictor test may be valid but the criterion test lacks validity, or (c) both tests lack validity. Since evidence concerning validity of the criterion test will negate interpretations (b) and (c), evidence for the validity of the criterion test becomes a significant undertaking in providing criterion-related evidence for validity. Much has been written concerning the development of criterion measures (Brogden & Taylor, 1950; Guion, 1978a; Gulliksen, 1950a). Since the logic of criterion-related evidence stems from the relationship of test scores as an approximation of criterion test scores, by definition the criterion measure should be the most accurate (albeit more time consuming, more costly, and/or less efficient) indicator of the characteristic being measured. If the criterion measure is the best available measure of a characteristic, it follows that evidence for the validity of the criterion cannot include computation of validity coefficients, because by definition there is no criterion with which to compare a criterion score. For example, to provide criterion-related evidence for a test of the tennis forehand groundstroke, a test developer may compare test scores with a criterion score consisting of the average of judges' ratings of each player's forehand ability. Evidence for validity of the criterion measure (i.e., judges' ratings) must be made on evidence other than criterion-related evidence, because there is no criterion with which to compare the judges' ratings. Use of invalid criterion measures will attenuate the validity coefficient, with the degree of attenuation depending, in part, on the validity of the criterion measure.

How then are criterion measures to be validated? Validation of criterion measures begins with identifying criterion elements that best reflect the predictor test scores and the purposes to which the scores will be put, followed by construction of instruments to measure each criterion element (Brogden & Taylor, 1950). During this process careful attention must be given to content (logical or rational) related evidence of each instrument and to the existence of bias or "any variable, except errors of measurement and sampling error, producing a deviation of obtained criterion scores for a hypothetical 'true' criterion score" (Brogden & Taylor, 1950, p. 161). Brogden and Taylor identify four classifications of bias that may affect criterion test scores:

- **criterion deficiency**: Failing to identify important elements of the criterion. For example, years of soccer playing experience used as a criterion for a test of soccer kicking ability fails to provide a measure of kicking ability (e.g., judges' ratings of kicking ability) as part of the criterion and thus is deficient;

- **criterion contamination**: Extraneous factors that are not directly related to the characteristic being measured are introduced into the criterion measure during the construction of test instruments. For example, several contaminating elements can affect judges' ratings of performance. **Halo effects** occur when judges rate performance based on previous and often unrelated knowledge of the performer, while errors of illation occur when judgments are based on appearance rather than performance (e.g., when judging gymnastics ability judges may tend to give higher ratings to those who look more athletic). Other forms of contamination include opportunity bias (e.g., in archery performance tests of accuracy from a fixed distance, women suffer from opportunity bias, because their arm-shoulder girdle strength forces them to use a bow with a lower draw weight), and the effect of systematic assignment of respondents to "tough" or "easy" raters;
- **criterion scale unit bias**: This occurs in the method used to score criterion tests. For example, in the use of rating scales, raters typically score examinees on the high end of the scale, thus biasing scores toward that end; and
- **criterion distortion**: If more than one criterion measure is employed, a common practice is to combine the scores into a single criterion composite score. If important elements of the criterion have been omitted, then these elements effectively have been given a weight of zero in the composite score, while criterion contaminants have been given a weight of one. Criterion scale unit bias can cause criterion distortion when judges fail to use scores on a rating scale, because these scores effectively are given a weight of zero.

In addition to content- (logical or rational) related evidence for criterion measures, Gulliksen (1950a) advocated evidence of *intrinsic content validity* and *intrinsic correlational validity*. Evidence for intrinsic content validity includes factor analysis of criterion measures, a rational comparison of the predictor/criterion intercorrelation matrix with expected relationships among various predictors and the criterion measure, and examination of pre-training and post-training test results administered to a sample of subjects. In contrast, evidence of intrinsic correlational validity is aimed at supporting a causal relationship between predictor and criterion. Safrit (1981) provides a humorous yet pointed example of such evidence:

> If a track coach suggested that the headstand is a good predictor of sprinting ability, his colleagues would probably look at him in disbelief. The track coach . . . produces data yielding a correlation coefficient of 0.82 between the ability to perform a headstand and sprinting ability. Other coaches might respond with a key question: Would improving headstand ability increase sprinting ability? (This question would have to be tested by another method.) If not, the headstand as a predictor lacks intrinsic [correlational] validity. (p. 63)

Cross-validation. To estimate the accuracy and stability of prediction in predictive validity designs, cross-validation procedures should be employed. Although cross-validation procedures for prediction equations are relatively straightforward and are described adequately elsewhere (e.g., Mosier, 1951), several pitfalls deserve highlighting.

Dorans and Drasgow (1980) pointed out that of two procedures commonly employed in cross-validation—one involving application of raw scores from the validation sample to raw-score regression weights from the derivation sample, the other applying standard scores from the validation sample to standardized regression weights from the derivation sample—only the former procedure is correct, because "a standard score of a given magnitude from the derivation sample is not equivalent to a standard score of the same magnitude in the validation sample, unless the validation sample and derivation sample raw score standard deviations are equal" (p. 729). To obtain a less biased estimate of predictive accuracy than the commonly used squared multiple correlation coefficient (R^2) computed from the derivation sample, Mosier (1951) introduced the double cross-validation procedure. Noting that R^2 tended to overestimate predictive accuracy, Mosier suggested developing prediction equations for both samples in a cross-validation study, then applying the regression weights from one sample to the raw predictor scores from the other sample to generate two cross-validation coefficients (R_{cv}), one for each sample. In essence the double cross-validation technique treats each sample as both a derivation sample and as a validation sample.

Correcting for attenuation. The relationship between relevancy and reliability was described briefly at the beginning of this chapter. Unreliability in the predictor test and/or the criterion measure serves to attenuate or lower the validity coefficient. Equation 2.3 (Nunnally, 1978) can be employed to obtain an estimate of the validity coefficient unaffected by errors of measurement (i.e., by unreliability in the predictor scores *and* in the criterion measures).

$$r^*_{xy} = \frac{r_{xy}}{\sqrt{r_{xx'}\, r_{yy'}}} \qquad\qquad (2.3)$$

where r^*_{xy} is the validity coefficient corrected for attenuation, r_{xy} is the sample validity coefficient, and $r_{xx'}$ and $r_{yy'}$ are the reliability coefficients for the predictor and criterion measures, respectively. Nunnally (1978) and others have aptly pointed out that such corrections in the validity coefficient are "handy fiction." Correcting the predictor scores for unreliability may mask the true operational value of these scores, because the predictor test scores, not estimated error-free scores, will be used in applied settings. Thus the following attenuation formula, which corrects only for unreliability in the criterion scores, is more appropriate for use in criterion-related validity designs:

$$r^*_{xy^*} = \frac{r_{xy}}{\sqrt{r_{yy'}}} \qquad\qquad (2.4)$$

In terms of classical test theory, r^*_{xy} has been interpreted as an estimate of ρ_{TxTy}, the correlation between predictor "true" scores and criterion "true" scores. Such an interpretation must be made with caution, because the magnitude of r^*_{xy} depends on the accuracy of the reliability coefficients employed (i.e., underestimating $r_{xx'}$ and/or $r_{yy'}$ results in an inflated estimate of ρ_{TxTy}) and on the sampling error of the observed validity coefficient r_{xy} (Winne & Belfry, 1982).

Restriction of range. A correlational approach often is employed in predictive validity studies. For example, suppose a college football coach developed a written psychological test instrument to predict the probability of success (measured by number of games played while in college) of incoming freshman athletes trying out for the football team. Typically, to examine the predictive validity of the instrument, all freshman athletes trying out for the team over a period of several years would take the test, the number of games played while in college would be recorded for those athletes selected for team membership, and the correlation between test results and number of games played would be computed to provide an index of the relationship between test scores and success in football. A major flaw in such designs is the explicit selection of a subsample of the population tested, resulting in a restriction in the range of the predictor test scores (x) and the attenuation of the validity coefficient (r_{xy}). In other words, all freshman athletes trying out for football were administered the predictor test; however, criterion data are only available for those who were selected for team membership. Truncation of the sample reduces the variance of the predictor scores, resulting in attenuation of the validity coefficient (Linn, Harnisch, & Dunbar, 1981). Several methods for correcting the validity coefficient for restriction of range have been offered. Under the assumptions of linearity of regression and homoscedasticity of error distributions, Gullicksen (1950b) presented the following correction formula[1]:

$$r_{xy} = \frac{S_x \, r_{x^*y^*}}{\sqrt{S_x^2 \, r_{x^*y^*}^2 + S_{x^*}^2 - S_{x^*}^2 \, r_{x^*y^*}^2}} \tag{2.5}$$

where S represents a standard deviation, x^* and y^* represent scores in the restricted group for the predictor and criterion variables, respectively, and x represents predictor scores for the total group.

Validity generalization (see chapter 5 in this text for a more complete description of the rationale and methodology of validity generalization). A question of some import regards the generalizability of criterion-related evidence across various subject populations, testing environments, and uses of test scores. For example, to what extent are scores from a submaximal test of aerobic capacity using a bicycle ergometer valid over different populations, such as college-aged men and women, middle-aged individuals, young boys and girls, or populations with various levels of physical fitness? Must criterion-related evidence be gathered for each new population or use of test scores, or can the relationship between criterion measures and predictor test scores evidenced in completed research be employed to generalize use of the test score across new situations? The validity generalization model first proposed by Schmidt, Hunter, and Urry (1976) employs meta-analytic concepts to explore the degree to which validity coefficients reflecting a common predictor/criterion relationship can be generalized to

---

[1]The methods outlined by Gulliksen (1950b) assume that the sample was truncated based on knowledge of the predictor scores. In some instances the sample is truncated relative to a third, often unknown, variable. Linn et al. (1981) offer restriction of range equations that include an estimation of the effect of these unknown variables.

new populations and/or testing situations. The first demonstration of validity generalization to criterion-related evidence in physical education was made by Safrit, Costa, and Hooper (1986). Applying the Schmidt and Hunter (1977) model to a restricted sample of concurrent validity studies dealing with distance run field tests of cardiorespiratory function in college-aged women, Safrit et al. concluded that "the validity generalization model holds considerable promise for making viable contributions toward a synthesis of the body of knowledge contained in a wide variety of studies in physical education and the exercise sciences" (p. 294).

Construct-Related Evidence of Validity

Definition and Assessment

Many measurement specialists (e.g., Cronbach, 1980; Guion, 1978a; Messick, 1975, 1980; Tenopyr, 1977) have made a convincing case against the division of validity into three types (content, criterion-related, and construct), arguing that "all validation is one, and in a sense all is construct validation" (Cronbach, 1980, p. 99). Subsequently, the 1985 *Standards for Educational and Psychological Testing* (American Psychological Association, 1985) reflected a turn toward a unified concept of validity and a methodology focusing on the gathering of evidence from various sources rather than the determination of various types of "validities." The origin of this position is the concept of *construct validity*, which first appeared in the 1954 *Technical Recommendations for Psychological Tests and Diagnostic Techniques* (American Psychological Association, 1954) and then was explicated in a seminal article by Cronbach and Meehl (1955), although its roots can be traced to the decade preceding the publication of these documents (Cronbach & Meehl, 1955). Construct validity evolved as a process for validating tests of more abstract characteristics such as (a) psychological states and traits (e.g., attitude toward physical activity—Kenyon, 1968, physical estimation and attraction—Sonstroem, 1978, sport competition anxiety—Martens, 1977); (b) abilities (e.g., playing ability in various sports—Safrit, 1981); and (c) physiological parameters such as endurance.

The 1974 *Standards for Educational and Psychological Tests* (American Psychological Association, 1974) defined a construct as "an idea developed or 'constructed' as a work of informed scientific imagination; that is, it is a theoretical idea developed to explain and to organize some aspects of existing behavior" (p. 29). Similarly, Cronbach and Meehl (1955) defined a construct as "some postulated attribute of people, assumed to be reflected in test performance" (p. 283). For example, a sport psychologist may notice that some children tend to be more involved than others in physical activity. The psychologist hypothesizes that these children have good feelings toward physical activity, decides to label these feelings "attitude toward physical activity", and develops a written test instrument to measure the extent to which children exhibit this characteristic. These hypothesized feelings could have been labeled *values* or *beliefs*; regardless of the label, the existence of "attitude toward physical activity" is only an abstraction which the psychologist has *constructed* to explain surrounding events.

Construct validity is the process of determining the degree to which a test measures the construct it was designed to measure. *Standards For Educational and Psychological Tests* (American Psychological Association, 1974) provides a clue for the method of construct validation when it further describes a construct as "more than a label; it is a dimension understood or inferred from its network of interrelationships" (p. 29). Construct validation involves three processes (Cronbach, 1971). First, the researcher explicitly defines the construct and the test that is purported to measure the construct. Second, the researcher develops a hypothesized network of interrelationships (the **nomological net**—Cronbach & Meehl, 1955, or conceptual framework—American Psychological Association, 1985) between the construct and other constructs and observable behaviors, then tests each branch in the nomological net via empirical research, employing the proposed test instrument. Third, and most important, counterhypotheses explaining results of the various studies are proposed and tested. It is crucial to explore the extent to which negative (i.e., unexpected) results are due to inadequate conceptualization of the construct or the nomological net, and/or inadequate measurement of the construct, and/or inappropriate experimental design. Equally important is reporting limitations regarding the interpretation of positive (i.e., expected) results (Cronbach & Meehl, 1955).

The more each link in the nomological net can be predicted and variability among scores explained, the stronger the claim for construct validity of the test instrument. Validation of constructs, then, is based on an accumulation of research findings and parallels the process of scientific theory building (Cronbach & Meehl, 1955). Figure 2.3 presents a hypothetical nomological net for exploring the construct *attitude toward physical activity* (*ATPA*). Assuming the construct has been defined adequately and a test instrument has been developed to measure the construct, investigators hypothesize interrelationships between the construct and observable behaviors and other constructs. For example, it may be hypothesized that the construct ATPA should have a moderate relationship with the construct *physical estimation and attraction* (a similar construct) but little relationship to a measure of a very different construct *general anxiety*. Studies could easily be designed to investigate these hypotheses. Similarly, one might reasonably hypothesize that a moderately high relationship exists between respondents' ATPA and their level of involvement in physical activity, while another study might explore the effect of a physical fitness program on the ATPA of a sedentary group of individuals evidencing initial low levels of ATPA.

The nomological net can be viewed as a slow-moving amoeba of ever-changing size and shape. In the early stages of construct validation, the amoeba is small, as few links in the nomological net have been validated. Through the formulation of counterhypotheses more links in the net are hypothesized, and the amoeba extends its boundaries. However, some links in the net may fail to generate results in the hypothesized direction, and the shape of the amoeba changes as the construct is revised. As the nomological net grows to explain a wide variety of hypothesized relationships, our faith in the existence of the construct grows. It is important to remember that the existence of a construct is not proven. Instead our faith in the existence of the construct, as measured by the test instrument, is strengthened or weakened by analysis of **construct-related evidence**. In addition, Cronbach and Meehl (1955) emphasize that "construct validation is possible only when some of the statements in the network lead to

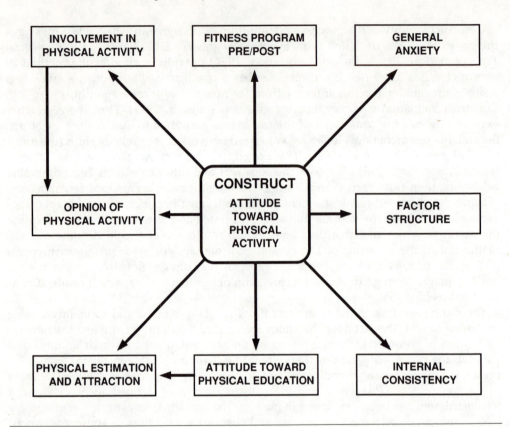

Figure 2.3 Hypothetical nomological net for exploring the construct validity of the construct *attitude toward physical activity.*

predicted relationships among observables. While some observables may be regarded as 'criteria,' the construct validity of the criteria themselves is regarded as under investigation'' (p. 300).

It is clear from Figure 2.3 that construct validation is a process that involves many planned research undertakings, including gathering content-related and criterion-related evidence, and that conceivably could take a significant period of time. The methodology of construct validation is varied and limited only by the imagination of the researcher; however, three categories of procedures have traditionally been identified (Cronbach, 1971): correlational procedures, experimental procedures, and judgmental/logical procedures. Use of these procedures in construct validation is treated adequately elsewhere (e.g., Cronbach, 1971; Cronbach & Meehl, 1955; Safrit, 1981); therefore, only brief descriptions of the procedures are given below. More recent developments in the assessment of construct-related evidence are treated in a separate section.

Correlational procedures. Correlational procedures can take one of several forms. Evidence of **convergent validity** is given when measures of the same or similar constructs reveal high to moderate correlations. In contrast, evidence of **discriminant validity** is revealed when measures of different constructs show low correlations. The hypothesized multidimensional nature of constructs can be confirmed with factor analytic techniques (see chapter 8 and Safrit, Wood, & Dishman, 1985), while the multitrait-multimethod approach (e.g., Campbell & Fiske, 1959; Douglass, 1979) can be employed to simultaneously explore convergent and discriminant validity, along with the degree to which similarity in the method of testing contributes to common variability in scores.

Experimental procedures. Cronbach and Meehl (1955) describe two experimental methods: the known-group differences method and studies of change over occasions. In the former method, the instrument presumed to measure the construct is administered to groups that are theoretically known to differ. Hypothesizing that athletes' responses regarding attitude toward the sport in which they were currently involved may differ from their responses to ATPA as measured by the Simon and Smoll (1974) adaption of Kenyon's (1968) ATPA inventory, Schutz, Smoll, and Wood (1981) investigated the meaning to children of the attitude object *physical activity*. They employed the group differences method with a sample of 550 young male and female athletes involved in different sports (e.g., basketball, volleyball, hockey, figure skating, swimming, soccer). Results of the investigation revealed that across all sports included in the study, children's ATPA were equivalent to their attitudes toward a specific sport, lending support to the term *physical activity* as a well-defined and stable attitudinal object.

Judgmental/logical procedures. Valid interpretation of test scores can be aided with evidence arising from subjective analysis of content (e.g., content-related evidence and content relevancy), interviews with respondents regarding the nature of the test, and evidence of internal consistency reliability (see chapter 3). It must be pointed out, however, that such evidence is supportive and not in itself conclusive evidence for validity. Counterhypotheses arising from such analyses should be tested empirically (Cronbach, 1971).

Discussion

The availability of inexpensive yet powerful computers, coupled with a recognition of the multidimensional nature of behavior and development of sophisticated multivariate statistical procedures, is changing the nature of construct validity. Embretson (1983) described the change in the field of psychology as a paradigm shift from *functionalism* (with emphasis on explaining antecedent/consequent relationships) to one of *structuralism* (with emphasis on explaining systems and underlying processes). Characterizing the latter is the development and empirical testing of formal theoretical models, presumed to underlie constructs, by employing concepts of linear structural equation modeling and item response theory. Such a shift has resulted in a redefinition of construct validity into two components: construct representation and nomothetic span (Embretson, 1983). *Construct representation* deals specifically with the "theoretical mechanisms which underlie task performance" (Embretson, 1983, p. 180), whereas *nomothetic span* parallels the more traditional concept of construct validity as the network of interrelationships of a measure in the nomological net. Assessing construct representation involves delineating a theoretical model (e.g. latent trait models) that relates test performance to characteristics of test items or tasks and comparing the fit of the model with the fit of competing models. Once the underlying constructs of the test are specified, linear structural equation models can be employed to judge the degree of relationship between the theorized constructs and other constructs and observables in an investigation of nomothetic span.

The impact of this redefinition of construct validity in exercise science remains to be seen; however, there are indications that an impact is being felt. The September 1987 issue of *Research Quarterly for Exercise and Sport* "Review and Commentary Series" provided the first explication of item response theory (IRT) in the exercise science literature, and chapter 11 in this text is devoted to IRT. If IRT concepts can be applied to tests of motor skill, it is likely that the concept of construct representation will be useful in the validation of motor skill tests. In contrast, linear structural equation modeling has already seen limited use in the sport psychology literature to explore nomothetic span (e.g., Weiss, Bredemeier, & Shewchuk, 1985). It is discussed below.

Linear structural equation modeling (also known as covariance structure modeling) is a series of multivariate statistical techniques that analyzes the relationships (i.e., the covariance structure) among a group of observed variables to discover underlying factors that may be contributing to these relationships. The underlying factors or latent variables are often interpreted as the constructs underlying observed scores. Several techniques for analyzing covariance structures have been proposed; LISREL (Jöreskog & Sörbom, 1981), a procedure named after the computer program developed to generate such models, has enjoyed widespread acceptance. Put simply, the method employs confirmatory factor analysis to determine the constructs underlying observed scores, then estimates mathematical relationships among these constructs.

Linear structural equation modeling offers several attractive features. An obvious strength of such procedures is the explicit *a priori* specification of hypothesized latent variables and the relationships among them, and the statistical test of fit of proposed models. In addition, the procedure allows for the estimation of the degree of measurement error.

Conclusion

Test validity is a unified concept consisting of evidence gathered from a variety of sources, using wide ranging methodologies. Because test validation is concerned with appropriate interpretation of test scores, it is an evolving process. It makes little sense to speak of a test as valid or not. Instead we must judge our degree of acceptance or faith in the use of test scores for a particular purpose under specified conditions. This chapter has taken a more technical approach to test validity, touching on both the concepts underlying the meaning of test validity and the methodology for presenting evidence for validity. That ethical and legal concepts of validity were not included in the discussion is by no means a reflection on the significance of these issues. Readers interested in such topics should explore the insightful discussions by Messick (1980), Kleiman and Faley (1985), Cole (1981), and Cronbach (1980).

References

Aiken, L.R. (1985). Three coefficients for analyzing the reliability and validity of ratings. *Educational and Psychological Measurement, 45*, 131–142.

Alexander, J.F., Liang, M.T.C., Stull, G.A., Serfass, R.C., Wolfe, D.R., & Ewing, J.L. (1984). A comparison of the Bruce and Liang equations for predicting $\dot{V}O_2$max in young adult males. *Research Quarterly for Exercise and Sport, 55*, 383–387.

American Psychological Association. (1954). *Technical recommendations for psychological tests and diagnostic techniques*. Washington, DC: Author.

American Psychological Association. (1974). *Standards for educational and psychological tests*. Washington, DC: Author.

American Psychological Association. (1985). *Standards for educational and psychological testing*. Washington, DC: Author.

Benson, J. (1981). A redefinition of content validity. *Educational and Psychological Measurement, 41*, 793–802.

Brogden, H.E., & Taylor, E.K. (1950). The theory and classification of criterion bias. *Educational and Psychological Measurement, 10*, 159–186.

Campbell, D.T., & Fiske, D.W. (1959). Convergent and discriminant validation by the multitrait-multimethod matrix. *Psychological Bulletin, 56*, 81–105.

Chapman, N.L. (1982). Chapman Ball Control Test—field hockey. *Research Quarterly for Exercise and Sport, 53*, 239–242.

Cole, N.S. (1981). Bias in testing. *American Psychologist, 36*, 1067–1077.

Cronbach, L.J. (1971). Test validation. In R.L. Thorndike (Ed.), *Educational measurement* (2nd ed.) (pp. 443–507). Washington, DC: American Council on Education.

Cronbach, L.J. (1980). Validity on parole: How can we go straight? In W.B. Schrader (Ed.), *New directions in testing and measurement No. 5* (pp. 99–108). San Francisco: Jossey-Bass.

Cronbach, L.J., & Meehl, P.E. (1955). Construct validity in psychological tests. *Psychological Bulletin, 52*, 281–302.

Dorans, N.J., & Drasgow, F. (1980). A note on cross-validating prediction equations. *Journal of Applied Psychology, 65*, 728–730.

Douglass, J.A. (1979). Comparison of two subjective rating systems for synchronized swimming. *Educational and Psychological Measurement, 39*, 411–415.

Durnin, J.V., & Womersly, J. (1974). Body fat assessed from total body density and its estimation from skinfold thickness: Measurements on 481 men and women aged from 16 to 72 years. *British Journal of Nutrition, 32*, 77–97.

Ebel, R.L. (1983). The practical validation of tests of ability. *Educational Measurement: Issues and Practice, 2*(2), 7–10.

Embretson, S. (1983). Construct validity: Construct representation versus nomothetic span. *Psychological Bulletin, 93,* 179–197.

Fitzpatrick, A.R. (1983). The meaning of content validity. *Applied Psychological Measurement, 7,* 3–13.

Getchell, L.H., Kirkendall, D., & Robbins, G. (1977). Prediction of maximal oxygen uptake in young adult women joggers. *Research Quarterly, 48,* 61–67.

Green, K.N., East, W.B., & Hensley, L.D. (1987). A golf skills test battery for college males and females. *Research Quarterly for Exercise and Sport, 58,* 72–76.

Guion, R.M. (1978a). "Content validity" in moderation. *Personnel Psychology, 31,* 205–213.

Guion, R.M. (1978b). Scoring of content domain samples: The problem of fairness. *Journal of Applied Psychology, 63,* 499–506.

Gulliksen, H. (1950a). Intrinsic validity. *The American Psychologist, 5,* 511–516.

Gulliksen, H. (1950b). *Theory of mental tests.* New York: Wiley.

Jackson, A.W., & Baker, A.A. (1986). The relationship of the sit and reach test to criterion measures of hamstring and back flexibility in young females. *Research Quarterly for Exercise and Sport, 57,* 183–186.

Jöreskog, K.G., & Sörbom, D. (1981). *LISREL V. User's Guide.* Chicago: National Educational Resources.

Katzell, R.A., & Dyer, F.J. (1977). Differential validity revived. *Journal of Applied Psychology, 62,* 137–145.

Kenyon, G.S. (1968). Six scales for assessing attitude towards physical activity. *Research Quarterly, 39,* 566–574.

Kleiman, L.S., & Faley, R.H. (1985). The implications of professional and legal guidelines for court decisions involving criterion-related validity: A review and analysis. *Personnel Psychology, 38,* 803–833.

Lawshe, C.H. (1975). A quantitative approach to content validity. *Personnel Psychology, 28,* 563–575.

Linn, R.L. (1978). Single-group validity, differential validity, and differential prediction. *Journal of Applied Psychology, 63,* 507–512.

Linn, R.L., Harnisch, D.L., & Dunbar, S.B. (1981). Corrections for range restriction: An empirical investigation of conditions resulting in conservative corrections. *Journal of Applied Psychology, 66,* 655–663.

Lohman, T.G. (1981). Skinfolds and body density and their relation to body fatness: A review. *Human Biology, 53,* 181–225.

Martens, R. (1977). *Sport Competition Anxiety Test.* Champaign, IL: Human Kinetics.

Messick, S. (1975). The standard problem: Meaning and values in measurement and evaluation. *American Psychologist, 30,* 955–966.

Messick, S. (1980). Test validity and the ethics of assessment. *American Psychologist, 35,* 1012–1027.

Morgan, W.P., & Johnson, R.W. (1978). Personality characteristics of successful and unsuccessful oarsmen. *International Journal of Sport Psychology, 9,* 119–133.

Mosier, C.I. (1947). A critical examination of the concepts of face validity. *Educational and Psychological Measurement, 7,* 191–205.

Mosier, C.I. (1951). Problems and designs of cross-validation. *Educational and Psychological Measurement, 11*, 5–11.

Nagle, F.J., Morgan, W.P., Hellickson, R.O., Serfass, R.C., Alexander, J.P. (1975). Spotting success traits in Olympic contenders. *The Physician and Sportsmedicine, 3*, 31–34.

Nevo, B. (1985). Face validity revisited. *Journal of Educational Measurement, 22*, 287–293.

Nichols, J.G., Licht, B.G., & Pearl, R.A. (1982). Some dangers of using personality questionnaires to study personality. *Psychological Bulletin, 92*, 572–580.

Nichols, J.G., Licht, B.G., & Pearl, R.A. (1983). On the validity of inferences about personality constructs: A response to Friedman and Spence and Helmreich. *Psychological Bulletin, 94*, 188–189.

Nunnally, J.C. (1978). *Psychometric theory* (2nd ed.). New York: McGraw-Hill.

Safrit, M.J. (1981). *Evaluation in physical education* (2nd ed.). Englewood Cliffs, NJ: Prentice-Hall.

Safrit, M.J. (1986). *Introduction to measurement in physical education and exercise science.* St. Louis: Times Mirror/Mosby.

Safrit, M.J., Costa, M.G., & Hooper, L.M. (1986). The validity generalization model: An approach to the analysis of validity studies in physical education. *Research Quarterly for Exercise and Sport, 57*, 288–297.

Safrit, M.J., & Wood, T.M. (1983). The Health-Related Fitness Test opinionnaire: A pilot survey. *Research Quarterly for Exercise and Sport, 54*, 204–207.

Safrit, M.J., Wood, T.M., & Dishman, R.K. (1985). The factorial validity of the Physical Estimation and Attraction Scales for adults. *Journal of Sport Psychology, 7*, 166–190.

Safrit, M.J., Wood, T.M., Ehlert, S.A., Hooper, L.M., & Patterson, P. (1985). The application of sequential probability ratio testing to a test of motor skill. *Research Quarterly for Exercise and Sport, 56*, 58–65.

Schmidt, F.L., & Hunter, J.E. (1977). Development of a general solution to the problem of validity generalization. *Journal of Applied Psychology, 62*, 529–540.

Schmidt, F.L., Hunter, J.E., & Urry, V.W. (1976). Statistical power in criterion-related validation studies. *Journal of Applied Psychology, 61*, 473–485.

Schutz, R.W., Smoll, F.L., & Wood, T.M. (1981). Physical activity and sport: Attitudes and perceptions of young Canadian athletes. *Canadian Journal of Applied Sport Sciences, 6*, 32–39.

Secolsky, C. (1987). On the direct measurement of face validity: A comment on Nevo. *Journal of Educational Measurement, 24*, 82–83.

Simon, J.A., & Smoll, F.L. (1974). An instrument for assessing children's attitudes toward physical activity. *Research Quarterly, 47*, 797–803.

Sonstroem, R.J. (1978). Physical estimation and attraction scales: Rationale and research. *Medicine and Science in Sports, 10*, 97–102.

Tenopyr, M.L. (1977). Content-construct confusion. *Personnel Psychology, 30*, 47–54.

Weiss, M.R., Bredemeier, B.J., & Shewchuk, R.M. (1985). An intrinsic/extrinsic motivation scale for the youth sport setting: A confirmatory factor analysis. *Journal of Sport Psychology, 7*, 75–91.

Winne, P.H., & Belfry, M.J. (1982). Interpretive problems when correcting for attenuation. *Journal of Educational Measurement, 19*, 125–134.

Supplementary Readings

Bynner, J.M., & Romney, D.M. (1985). LISREL for beginners. *Canadian Psychology, 26*,
43–49.
Cascio, W.F., Valenzi, E.R., & Silbey, V. (1980). More on validation and statistical power.
Journal of Applied Psychology, 65, 135–138.
Claudy, J.G. (1978). Multiple regression and validity estimation in one sample. *Applied
Psychological Measurement, 2*, 595–607.
Lee, R., Miller, K.J., & Graham, W.K. (1982). Corrections for restriction of range and
attenuation in criterion-related validation studies. *Journal of Applied Psychology, 67*,
637–639.
Long, J.S. (1983a). *Confirmatory factor analysis: A preface to LISREL*. Beverly Hills, CA:
Sage.
Long, J.S. (1983b). *Covariance structure models: An introduction to LISREL*. Beverly Hills,
CA: Sage.
Marsh, H.W., & Hocevar, D. (1983). Confirmatory factor analysis of multitrait-multi-
method matrices. *Journal of Educational Measurement, 20*, 231–248.
Wainer, H., & Braun, H.I. (Eds.) (1988). *Test validity*. Hillsdale, NJ: Lawrence Erlbaum.

CHAPTER 3

Norm-Referenced Measurement: Reliability

Ted A. Baumgartner
University of Georgia

Two essential characteristics of any test or measuring instrument are validity and reliability. Validity was discussed in chapter 2. **Reliability** will be discussed thoroughly in this chapter. Reliability is an important characteristic of a test, because it influences the validity of a test and because without reliability no faith can be put in scores from a test.

If a test or measuring instrument is reliable, it consistently will provide the same measurement of a person. If a measurement instrument is totally reliable, it can be administered several times in one day or on several different days, and each time a person would obtain the same score. This is important, because the score obtained is expected to be a good indicator of the person's true ability. If the score contained substantial error, it would change when the person was measured again that day or several days later—the test would be unreliable.

Reliability influences the validity of a test. For a test to be valid it must be reliable, because a test that measures what it is supposed to measure must consistently provide the same information about a person. However, a reliable test may not be valid. A highly reliable test could be used in the wrong situation, and it would not be valid. For example, the pull-up test is quite reliable, but it is not a valid measure of leg strength.

There are two general types of reliability: relative and absolute. **Relative reliability** is estimated by using some type of correlation coefficient. It is an indication of the degree to which people maintain their position within a group, for example, from trial to trial within a day, day to day, or rater to rater. Three kinds of relative reliability are used frequently in physical education and exercise science. **Internal consistency reliability** is the degree to which people are consistent in their performance from trial to trial within a day. **Stability reliability** is the degree to which the performance of people is unchanging or stable from day to day. *Rater reliability* or **objectivity** is the degree to which the performance of a person is scored the same by two or more raters. Each of these three kinds of reliability indicates different characteristics of measurement instruments. It is important to calculate the correct estimate in determining the reliability of a measuring instrument or to require the correct estimate before using an instrument that already has established reliability.

Absolute reliability, the other general type, is estimated by using a measure of variability that indicates the degree to which people's scores did not change in magnitude or value. In other words, it is the amount of variability to be expected in a person's score if the person were tested again that day or several days later.

Reliability Theory

In theory, the score recorded for a person, which is called the *obtained score* (*x*), consists of two components, known as the *true score* (*t*) and the *error score* (*e*):

$$x = t + e \tag{3.1}$$

This is a theoretical formula, because the true score of a person is never known. For example, if a person's true ability to run 100 yd is 11.5 sec but the score is recorded as 11.7 sec, the error is .2 (11.7 = 11.5 + .2). If the 100-yd dash is run again, the recorded score might be 11.4 sec, so the error is −.1 (11.4 = 11.5 + −.1). Error can be caused by a variety of factors. The person might have been inconsistent in performance, might not have lined up exactly on the start line, and so forth. Perhaps the tester did not start or stop the timing clock correctly, did not read the timing clock correctly, and so forth.

Mathematically it can be shown that the variance of the obtained scores of a group is equal to the variance of their true scores plus the variance of their error scores:

$$\sigma_x^2 = \sigma_t^2 + \sigma_e^2 \tag{3.2}$$

In terms of relative reliability, reliability is defined as true score variance divided by obtained score variance:

$$\text{Reliability} = \sigma_t^2 / \sigma_x^2 \tag{3.3}$$

Notice in Equation 3.2 that if there is no error in each person's score, $\sigma_e^2 = 0$ and $\sigma_x^2 = \sigma_t^2$, so from Equation 3.3 the maximum value of reliability equals 1.0. Similarly, if each person's score consists only of error, $\sigma_I^2 = 0$, and the minimum value of reliability equals 0.0. Since the true score of each person is not known, the calculation of σ_I^2 is impossible; thus, it is impossible to calculate reliability directly. As is shown later in this chapter, estimates of σ_I^2 and σ_X^2 can be obtained, so reliability can be estimated.

With regard to absolute reliability, our interest concerns how much error to expect in a person's obtained score. We can approximate a person's true score by measuring the person a large number of times and calculating a mean score. The variability (standard deviation) in this large number of measures is the amount of variability to expect typically in the person's obtained score. Because it is not possible to obtain a large number of independent measures for each person in a group, a single measure is obtained for each person, and a measure of variability or expected obtained score error is estimated based on the variability in the measures of the group.

Methods of Estimating Reliability

Old Methods No Longer Appropriate

Before 1970 most physical educators, exercise scientists, and researchers estimated the reliability of physical performance measures by calculating a Pearson Product-Moment (PPM) correlation coefficient. To use this procedure, it was necessary to obtain two scores, X and Y, for each person. For example, the X score could be a score from one day and Y score from another day, or the X score the first trial and the Y score the second trial of a test administered within a day. If more than two scores were available for each person, such as scores on three or more trials of a test, the scores were divided into two parts—usually the sum of the odd-numbered trials and the sum of the even-numbered trials. Then the PPM correlation coefficient was calculated, using the two sums for each person as the X and Y scores. Finally, the obtained PPM coefficient was corrected by using the **Spearman-Brown prophecy formula** (see chapter 12). This was called the split-half technique.

There were problems in using the split-half technique, particularly if the number of trials or days was an odd number. But the biggest problem was with the use of the PPM correlation coefficient. It is a *bivariate* statistic, or **interclass correlation coefficient,** designed to be used when the X and Y scores represent *different variables* and not *repeated administrations* of the same test. Multiple administrations of one test is a *univariate* situation. Further, the PPM coefficient is not affected by change in the mean performance of the group from the X to the Y score. For example, if each subject's score increased three units from one testing period to another, the correlation coefficient would be perfect ($r = 1.0$). This suggests perfect reliability, but conceptually perfect reliability exists when there is no change in a subject's score from trial to trial within a day or from day to day.

The appropriate statistical technique for estimating reliability of repeated measures is called the **intraclass correlation coefficient** (R). It is a univariate statistic that takes

Subject 1	Subject 2	• • •	Subject n
X	X		X
X	X		X
•	•		•
•	•		•
•	•		•
scores of	scores of		scores of
subject 1	subject 2		subject n
•	•		•
•	•		•
•	•		•
X(score K)	X(score K)		X(score K)

n = number of subjects

K = number of scores per subject

Figure 3.1   One-Way ANOVA Model for Reliability Purposes

into account change in the mean of a group from trial to trial or day to day. It will also handle more than two scores per person. Kroll (1962) discusses the intraclass correlation coefficient in greater detail.

Intraclass Coefficient with One-Way ANOVA Model

The values needed in Equation 3.3 to estimate the reliability of a test cannot be obtained, so they must be estimated. Just as the variance in obtained scores can be separated into true score variance and error score variance (see Equation 3.2), the total variability in a set of scores can be divided into several components, by using analysis of variance (ANOVA) techniques (Ferguson, 1981; Glass & Stanley, 1970; Roscoe, 1975). Among the many ANOVA models is one called *Simple ANOVA, One-Way ANOVA,* or *Random Groups ANOVA.* Researchers typically use this ANOVA model to determine if there is a difference among groups in mean performance. Scores for a group are organized into a column, with the number of columns equal to the number of groups. For reliability purposes each subject is treated as a group, so the scores of a subject are organized into a column of scores (see Figure 3.1). Notice in Figure 3.1 that n represents the number of subjects measured and K represents the number of scores obtained for each subject. The scores represent multiple trials within a day, if internal consistency reliability is of interest; multiple days, if stability reliability is desired; or multiple raters, if objectivity is to be estimated.

An overview of the ANOVA process and the reliability coefficient calculation will be helpful before presenting the necessary computational equations and a sample calculation. The total variability in all the scores (there are K times n scores, because each of the n subjects has K scores), called *sum of squares total* (SS_T), is divided into *sum of squares between subjects* (SS_s) and *sum of squares within subjects* (SS_w). Sum of squares *between* subjects is an indication that all subjects do not have the same mean score and is used as an indication of true score variance (see Equation 3.2). Sum of squares *within* subjects is an indication that scores vary within a subject for some or all of the subjects and is used as an indication of error score variance (see Equation 3.2). After these sums of squares values are calculated, a *degrees of freedom* (df) value is calculated for each of the three sum of squares values. Next, each sum of squares value is divided by its degrees of freedom value to obtain a *mean square* value. Finally, these mean square values are used in an equation to obtain a reliability coefficient.
Necessary equations:

$$SS_T = \Sigma X^2 - \frac{(\Sigma X)^2}{(n)(K)} \tag{3.4}$$

$$SS_s = \frac{\Sigma T_i^2}{K} - \frac{(\Sigma X)^2}{(n)(K)} \tag{3.5}$$

$$SS_w = \Sigma X^2 - \frac{\Sigma T_i^2}{K} \tag{3.6}$$

$$df_T = (n)(K) - 1 \tag{3.7}$$

$$df_s = n - 1 \tag{3.8}$$

$$df_w = (n)(K-1) \tag{3.9}$$

$$MS_s = SS_s/df_s \tag{3.10}$$

$$MS_w = SS_w/df_w \tag{3.11}$$

$$R = (MS_s - MS_w)/MS_s \tag{3.12}$$

where ΣX^2 is the sum of the squared scores, ΣX is the sum of the scores, n is the number of subjects, K is the number of scores per subject, T_i is the sum of the scores for subject i, SS_T is the sum of squares total, SS_s is the sum of squares between subjects, SS_w is the sum of squares within subjects, df is degrees of freedom, MS is mean square, and R is the intraclass correlation coefficient—the reliability of the mean score for each subject.

Computational Example 1. Five subjects were administered three trials of a sit-and-reach test on the same day. Each trial was scored to the nearest inch. The scores are presented in Table 3.1.

Table 3.1   One-Way ANOVA Data from 3 Trials of a Test

Subject 1	Subject 2	Subject 3	Subject 4	Subject 5
15	11	9	10	17
16	10	11	11	16
18	11	14	8	16

Step 1: Obtain ΣX^2, ΣX, and the sum of the scores, T, for each subject.

$$\Sigma X^2 = 15^2 + 16^2 + 18^2 + 11^2 + 10^2 + 11^2 + \ldots + 17^2 + 16^2 + 16^2$$
$$= 2631$$

$$\Sigma X = 15 + 16 + 18 + 11 + 10 + 11 + \ldots + 17 + 16 + 16$$
$$= 193$$

Sum for Subject 1 $(T_1) = 15 + 16 + 18 = 49$
Sum for Subject 2 $(T_2) = 11 + 10 + 11 = 32$
Sum for Subject 3 $(T_3) = 9 + 11 + 14 = 34$
Sum for Subject 4 $(T_4) = 10 + 11 + 8 = 29$
Sum for Subject 5 $(T_5) = 17 + 16 + 16 = 49$

Step 2: Calculate the three sum of square values.

$$SS_T = \Sigma X^2 - \frac{(\Sigma X)^2}{(n)(K)} = 2631 - \frac{(193)^2}{(5)(3)} = 2631 - \frac{37249}{15}$$
$$= 2631 - 2483.27 = 147.73$$

$$SS_s = \frac{\Sigma T_i^2}{K} - \frac{(\Sigma X)^2}{(n)(K)}$$
$$= \frac{49^2 + 32^2 + 34^2 + 29^2 + 49^2}{3} - \frac{(193)^2}{(5)(3)}$$
$$= \frac{7823}{3} - \frac{37249}{15}$$
$$= 2607.67 - 2483.27$$
$$= 124.40$$

$$SS_w = \Sigma X^2 - \frac{\Sigma T_i^2}{K}$$
$$= 2631 - \frac{7823}{3}$$
$$= 2631 - 2607.67$$
$$= 23.33$$

Step 3: Calculate the three degrees of freedom values.

$df_T = [(n)(K)] - 1 = [(5)(3)] - 1 = 15 - 1 = 14$
$df_s = n - 1 = 5 - 1 = 4$
$df_w = (n)(K-1) = (5)(3-1) = (5)(2) = 10$

Step 4: Check the calculations.

$SS_T = SS_s + SS_w$
$147.73 = 124.40 + 23.33$
$147.73 = 147.73$
$df_T = df_s + df_w$
$14 = 4 + 10$
$14 = 14$

Step 5: Calculate *MS* for between and within.

$$MS_s = \frac{SS_s}{df_s} = \frac{124.40}{4} = 31.10$$

$$MS_w = \frac{SS_w}{df_w} = \frac{23.33}{10} = 2.33$$

Step 6: Calculate the *R*.

$$R = \frac{MS_s - MS_w}{MS_s}$$
$$= \frac{31.10 - 2.33}{31.10} = .93$$

The intraclass correlation coefficient varies from zero to one. In terms of reliability, an *R* of zero indicates absolutely no reliability. Because *R* indicates the reliability of the mean score for each subject, the mean score for each subject in Table 3.1 is quite reliable.

Sometimes the reliability of a single score is of more interest than the mean score for each subject. For example, a test might be administered on each of two days to calculate stability reliability, but in the future the test will be administered on only one day. How reliable is that single score? The formula for the reliability of a single score is:

$$R = \frac{MS_s - MS_w}{MS_s + (K/K' - 1)(MS_w)} \tag{3.13}$$

where *K* is the number of repeated measures administered and *K'* is the number of repeated measures for which *R* is estimated.

Computational Example 2. Using the mean square values from computational example 1:

$$R = \frac{MS_s - MS_w}{MS_s + (K/K' - 1)(MS_w)} = \frac{31.10 - 2.33}{31.10 + (3/1-1)(2.33)} = .80$$

In many situations this reliability coefficient is high enough to justify the use of one score rather than the mean of several scores for each subject.

With the one-way ANOVA model, all sources of variation other than differences between subjects are considered error (lack of reliability). For example, change in the mean performance of the subjects from trial to trial or day to day is considered lack of reliability. If before testing the mean performance was expected to change (due to warm-up, practice, or fatigue), this should not always be considered unreliability. A different ANOVA model allows the tester to look at the various sources of variation in a different way.

Intraclass Coefficient with Two-Way ANOVA Model

In the one-way ANOVA model just presented, only the column (subject) a score belonged to was important. Scores of a subject could be written in any order without affecting the sums of squares. The two-way ANOVA model presented here is one of several two-way ANOVA models. Often it is called a *random blocks* ANOVA or a *two-way repeated measures* ANOVA. In this model, rows (subjects) and columns (repeated measures) are important in the data analysis. Repeated measures could be scores from multiple trials within a day, multiple days, or multiple raters. The score arrangement for this ANOVA design is presented in Figure 3.2. Again, n represents the number of subjects measured and K represents the number of scores for each subject. With this score arrangement the sum of squares total can be divided into sum of squares between subjects (SS_s); sum of squares between repeated measures (SS_m); and sum of squares interaction (SS_i). Sum of squares between subjects is an indication that all subjects do not have the same mean score and is used as an indication of true score variance. Sum of squares between measures is an indication that all repeated measures do not have the same mean score (if trials are the repeated measures, all trial means are not equal). Sum of squares interaction is an indication that all subjects did not score in the same pattern on the repeated measure and is used as an indication of error variance (lack of reliability).

Necessary equations:

$$SS_T = \Sigma X^2 - \frac{(\Sigma X)^2}{(n)(K)} \tag{3.14}$$

$$SS_s = \frac{\Sigma(T_i)^2}{K} - \frac{(\Sigma X)^2}{(n)(K)} \tag{3.15}$$

$$SS_m = \frac{\Sigma(T_j)^2}{n} - \frac{(\Sigma X)^2}{(n)(K)} \tag{3.16}$$

$$SS_i = \Sigma X^2 + \frac{(\Sigma X)^2}{(n)(K)} - \frac{\Sigma(T_i)^2}{K} - \frac{\Sigma(T_j)^2}{n} \tag{3.17}$$

$$df_T = (n)(K) - 1 \tag{3.18}$$

	Subject		Repeated Measure				
			1	2	3	$\bullet\bullet\bullet$	K
	1		X_{11}	$X_{12}{}^{*}$	X_{13}	$\bullet\bullet\bullet$	X_{1K}
	1		X_{21}	$X_{22}{}^{*}$	X_{23}	$\bullet\bullet\bullet$	X_{2K}
	1		X_{31}	$X_{32}{}^{*}$	X_{33}	$\bullet\bullet\bullet$	X_{3K}
	$\bullet$		$\bullet$	$\bullet$	$\bullet$	$\bullet$	
	$\bullet$		$\bullet$	$\bullet$	$\bullet$	$\bullet$	
	$\bullet$		$\bullet$	$\bullet$	$\bullet$	$\bullet$	
	n		X_{n1}	$X_{n2}{}^{*}$	X_{n3}	$\bullet\bullet\bullet$	X_{nK}

n = number of subjects

K = number of scores per subject

*X_{12}, the second score of subject one

Figure 3.2   Two-Way ANOVA Model for Reliability Purposes

$$df_s = n - 1 \tag{3.19}$$

$$df_m = K - 1 \tag{3.20}$$

$$df_i = (n-1)(K-1) \tag{3.21}$$

$$MS_s = SS_s/df_s \tag{3.22}$$

$$MS_m = SS_m/df_m \tag{3.23}$$

$$MS_i = SS_i/df_i \tag{3.24}$$

where ΣX^2 is the sum of the squared scores, ΣX is the sum of the scores, n is the number of subjects, K is the number of scores per subject, T_i is the sum of the scores for subject i, T_j is the sum of the scores for measure j, SS_T is the sum of squares total, SS_s is the sum of squares subjects, SS_m is the sum of squares repeated measure, SS_i is the sum of squares interaction, df is degrees of freedom, MS is mean square, and R is the intraclass correlation coefficient—the reliability of the mean score for each subject.

Computational Example 3.   The scores from computational example 1 are used again and presented in Table 3.2.

Table 3.2 Two-Way ANOVA Data from 3 Trials of a Test

		Data	
Subject	Trial 1	Trial 2	Trial 3
1	15	16	18
2	11	10	11
3	9	11	14
4	10	11	8
5	17	16	16

Step 1: Obtain ΣX^2, ΣX, the sum of the scores for each subject (T_i), and the sum of the scores for each repeated measure (T_j).

$$\Sigma X^2 = 15^2 + 16^2 + 18^2 + 11^2 + 10^2 + 11^2 + \ldots + 17^2 + 16^2 + 16^2$$
$$= 2631$$
$$\Sigma X = 15 + 16 + 18 + 11 + 10 + 11 + \ldots + 17 + 16 + 16$$
$$= 193$$

Sum for Subject 1 = 15 + 16 + 18 = 49
Sum for Subject 2 = 11 + 10 + 11 = 32
Sum for Subject 3 = 9 + 11 + 14 = 34
Sum for Subject 4 = 10 + 11 + 8 = 29
Sum for Subject 5 = 17 + 16 + 16 = 49
Sum for Trial 1 = 15 + 11 + 9 + 10 + 17 = 62
Sum for Trial 2 = 16 + 10 + 11 + 11 + 16 = 64
Sum for Trial 3 = 18 + 11 + 14 + 8 + 16 = 67

Step 2: Calculate the four sum of squares values.

$$SS_T = \Sigma X^2 - \frac{(\Sigma X)^2}{(n)(K)} = 2631 - \frac{(193)^2}{(5)(3)} = 2631 - \frac{37249}{15}$$
$$= 2631 - 2483.27 = 147.73$$

$$SS_s = \frac{\Sigma (T_i)^2}{K} - \frac{(\Sigma X)^2}{(n)(K)}$$
$$= \frac{49^2 + 32^2 + 34^2 + 29^2 + 49^2}{3} - \frac{(193)^2}{(5)(3)}$$
$$= \frac{7823}{3} - \frac{37249}{15} = 2607.67 - 2483.27 = 124.40$$

$$SS_m = \frac{\Sigma (T_j)^2}{n} - \frac{(\Sigma X)^2}{(n)(K)} = \frac{62^2 + 64^2 + 67^2}{5} - \frac{(193)^2}{(5)(3)} = \frac{12429}{5} - \frac{37249}{15}$$
$$= 2483.80 - 2483.27 = 2.53$$

$$SS_i = \Sigma X^2 + \frac{(\Sigma X)^2}{(n)(K)} - \frac{\Sigma (T_i)^2}{K} - \frac{\Sigma (T_j)^2}{n}$$

$$= 2631 + \frac{(193)^2}{15} - \frac{7823}{3} - \frac{12429}{5}$$

$$= 2631 + 2483.27 - 2607.67 - 2485.80 = 20.80$$

Step 3: Calculate the four degrees of freedom values.

$$df_T = [(n)(K)] - 1 = [(5)(3)] - 1 = 14$$

$$df_s = n - 1 = 5 - 1 = 4$$

$$df_m = K - 1 = 3 - 1 = 2$$

$$df_i = (n-1)(K-1) = (5-1)(3-1) = 8$$

Step 4: Check the calculations.

$$SS_T = SS_s + SS_m + SS_i$$
$$147.73 = 124.40 + 2.53 + 20.80$$

$$df_T = df_s + df_m + df_i$$

$$14 = 4 + 2 + 8$$

Step 5: Calculate MS for subjects, measures, and interaction.

$$MS_s = \frac{SS_s}{df_s} = \frac{124.4}{4} = 31.10$$

$$MS_m = \frac{SS_m}{df_m} = \frac{2.53}{2} = 1.27$$

$$MS_i = \frac{SS_i}{df_i} = \frac{20.80}{8} = 2.60$$

Step 6: Calculate R.
There are several different approaches to calculating a reliability estimate (R) at this point. One approach is presented here; several others are presented later in the chapter.

$$R = \frac{MS_s - MS_i}{MS_s} = \frac{31.10 - 2.60}{31.10} = .92 \tag{3.25}$$

As with the R from the one-way ANOVA model presented previously, R is an estimate of the reliability of the mean score for each subject. The value of .92 indicates that the mean score for each subject is quite reliable.

Notice that in Equation 3.25, which was $R = (MS_s - MS_i)/MS_s$, the mean square for repeated measures (MS_m) does not appear. This equation is mathematically correct; but the omission of the mean square for repeated measures might suggest that it is an indication of neither true score nor error score variance (see Equations 3.2 and 3.3).

The mean square for repeated measures is greater than zero when the mean performance of a group changes from repeated measure to repeated measure (e.g., trial to trial, day to day, or rater to rater). Since the mean square for repeated measures is not in Equation 3.25, this source of variation is not considered error score variance or lack of reliability. In situations where the subjects were expected to change from repeated measure to repeated measure (e.g., through the effect of warm-up or fatigue) or in situations where the repeated measures are ratings of different judges and all judges are not expected to use the same standards, this seems quite appropriate. However, based on the definition of reliability (consistency of performance) given at the beginning of the chapter, it would seem that any change from repeated measure to repeated measure should be considered lack of reliability. The equation for R using a one-way ANOVA model, Equation 3.12, treats this change as lack of reliability.

As indicated earlier, sometimes the reliability of a single score is more important than the reliability of the mean score. With a two-way ANOVA model, the reliability of a single score is estimated with the equation:

$$R = \frac{MS_s - MS_i}{MS_s + (K/K'-1)(MS_i)} \qquad (3.26)$$

where K is the number of repeated measures administered and K' is the number of repeated measures for which R is estimated.

Computational Example 4. Using the mean square values from computational example 3:

$$R = \frac{MS_s - MS_i}{MS_s + (K/K'-1)(MS_i)} = \frac{31.10 - 2.60}{31.10 + (3/1-1)(2.60)} = .79$$

As a stability reliability coefficient, $R = .79$ often would be acceptable. As an internal consistency reliability coefficient, it probably would be considered too low.

Other Approaches to Reliability Using a Two-Way ANOVA Model

Baumgartner (1969) and Baumgartner and Jackson (1987) suggested that a teacher, exercise scientist, or researcher should attempt to find a measurement schedule consisting of a sequence of multiple trials that was highly reliable and that at the same time tended to maximize the mean performance of the group tested. Underlying this approach is the assumption that a criterion score based on multiple trial scores is better than a single score. This approach was utilized by Baumgartner and Jackson (1970). The first step is to perform a two-way ANOVA on the multiple trial data. The second step is to determine if there seems to be a difference among the trial means. One way this could be done is by conducting an F-test: $F = MS$ trials$/MS$ interaction, with degrees of freedom $(K-1)$ and $(n-1)(K-1)$. A table of the F distribution must be consulted to determine whether this value is significant. If it is significant, there is a difference among the trial means. The other way to determine if there seems to be a

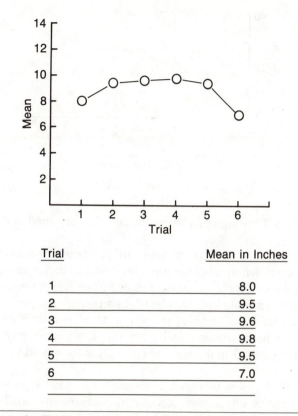

Trial	Mean in Inches
1	8.0
2	9.5
3	9.6
4	9.8
5	9.5
6	7.0

Figure 3.3   Graphing the Trial Means of a Sit-and-Reach Test

difference among the trial means is to graph the means. Based on a visual inspection of the graph, an investigator decides whether the trial means seem to differ. Some people first conduct an *F*-test and, if it is significant, then graph the trial means. Others just graph the trial means. Either approach is acceptable. An example of graphing the trial means is presented in Figure 3.3.

The third step is to decide whether to keep all of the trial data or eliminate certain trials. Remember, at this point a person is looking for a sequence of trials that are similar in mean score and tend to maximize the mean performance of the group. In Figure 3.3 it seems that trials 1 and 6 should be eliminated, because they are not similar to the other trials in mean score. There seems to have been an increase from trial 1 to trial 2 due to a practice and/or warm-up effect and a decrease from trial 5 to trial 6 due to a fatigue effect.

The fourth step is to calculate the reliability of the test using the trials retained. If no trials were eliminated, the ANOVA conducted at step 1 is used. If trials were eliminated, a two-way ANOVA must be conducted on the scores of the trials retained. For the sit-and-reach test presented in Figure 3.3, the ANOVA would be conducted

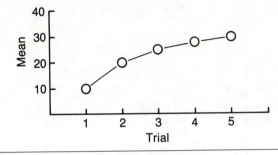

Figure 3.4   Another Example of Graphing the Trial Means

on the scores for trials 2 through 5. The reliability value obtained at this step is usually quite acceptable.

Based on the outcome of step 4, a test user could decide on the measurement schedule to follow in the future when administering the test to similar groups. For example, consider the sit-and-reach test data presented in Figure 3.3. A person could decide in the future to administer 5 trials and consider trial 1 a practice and/or warm-up, resulting in a criterion score that is the mean of the scores on trials 2 through 5. Alternatively, since the trial means were almost equal after trial 1, a person might decide to save testing time by giving only 3 trials, and the criterion score would be the mean of trials 2 and 3.

The pattern the trial means followed in Figure 3.3 is quite typical for many tests— warm-up and/or practice effect, then stable performance, and finally a fatigue effect. Another pattern is presented in Figure 3.4, along with a suggestion as to which trials to use to calculate the criterion score.

In Figure 3.4 it appears the subjects were not ready to be tested, because they continued to improve from trial to trial. The best course of action is to throw all the data away, give the subjects more exposure to the test to make sure they understand the test procedure so that their trial means will stabilize upon retesting, and then retest the subjects. If the data presented in Figure 3.4 must be used, only the last 2 trials should be retained.

The intraclass reliability coefficients from both a one-way ANOVA model (Equation 3.12) and a two-way ANOVA model (Equation 3.25) are appropriate estimates of the reliability of the mean score for each person. The two reliability coefficients differ in how error variance (lack of reliability) is defined, so selection of the appropriate coefficients is important. The choice between the two coefficients is mostly a philosophical one.

If a test developer is interested in knowing as much as possible about the characteristic of the test and particularly if a computer is used to run the ANOVA, a two-way ANOVA should be calculated initially, because it can always be collapsed to a one-way ANOVA. The relationship between the values from a one-way and two-way ANOVA is presented in Table 3.3. To obtain the values for a one-way ANOVA from a two-way ANOVA,

Table 3.3   Relationship Between a One-Way and a Two-Way ANOVA

One-Way ANOVA value	Equivalent Two-Way ANOVA value
Sum of squares total (SS_T)	Sum of squares total (SS_T)
Sum of squares subjects (SS_s)	Sum of squares subjects (SS_s)
Sum of squares within (SS_w)	Sum of squares repeated measure (SS_m) + sum of squares interaction (SS_i)
Degrees of freedom total (df_T)	Degrees of freedom total (df_T)
Degrees of freedom subjects (df_s)	Degrees of freedom subjects (df_s)
Degrees of freedom within (df_w)	Degrees of freedom repeated measure (df_m) + degrees of freedom interaction (df_i)

only the sum of squares, degrees of freedom, and mean square for within must be calculated. The equations for doing this are:

$$SS_w = SS_m + SS_i \tag{3.27}$$

$$df_w = df_m + df_i \tag{3.28}$$

$$MS_w = \frac{SS_w}{df_w} \tag{3.29}$$

To calculate the R as if a one-way ANOVA model had been used instead of a two-way ANOVA model, Equation 3.12 is utilized:

$$R = \frac{MS_s - MS_w}{MS_s}$$

One of the major advantages of first using a two-way ANOVA model, particularly with a computer, is that it is possible to determine if there seems to be a difference among the repeated measure (trials, days, or raters) means, and at the same time not be limited to using only one of the two intraclass R equations (Equation 3.12 or 3.25). If there seems to be a difference among the means of the repeated measure, the researcher can classify the difference as undesirable error and use Equation 3.12, consider it to be an expected source of variance and use Equation 3.25, or eliminate certain repeated measures so that the remaining repeated measures will be equal in mean value.

Other Reliability Approaches

Intraclass reliability coefficients can be calculated from ANOVA designs other than one-way and two-way. Feldt and McKee (1958) present a three-way ANOVA design for estimating reliability when a group of subjects has been administered multiple trials of a test on each of several days. The report by Safrit, Atwater, Baumgartner, and West (1976) is an excellent reference on reliability of motor performance measures and various ANOVA designs from which an intraclass reliability coefficient can be calculated.

Particularly with ordinal data, reliability coefficients other than the intraclass coefficient can be utilized. Stamm (1976) and Stamm and Safrit (1977) suggest a few alternative coefficients.

Some test developers and users are interested in how much of the variance in a set of scores is due to each of several sources. These variance components and the proportion of the total variance associated with each source can be determined by using the mean square values utilized in the R equations previously discussed. Safrit et al. (1976) and Safrit (1981) are excellent references on this topic.

ANOVA Values From the Computer

The necessary mean square values to calculate an intraclass reliability coefficient can be obtained easily from the computer by using any one of many different computer programs. One-way and two-way ANOVA computer programs are quite plentiful for both mainframe computers and microcomputers. Two-way ANOVA programs usually provide means for the repeated measure.

Mainframe Computer Programs

The mainframe version of SPSS is discussed here because of its great popularity and accessibility. In the SPSS package of computer programs there is a one-way ANOVA program called ONEWAY. There is no two-way ANOVA program in the package that will handle repeated measures, but starting with Version 7 of SPSS there is a program called RELIABILITY that will calculate an intraclass R from a two-way ANOVA model $[R = (MS_s - MS_i)/MS_s]$. The form of SPSS statements to the computer changed with Version 10 (SPSS^X), but statements in Versions 7 through 9 are quite similar to Version 10 statements. Each program in Versions 7 through 9 is explained in a manual (Nie, Hull, Jenkins, Steinbrenner, & Bent, 1975). All SPSS examples in this chapter are for Version 10 on a mainframe computer. Each program in Version 10 is explained in a manual (SPSS, 1983). SPSS^X examples are presented in appendix 3-A.

Microcomputer Programs

A number of packages of statistical programs for microcomputers exist, including several nationally distributed packages originally designed for mainframe computers (e.g., BMDP—Dixon & Brown, 1981; SAS, 1982; SPSS, 1983). The microcomputer versions of the mainframe programs are quite complete, relatively expensive, and very good. Other packages are not very complete or particularly good, although they still may be expensive. Discussed in this part of the chapter are a few computer program packages and one computer program, all of which are quite good and not very expensive.

Microcomputer programs are stored on floppy disks or, in a few cases, on cassette tapes. Disks for one brand of microcomputer will seldom work in another brand of computer, although many computers are compatible with the IBM-PC. When selecting a computer program it is beneficial if (a) the program has the ability to save the data in case another analysis is required and (b) it will print the results of the analysis to either the computer screen or a printer. Certainly a program that is user-friendly, with good prompts and error messages, is most desirable.

A package of computer programs for use with either an Apple or IBM microcomputer called *Statistics With Finesse* (Bolding, 1985) is user-friendly, inexpensive, and capable of building files and saving the data. The manual and computer prompts are easy to follow. After the computer reads the program disk, a menu appears so the user can select a particular program. The *One-Way* program computes a one-way ANOVA, and the *Repeated Measures* calculates a two-way ANOVA for repeated measures.

A package of computer programs for the Apple microcomputer by Steinmetz, Romano, and Patterson (1981) is referenced extensively and discussed by Thomas and Nelson (1985). It is user-friendly, inexpensive, and capable of saving data. The computer prompts are good. The *One-Way* program computes a one-way ANOVA, and a program called *Random Blocks Analysis* performs a two-way ANOVA for repeated measures. When the program first starts, it displays a menu so the user can select a particular program. One limitation of the package of programs is that all programs in the package do not save the data in the same manner, so data saved under one program cannot always be used with another program.

A program called *Intraclass Reliability* was written for an Apple II computer and is available from the author of this chapter. The program is very user-friendly with good computer prompts, and it will save data. A short manual accompanies the program. The program computes an intraclass R for the mean score of a person from both a one-way and two-way ANOVA model. The results can be displayed on the computer screen or printed on paper. An example of this program is presented in appendix 3-B.

Absolute Estimates of Reliability

As indicated at the beginning of this chapter, the two basic types of reliability are *relative* and *absolute*. Relative reliability has been discussed in great detail; absolute reliability is discussed in the following section.

Absolute reliability focuses on the amount of error to expect in a person's recorded score. One way to determine this would be to measure the person independently many times in one day or on several days. The standard deviation for the person's multiple measures would be the amount of error to expect in a person's recorded score. Obviously, to do this for every person in a group would be impossible, so a measure of the average error to expect in a person's recorded score is estimated by using the scores of a group. This measure is called the **standard error of measurement**.

The standard error of measurement (SEM) is in the actual score units of the data. It is the amount of error to expect in any person's obtained score. The equation for the SEM is determined as follows:

$$\text{SEM} = s_x \sqrt{1 - r_{xx'}} \tag{3.30}$$

where s_x is the group standard deviation for the test scores and $r_{xx'}$ is the reliability for the test.

Computational Example 4. A mile-run test was administered to a group of boys. The reliability of the test was .90 and the standard deviation was 20 seconds. What is the standard error of measurement?

$$\text{SEM} = s_x \sqrt{1 - r_{xx'}} = 20 \sqrt{1 - .90} = 20 \sqrt{.10} = (20)(.32) = 6.40$$

The standard error of measurement is like a test score standard deviation. In a normal curve, approximately 68% of the scores are within ± 1 standard deviation of the mean. The mean in this case is a test score, and the standard deviation is the standard error of measurement.

If in computational example 4 a person received a score of 360 seconds on the mile run, the chances are 68% that if the person were tested again before a change in ability level, a ± 1 SEM band would span the person's true score. This band is 353.60 (360 − 6.40) and 366.40 (360 + 6.40). If the same classification results if a person has a true score as low as 353.60 or as high as 366.40, then the limits of the confidence band are acceptable, and the person's score is utilized with faith that it is a good indication of the person's true ability. A perceived difference between 353.60 and 366.40, however, would limit the usefulness of the score 360.

A common interpretation of the standard error of measurement is that the smaller the standard error of measurement the more reliable the test is. Note in Equation 3.30 that the standard error of measurement is influenced by the standard deviation for the test. Since the standard deviation is influenced by the difference between the maximum and minimum scores possible on a test, all tests will not have the same standard deviation and, therefore, will not have the same standard error of measurement. Only if the reliability of a test is 1.0 will the standard error of measurement be zero.

The ± 1 SEM confidence band can be useful when comparing the performance of two students. Although their test scores may not seem similar, their confidence bands may overlap considerably. Only if their confidence bands do not overlap is it quite safe to say that the two students differ in ability. For additional discussion of the standard error of measurement, see Safrit (1981) or Ferguson (1981).

Factors Affecting Reliability Coefficients

One factor affecting the magnitude of the reliability coefficient is the type of reliability coefficient. Generally, the internal consistency reliability coefficient for a group will be higher than its stability coefficient. This is because there are fewer potential sources of change in a person's score from trial to trial than from day to day. For example, in a stability reliability coefficient the good-day/bad-day phenomenon can be operating, but it cannot affect an internal consistency reliability coefficient. In fact, whether a one-way ANOVA model or two-way ANOVA model was used to calculate the intraclass R makes a difference in the magnitude of the reliability coefficient. Thus, it is very important to report the type of reliability coefficient and the ANOVA model utilized after determining reliability.

Another factor that will affect the magnitude of the reliability coefficient is the homogeneity/heterogeneity of the data. This can be considered in two different ways. First, if the group is more homogeneous or heterogeneous than is typical this will tend to affect the magnitude of the reliability coefficient. Homogeneity tends to deflate, and heterogeneity tends to inflate the magnitude of the reliability coefficient. Looking at the intraclass reliability equations (Equations 3.12 and 3.25), as heterogeneity of the subjects, and thus their scores, increases, the mean square subjects (MS_s) increases too. If the mean square within (MS_w) in Equation 3.12 or the mean square interaction (MS_i) in Equation 3.25 is unchanged, the reliability increases. Second, the larger the potential spread or range in the test scores, the larger the reliability coefficient may be. Often tests with a very limited number of potential scores (like target-type tests) are not very reliable. Of course, if most of the potential range of the test scores is not used or other problems exist in the test, the reliability may still be low.

The size of the group may affect the magnitude of the reliability coefficient. When estimating the reliability of a test, the group should be large enough that most, if not all, abilities are represented. Sometimes small groups are more homogeneous or heterogeneous than is typical, because all abilities are not represented. Some test developers recommend that the group size be several hundred. Often a group size of 30 to 50 is used to estimate the reliability of a test. It is certainly more economical to test this group size. If a group seems typical, there is no harm in estimating reliability with small group sizes of 30 to 50.

The age, gender, and experience level of the subjects also may affect the magnitude of the reliability coefficient. Although these characteristics may have absolutely no effect, there is no guarantee of this. It is unwise to assume that a test that is reliable for one gender, age, or experience level is automatically reliable for another gender, age, or experience level.

A big factor in the reliability of a test is whether the subjects are ready to be tested. Usually for a test to be reliable the subjects must have had experience with the test before the day they are tested so they understand the test, know the testing procedure, use the best possible form, and so forth. They also need to know when they will be tested so they are ready physiologically and psychologically. If a person who has never run a mile before is suddenly tested, without prior warning, how reliable will the score be? Finally, the subjects need adequate time to warm up and/or practice on the day of the test.

A sixth factor that can affect the magnitude of the reliability coefficient is characteristics of the tester or rater. One reason the scores of a subject could differ from trial to trial or day to day is that the scorer is not consistent in administering or scoring the test, i.e., there is a lack of objectivity. Similarly, the scores assigned by several raters may differ because the raters are not using the same standards. If testers or raters are qualified and clearly understand how a test should be administered and scored, this factor should have a very minor effect on the magnitude of the reliability coefficient.

Test characteristics also affect the magnitude of the reliability coefficient. All tests do not have the same potential for high reliability, even if everything is done correctly. Some attributes are easier to measure than others. Generally, physical fitness tests are more reliable than sports skills tests. Objective measures are usually more reliable than subjective measures. The number of different scores possible on a test and whether scores tend to cluster at certain points both have an effect on the magnitude of the reliability coefficient. Much of what was said earlier about homogeneity and heterogeneity of the data applies here.

The number of measures in the criterion score will affect the magnitude of the reliability coefficient. Generally, the more measures in a criterion score, the more reliable the criterion score will be. Unless fatigue sets in, a three-trial test with the criterion score being the mean of the three trials will be more reliable than a one-trial test. The increase in the reliability of a test as it is increased in length can be predicted by the **Spearman-Brown prophecy formula:**

$$r_{xx'}^* = \frac{K(r_{xx'})}{1 + [(K-1)(r_{xx'})]} \tag{3.31}$$

where K is number of times the length of the test has been increased, $r_{xx'}$ is the present reliability of the test, and $r_{xx'}^*$ is the estimated reliability of the lengthened test.

Computational Example 5. The reliability of a one-trial sit-and-reach test is .82. What would be the reliability of a three-trial test?

In this case $K = 3$, because the number of trials has been tripled:

$$r_{xx'}^* = \frac{3(.82)}{1 + [(3-1)(.82)]} = \frac{2.46}{2.64} = .93$$

A reliability of .93 is quite good and should be interpreted as the maximum reliability that might be obtained if three trials were administered and the criterion score of each person was the mean or sum of the three trial scores.

The discussion of the Spearman-Brown Prophecy Formula introduced the issue of the **criterion score**, i.e. the score for a person when multiple trials of a test are administered. Two commonly used criterion-score options are the *best score* and the *mean score*. Note that the sum of the scores is the same as the mean score, because each person's sum is divided by the same number. Many investigators have published articles concerned with selecting the criterion score (Baumgartner, 1974; Berger & Sweney, 1965; Henry, 1967; Hetherington, 1973; Johnson & Meeter, 1977). The decision as to which one to use is based on the situation and what the criterion score is supposed to indicate. The directions for many tests will indicate that the best score should be used, although the directions for some of the most recent fitness tests and sports skills tests suggest using the mean score. One advantage of using the best score is that each trial may not have to be measured, as in the discus throw during a track meet. Even if all the trials are measured, a mean score or sum of the scores will not have to be calculated. From a philosophical position, if the criterion score is supposed to indicate the maximum performance of a person at the time the test is administered, the criterion score should be the best score. This philosophical position is common in athletic contests. However, the best score can be a fluke score, which the person seldom if ever accomplishes again.

The mean score or sum of the trial scores is more reliable than the best score. If the intent of the test is to obtain the best indication of the person's typical performance, the mean score or sum of the trial scores should be used. The intent of most testing situations in physical education, exercise science, and research is to obtain the best indication of the true score or typical score of a person. It is interesting to note that if a test is totally reliable there is no need for multiple trials, because all the scores of a person are equal and the best score is the mean score. A test's low stability reliability can be improved by using as the criterion score the mean score or sum of the scores from several days. A criterion score that is the mean score or sum of the scores from multiple trials on multiple days is another way to try to obtain a reliable criterion score.

Early in this chapter under the topic heading "Reliability Theory" it was stated that the criterion score or obtained score consists of two components: the true score and the error score. The true score of a person often is defined as the mean of an infinite number of trial scores. The error score is the amount of measurement error in an obtained score. Also, there is a natural phenomenon called the *regression effect*, which is the tendency for a person who scores particularly high or low on one measure to score closer to the mean performance of the group on another measure. In the case of multiple trial data, the regression effect would be the tendency for a person with a large error score on one trial to score closer to his or her true score on another trial. In theory the distribution of a person's obtained scores on multiple trials of a test would be normally distributed around the person's true score, the mean of the person's obtained scores. This suggests that the mean score is a better estimate of a person's true score and is more reliable than the best score. It might suggest that using the worst score makes as much sense as using the best score as an estimate of true score. Chapter 10 contains additional information on this topic.

Conclusion

Reliability has been discussed extensively in this chapter. From studying this chapter, the reader should have a good understanding of reliability and the difference between internal consistency and stability reliability.

The ability to calculate a reliability coefficient from either a one-way or two-way ANOVA model is an important outcome of this chapter. In addition, a clear understanding of the advantages of each ANOVA model to calculate the intraclass R should be obtained from this chapter.

The reader should recognize that relative reliability is used more commonly than absolute reliability, but there are situations where an indication of absolute reliability is necessary.

The use of the computer to calculate intraclass reliability coefficients should not be taken lightly and should not be considered non-essential information. Although a reliability coefficient can always be calculated by hand, it is inefficient to take the time to do so.

Finally, a good understanding of the factors affecting the size of the reliability coefficient is important if a person is constructing or using a test. To construct a good test or to improve an existing one, a person must be aware of the factors that influence reliability.

References

Baumgartner, T.A. (1969). Estimating reliability when all test trials are administered on the same day. *Research Quarterly, 40*, 222–225.

Baumgartner, T.A. (1974). Criterion score for multiple trial measures. *Research Quarterly, 45*, 193–198.

Baumgartner, T.A., & Jackson, A.S. (1970). Measurement schedules for tests of motor performance. *Research Quarterly, 41*, 10–17.

Baumgartner, T.A., & Jackson, A.S. (1987). *Measurement for evaluation in physical education and exercise science* (3rd ed.). Dubuque, IA: Wm. C. Brown.

Berger, R.A., & Sweney, A.B. (1965). Variance and correlation coefficients. *Research Quarterly, 36*, 368–370.

Bolding, J. (1985). *Statistics with finesse.* Fayetteville, AR: Author.

Dixon, W.J., & Brown, M.B. (1981). *BMDP statistical software 1981 manual.* Berkeley, CA: University of California Press.

Feldt, L.S., & McKee, M.E. (1958). Estimating the reliability of skill tests. *Research Quarterly, 29*, 279–293.

Ferguson, G.A. (1981). *Statistical analysis in psychology and education* (5th ed.). New York: McGraw-Hill.

Glass, G.V., & Stanley, J.C. (1970). *Statistical methods in education and psychology.* Englewood Cliffs, NJ: Prentice-Hall.

Henry, F.M. (1967). Best versus average individual score. *Research Quarterly, 38*, 317–320.

Hetherington, R. (1973). Within subject variation, measurement error, and selection of a criterion score. *Research Quarterly, 44*, 113–117.

Johnson, R., & Meeter, D. (1977). Estimation of maximum physical performance. *Research Quarterly, 48*, 74–84.

Kroll, W. (1962). A note on the coefficient of intraclass correlation as an estimate of reliability. *Research Quarterly, 33*, 313–316.

Nie, N.H., Hull, C.H., Jenkins, J.G., Steinbrenner, K., & Bent, D.H. (1975). *Statistical package for the social sciences* (2nd ed.). New York: McGraw Hill.

Roscoe, J.T. (1975). *Fundamental research statistics for the behavioral sciences* (2nd ed.). New York: Holt, Rinehart, and Winston.

Safrit, M.J. (1981). *Evaluation in physical education* (2nd ed.). Englewood Cliffs, NJ: Prentice-Hall.

Safrit, M.J., Atwater, A.E., Baumgartner, T.A., & West, C. (1976). *Reliability theory appropriate for motor performance measures.* Washington, DC: AAHPERD.

SAS Institute Inc. (1982). *SAS user's guide: Statistics* (rev. ed.). Cary, NC: Author.

SPSS Inc. (1983). *SPSS^X user's guide.* New York: McGraw-Hill.

Stamm, C.L. (1976). An alternative method for estimating reliability. *JOPERD, 47,* 66–67.

Stamm, C.L., & Safrit, M.J. (1977). Comparisons of two nonparametric methods for estimating the reliability of motor performance tests. *Research Quarterly, 48,* 169–176.

Steinmetz, J.E., Romano, A.G., & Patterson, M.M. (1981). Statistical programs for the Apple II microcomputer. *Behavior Research Methods and Instrumentation, 15*(5), 702.

Thomas, J.R., & Nelson, J.K. (1985). *Introduction to research in health, physical education, recreation, and dance.* Champaign, IL: Human Kinetics.

Supplementary Readings

Baumgartner, T.A. (1969). Stability of physical performance test scores. *Research Quarterly, 40,* 257–261.

Disch, J. (1975). Considerations for establishing a reliable and valid criterion measure for a multiple trial motor performance test. In T.A. Baumgartner (Ed.), *Proceedings of the C.I.C. symposium on measurement and evaluation in physical education.* Bloomington, IN: Indiana University.

Feldt, L. (1975). Estimating reliability when the parts of the total test differ in length. In T.A. Baumgartner (Ed.), *Proceedings of the C.I.C. symposium on measurement and evaluation in physical education.* Bloomington, IN: Indiana University.

Nunnally, J.C. (1967). *Psychometric Theory.* New York: McGraw-Hill.

Appendix 3-A
SPSS^X Examples

ONEWAY in Version 10 of SPSS computes a one-way ANOVA. To use this program, each subject must be considered a group and the repeated measure scores of the subject must be considered the scores for the group. A group identification number must accompany each score entered as data. The SPSS commands and data to obtain a one-way ANOVA on the data from Table 3.2 are presented in Figure 3.5. The printout for this analysis is presented in Figure 3.6.

In Figure 3.5, TITLE identifies that the title to appear at the top of each page of the computer printout is that which is in double quotation marks. The DATA LIST statement

TITLE   "ANALYSIS OF TABLE 3.2 DATA USING ONEWAY IN SPSS VERSION 10"

DATA LIST   / GROUP 1 SCORE 3-4

ONEWAY   SCORE BY GROUP (1,5)/

STATISTIC   1

BEGIN DATA

1*   15**

1   16

1   18

1   11

2   11

2   10

2   11

.   .

.   .

.   .

5   17

5   16

5   16

END DATA

FINISH

---

* Group (Subject) Number
** A score value

Figure 3.5   Input Statements for ONEWAY in SPSS Version 10, Using The Data in Table 3.2

Variable SCORE By Variable GROUP

ANALYSIS OF VARIANCE

Source	D.F.	SS	MS	F	F Prob.
Between Groups	4	124.40	31.10	13.33	.0005
Within Groups	10	23.33	2.33		
Total	14	147.73			

GROUP	COUNT	MEAN	S.D.	S.E.	MIN.	MAX.
1	3	16.33	1.53	.88	15.00	18.00
2	3	10.67	.58	.33	10.00	11.00
3	3	11.33	2.52	1.45	9.00	14.00
4	3	9.67	1.53	.88	8.00	11.00
5	3	16.33	.58	.33	16.00	17.00
TOTAL	15	12.87	3.25	.84	8.00	18.00

Figure 3.6 Computer Output for the Input Statements in Figure 3.5

communicates to the computer that the data follows the SPSS statements, there are 2 values per line, the group number (GROUP) is in column 1, and the score of a subject (SCORE) is in columns 3 and 4. The names GROUP and SCORE were chosen arbitrarily. ONEWAY indicates that the one-way ANOVA procedure is to be used with the data called SCORE and the five groups formed by the score GROUP (1,5). STATISTIC 1 indicates that certain statistics are desired (see p. 471 in the SPSS[x] manual). BEGIN DATA and END DATA go before and after the data. FINISH indicates that the analysis is finished.

The SPSS commands and data to obtain an intraclass R based on a two-way ANOVA model using RELIABILITY in SPSS Version 10 are presented in Figure 3.7. The printout for this analysis is presented in Figure 3.8.

The RELIABILITY statement in Figure 3.7 indicates to the computer that the reliability procedure should be used to analyze the data. For this analysis, the three scores per subject arbitrarily were named SCORE1, SCORE2, and SCORE3. VARIABLES indicates that these three scores are available for an analysis. SCALE indicates which of the variables will be used in the analysis. In this case, it is all variables from SCORE1 through SCORE3. The RCOEFF after SCALE is an arbitrary name. MODEL = ALPHA indicates that the alpha reliability model should be used to analyze the data.

TITLE	"ANALYSIS OF TABLE 3.2 DATA USING RELIABILITY IN SPSS VERSION 10"
DATA LIST	/ SUBJECT 1 SCORE1 3-4 SCORE2 6-7 SCORE3 9-10
RELIABILITY	VARIABLES = SCORE1 SCORE2 SCORE3/SCALE (RCOEFF) SCORE1 TO SCORE3/MODEL = ALPHA
STATISTIC	1

BEGIN DATA

1*   15   16   18**

2   11   10   11

3   09   11   14

4   10   11   08

5   17   16   16

END DATA

FINISH

---

*Subject number

**Third score of subject 1

Figure 3.7   Input Statements for RELIABILITY in SPSS Version 10, Using the Data in Table 3.2

Appendix 3-B
Intraclass Reliability Microcomputer Program Example

When the program is started, a menu is displayed with the options:

(1) Create a Data File.
(2) Add a Subject to a File.
(3) Edit an Existing File.
(4) Print an Existing File.
(5) Compute Reliability.
(6) Exit.

RELIABILITY ANALYSIS - SCALE (RCOEFF)

1. SCORE1

2. SCORE2

3. SCORE3

	MEAN	STD DEV	CASES
1. SCORE1	12.40	3.44	5.0
2. SCORE2	12.80	2.95	5.0
3. SCORE3	13.40	3.97	5.0

RELIABILITY COEFFICIENTS

N OF CASES = 5.0   N OF ITEMS = 3

ALPHA* = 0.92

---

*Alpha $= R = (MS_s - MS_i)/MS_s$

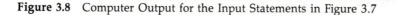

Figure 3.8   Computer Output for the Input Statements in Figure 3.7

The program requires that the data be saved on disk, so the first thing a user does is select option 1, "Create a Data File." Following prompts from the computer, the user enters the data and the computer saves the data. The user returns to the menu to select another option. Many users will select option 4 in order to check their data and, if any errors in the data are detected, select option 3. There is nothing wrong with selecting option 5 right after option 1. Eventually all users will select option 5, because it calculates the intraclass R values. The output from *Intraclass Reliability* for the data in Table 3.2 is presented in Figure 3.9.

In Figure 3.9 all the essential information is available no matter what reliability model is desired. In the two-way ANOVA table, under source, the terms will always be subject, trial, and inter. (interaction), regardless of whether the repeated measure is trials, days, or raters.

One-Way ANOVA Table

SOURCE	DF	SS	MS
Among	4	124.400	31.100
Within	10	23.333	2.333
Total	14	147.733	

One-Way Reliability*   0.924

Two-Way ANOVA Table

SOURCE	DF	SS	MS
Subject	4	124.400	31.100
Trial	2	2.533	1.266
Inter.	8	20.799	2.599
Total	14	147.733	

Two-Way Reliability**   0.916

TRIAL	MEAN
1	12.400
2	12.800
3	13.400

$*R = (MS_s - MS_w)/MS_s$
$**R = (MS_s - MS_i)/MS_s$

Figure 3.9   Output from Intraclass Reliability microcomputer program, using the data in Table 3.2

Generalizability Theory

James R. Morrow, Jr.
University of Houston

Why Generalizability Theory?

The purpose of this chapter is to describe an extension of reliability theory, termed **generalizability theory** (G-theory), provide step-by-step procedures for conducting research with generalizability theory models, and give examples of its use.

Interclass reliability models (e.g., test-retest, parallel forms) can use only *two* scores when computing a reliability coefficient. In contrast, the use of intraclass models permits *unlimited* scores or repeated measures to be used when determining the reliability of a measurement protocol. This is obviously a desirable feature, in that the reliability of a test improves as the number of scores increases. That is, the mean of two scores is more reliable than a single score. Thus, using intraclass models in classical test theory, reliability coefficients can be estimated for both an unlimited number of students and an unlimited number of scores.

But it is possible to extend this measurement schedule still further. Consider the assessment of subcutaneous skinfold fat. Several factors might affect the reliability of skinfold measures: the students, the caliper, the tester, the amount of training obtained by the tester, the experience of the tester with skinfold measurement, the gender of the student, and the location of the skinfold fat. All of these sources of variation contribute to either true variation in subjects or measurement error. Generalizability theory analysis can be used to incorporate all of the above factors (and others as well) into a model that estimates reliability when multiple sources of error can potentially be identified.

Comparison with Classical Test Theory

According to classical test theory, an obtained score can be partitioned into a true score and an error score. Assume that the reliability, $r_{xx'}$, equals .60. Under classical test theory, 60% of the observed score variance is assumed to be true score variance (σ_t^2) among people, whereas the remaining 40% is assumed to be error score variance (σ_e^2). Although intraclass models offer more flexibility than interclass models in estimating test reliability, neither approach allows differentiation of the random error component. Which factors might contribute to the error score variance? In classical test theory, there are only three quantifiable sources of variance (i.e., people, scores, and people $\times$ scores). Variance among people is always considered observed score variance. The error score variance depends upon the model chosen and the researcher's definition(s) of error (e.g., error may be defined as *all* variance not attributable to differences in people, i.e., scores and people $\times$ scores, or as only people $\times$ scores). Thus, only *two* sources of variation can be defined as error. This may be inadequate, because other factors might have contributed to the potentially large amounts of error in the measurement protocol. Classical test theory groups all of the error together into an undifferentiated error term. Generalizability theory analysis permits the researcher to partition the undifferentiated error by identifying an unlimited number of factors (facets) when determining the reliability of the data. The term **facet** represents a dimension on which measures are taken (e.g., days, classes, weeks). A facet is a "set of similar conditions of measurement" (Brennan, 1983, p. 2). Therefore, subjects is a source of variance, but technically is not considered a facet in a **G study**. G-theory can be used to partition the total variance and to estimate the contribution of each facet (and subjects) or combinations of facets in the model to the reliability (or lack of reliability) found within the model.

Safrit, Atwater, Baumgartner, and West (1976) indicate that in

> generalizability theory, the "true score" is replaced with the "expected value" of the score in the population of values from which the sample score was drawn. There is only one true score for a given person on a specified measure in the classical test framework, but there may be many universe scores in generalizability theory. (p. 36)

The different universe scores depend on the number of facets that are generalized. Once the researcher has ascertained which facets contribute most toward error, these facets can be controlled in a variety of ways (e.g., elimination of facets from the model, training observers, increasing the number of levels of the facets). As the levels of facets change (randomly) from one sampling to another, the precision of the measurement will be affected. With generalizability theory, the sample of facet levels can be used to generalize to the universe of facet levels available. This is referred to as the *universe of inference*. Since a large number of universes can be identified, there can be a large number of different reliability (generalizability) coefficients.

An Application: Volleyball Ratings

Consider a reliability study in which different physical education teachers rate the volleyball playing ability of students over several days. By examining the agreement among teachers, the objectivity (inter-rater reliability) of the observations can be determined effectively. But, it is reasonable to expect that along with the observations that vary as a function of the students (i.e., all do not have the same abilities and skills) observational ratings might also vary, as a function of both the teachers and the day on which the students are observed. A number of other facets could also be included in the model. For example, court position, the game, and whether the team is ahead or behind are only three of a number of facets that might influence the ratings assigned by teachers.

The facets in this study are days and teachers. Each of the three teachers rates the overall volleyball playing ability of ten students on each of four observational days. The reliability of observations across different teachers and across different days is of interest. Both teachers and days can be perceived as **randomly representative** of the potential universe of teachers and days that could have been chosen for observation. These *random* facets can be differentiated from *fixed* facets. In the present example, interest centers on estimating the reliability (i.e., generalizability) of the ratings for the potential universe of days and for the potential universe of teachers. Thus, differences in days and teachers might contribute to measurement error.

If each possible position played was included within the model, *position* would be termed a *fixed facet*, because there are no other levels of this facet to which the researcher can generalize. In effect, the universe of positions has now been exhausted with the model. In this chapter, **fully crossed random models** are described for which *all* of the facets are considered random, and all subjects are crossed with all other facets in the model. *Mixed models*, in which some facets are random and some are fixed, and *nested models*, in which some facets are *nested* (i.e., *not* crossed) within other facets, can also be used in generalizability theory. Such models involve slight modifications in the procedures presented in this chapter. The reader seeking additional information on mixed models should review Brennan (1977, 1983); Cardinet, Tourneur, and Allal (1976, 1981); and Godbout and Schutz (1983).

Generalizability Theory

G-theory is an extension of the intraclass reliability model. G-theory is perhaps the most appropriate methodology for estimating test reliability available today, because of its ability to identify numerous sources of error variation within a single model. G-theory is one of the few theories based on a mathematical framework that is sufficiently well developed to support practical test development. Deeper insight into the use of generalizability theory requires familiarity with (a) multifactor analysis of variance (**ANOVA**) procedures, including random, fixed, and mixed effects; (b) development of **expected mean squares** for any ANOVA model; and (c) use of expected mean squares to obtain estimates of **variance components**. The first of these three steps was described briefly above. The latter two steps are described fully with examples in this chapter.

G Study

G-theory differentiates between two types of studies: G Study and D Study. The G Study is based on the use of repeated measures analysis of variance (ANOVA) to quantify the amount of variance associated with each facet and its interactions within the ANOVA model. Expected mean squares are determined for each source of variance, and variance components are estimated for each source of variation based on the calculated mean square values and expected mean squares. The variance components are used to calculate the percentage of total variance represented by each source in the model. These percentages provide the most valuable information from a G Study. G Studies are useful when many facets are involved in a study and stable variance component estimates of the potentially large number of facets and interactions can be determined. The G Study can help the researcher determine which sources of variance contribute to measurement error. Decisions are then made regarding the manipulation or control of error sources. Subsequently, the investigator can conduct studies with models that examine important and large amounts of variation.

D Study

The **D (Decision) Study** provides data used to make substantive decisions about a measurement protocol. The results of a D Study are generalizability coefficients (Gs), which can be interpreted as reliability coefficients across the universe(s) of various facets in a study. Note that many different G coefficients can be obtained for a study, depending on the number of facets in the design and the various universes of generalization. For example, a researcher might want to generalize to the universe of potential teachers who perform ratings, the universe of days, or both. The Gs are determined by differentiation of error sources in those universes.

The results of the G and D studies are combined to determine the optimal measurement scheme or protocol to be used in collecting data. For example, does the researcher need to increase the number of observation days and/or teacher observers to obtain adequate reliabilities (G coefficients)? A G coefficient can be estimated for any number of days or observers. As would be expected, the G coefficients increase (assuming they were non-zero in the beginning) with an increase in the number of measures. Alternatively, the researcher could also estimate the effect of increasing the number of observations and decreasing the number of teacher observers (or vice versa).

This methodology, used to determine the best measurement protocol to follow, has been termed *optimization* or *forecasting* (Cardinet, Tourneur, & Allal, 1981).

Additional Statistics

Two additional calculations are helpful in generalizability theory. The **index of reliability** (generalizability) is the square root of the G coefficient and is interpreted as the theoretical correlation between the observed scores for people and their universe scores (i.e., the mean scores across the universe[s] of generalization) (Hopkins, 1983).

The absolute error variance is obtained by summing all of the variance components except that for the object of measurement. This is the "expected value of the squared differences between observed and universe scores for the objects of measurement" (Brennan, 1983, p. xii), which is an estimate of the error variance associated with an observed score. The square root of this error variance is the standard error of measurement (SEM) for the scores. This value is interpreted the same as the standard error of measurement used in classical test theory.

Expected Mean Squares

A basic knowledge of expected mean squares (EMS) is essential for a more thorough understanding of G-theory. *Mean square* is simply another name for a variance estimate. Classical test theory (as well as generalizability theory) involves the partitioning of observed score variance into portions associated with various facets in the reliability study. An *expected* mean square consists of those facets within the design that contribute to the numerical value of the calculated mean square. That is, each mean square value can be perceived as consisting of sources of variation (components) that contribute to the numeric value of the mean square.

Determining expected mean squares can be quite cumbersome for studies with a large number of facets. However, it is important to understand a method for determining them. Glass and Hopkins (1984) and Hopkins (1976) provide step-by-step methods for determining expected mean squares. Additionally, a *cookbook* approach to determining EMS for any model is presented in Table 4.1. Each of the suggested procedures involves familiarization and practice with a number of general rules. Whatever method is chosen for determining expected mean squares, the overall concept is perhaps best summarized by Glass and Hopkins (1984):

> The *components* (addends) of expected mean square for any source of variation are the specified effect (a main effect or interaction, i.e., source of variation), plus (a) the interaction of the specified effect with any random effect (including combinations of random effects) and (b) any random effect nested within the specified effect. (p. 479)

The **BMDP8V** (Dixon & Brown, 1983) computer program illustrated in Figures 4.1 and 4.2 can be used to obtain expected mean squares for the researcher. However, a deeper understanding of the processes involved can be obtained by studying Table 4.1.

Table 4.1   Steps for Calculating Expected Mean Squares for Any Model

1. Write each of the sources of variation in a single column. Use a *unique* upper case letter to designate each effect. Nested effects are noted with brackets (e.g., subjects nested within gender by treatment would be noted as $S[G \times T]$). See Tables 4.2 and 4.5 for calculation examples.

2. Write the unique subscripts in lower case letters for each main effect across the top of the page. There will be as many columns as there are main effects (i.e., facets) within your design. The trials source of variation could be designated "T" and the number of levels of trials would be designated with a "t."

3. Write FIXED (F) or RANDOM (R) above each of the unique subscripts at the top of each column. Subjects are always considered "random."

4. Write the number of levels associated with each effect under the subscript at the top of the page.

Complete the chart by following steps 5 through 7.

5. Complete each column first. For each source of variation in the model, bring down the number of levels of the facet provided that the source of variation does *not* appear in the row. Do this for each column, separately.

6. Now consider each row containing terms within brackets. For each term within brackets, put a "1" in the column with that subscript.

7. Now fill in the remainder of the chart by column. If an effect is "fixed" put a "0" and if it is "random" put a "1."

Compute each Row's EMS with steps 8 through 10.

8. Cover the subscript(s) (i.e., the column[s]) associated with the effect for which you are determining the EMS. Multiply the numbers in the remaining columns to arrive at the coefficient for that source of variation.

9. Provided that *all* of the subscripts for the source of variation you are completing are in the left-most column and the coefficient is *not* zero, this source of variation will be part of the expected mean square you are developing.

10. Repeat for all sources of variation. When determining which columns to cover with nested effects, you should cover all non-bracketed terms.

Computer Programs

Whereas programs for conducting generalizability theory analyses are not generally available (cf. Crick & Brennan, 1982; Bell, 1985), repeated measures ANOVA programs can be utilized to obtain mean square values. However, *none* of the generally available programs are specifically written for generalizability analyses; thus the necessary values must be taken from the output. Programs from BMDP8V (Dixon & Brown, 1983) and **SPSS^x** (SPSS^x, 1983) are demonstrated in this chapter. **SAS** (1979) programs can also be used to develop the required statistics (e.g., PROC ANOVA and PROC VARCOMP). The BMDP output is most easily followed and also presents expected mean squares and variance components. But caution must be used in interpreting the variance components from BMDP8V, as illustrated in example 2 in this chapter.

The SPSS^X MANOVA output is much more convoluted for the present purposes because, depending on the complexity of the model, numerous *within-cells* sources of variation must be collected to build the ANOVA source table. In general, the within-cells variation associated with the constant represents the highest level interaction. The subsequent within-cells sources of variation are actually the interactions between people and the respective within-subject facet(s) presented on the SPSS^X output. Familiarity with degrees of freedom and the appropriate ANOVA source table helps to obtain the proper mean squares for the model from the SPSS^X output.

Procedural Steps for a Generalizability Study

In summary, the procedural steps for completing a G-theory analysis are:

Step 1: Choose the facets for the design. Variance components should be estimated as accurately as possible, which necessitates as many levels of each facet as possible (and reasonable).

Step 2: Determine expected mean square values for each source of variation in the model. Typically the facets will be random.

Step 3: Determine the mean square for each source of variation.

Step 4: Calculate variance components for each source of variation in the model, either by hand or by computer.

Step 5: Conduct the G Study phase by determining the percentage of variance associated with each source of variation.

Step 6: Conduct the D Study phase by calculating G coefficients for the universes of interest.

Step 7: Determine the best measurement protocol to utilize by investigating the percentages of variance, G coefficients, indices of reliability, and SEMs.

Example 1: Classical Test Theory and Generalizability Theory

Two examples will be given to illustrate the steps above and the use of G-theory. Both examples are similar to the volleyball rating example presented previously. In example 1, assume that the teacher is using the average of three teacher raters on each of four days (i.e., ten subjects across four days *without* consideration of the different teachers).

The volleyball rating example with a sample data set, the associated expected mean squares, and ANOVA table are presented in Table 4.2. The scores presented are the average values across three different teachers on *each* of the four days. BMDP8V and SPSS^X computer commands are presented in Figure 4.1.

Table 4.2 Example Data Set 1, Expected Mean Squares, and ANOVA Table

	Days (D) with 4 (d) levels				Total
	5	4	3	4	16
	5	3	3	1	12
	5	4	4	3	16
	3	2	1	2	8
Subjects (S)	4	2	2	3	11
with	2	2	1	1	6
10 (s)	2	1	2	2	7
levels	2	2	1	2	7
	3	4	2	3	12
	2	2	1	3	8
Total	33	26	20	24	103

Calculation of Expected Mean Squares

	R s 10	R d 4	Expected Mean Square
S	1	4	$4 \sigma^2 S + \sigma^2 S \times D$
D	10	1	$10 \sigma^2 D + \sigma^2 S \times D$
S×D	1	1	$\sigma^2 S \times D$

ANOVA Source Table — Example 1

Source of Variation	Degrees of Freedom	Sum of Squares	Mean Square
Subjects	9	30.5250	3.3917
Days	3	8.8750	2.9583
Subjects × Days	27	14.3750	0.5324
Total	39	53.7750	

Classical Test Theory Statistics

Calculating the intraclass reliability coefficient using Equation 4.1 (alpha or KR 20) on the ANOVA output presented in Table 4.2 results in a reliability of .843:

$$R_{xx'} = \frac{MS_s - MS_i}{MS_s}$$

$$.843 = \frac{3.3917 - .5324}{3.3917}$$

(4.1)

```
                          BMDP8V
PROBLEM TITLE IS 'Example 1 BMDP8V'./
INPUT VARIABLES ARE 4.
       FORMAT IS '(4F2.0)'./
DESIGN LEVELS ARE 10,4.
       NAMES ARE S,D.
       RANDOM IS S,D.
       MODEL IS 'S,D'.
       DEPEND = 1 TO 4.
       PRINT = SD./
END/
5 4 3 4
5 3 3 1
5 4 4 3
3 2 1 2
4 2 2 3
2 2 1 1
2 1 2 2
2 2 1 2
3 4 2 3
2 2 1 3
                              SPSSx
TITLE 'Example 1 SPSSx MANOVA'
DATA LIST/D1 TO D4 1-8
MANOVA D1 TO D4/
       WSFACTORS = DAYS(4)/
       WSDESIGN = DAYS/
       ANALYSIS(REPEATED) = D1 TO D4/
       DESIGN/
BEGIN DATA
5 4 3 4
5 3 3 1
5 4 4 3
3 2 1 2
4 2 2 3
2 2 1 1
2 1 2 2
2 2 1 2
3 4 2 3
2 2 1 3
END DATA
FINISH
```

Figure 4.1 Computer Set-Up for Example 1

If the number of days is increased to eight, utilization of the intraclass correlation coefficient equation (see chapter 3), which is algebraically equivalent to the Spearman-Brown prophecy formula, to estimate the reliability results in a predicted reliability of .915:

$$M_{KK'} = \frac{MS_s - MS_i}{MS_s + \left[\left(\dfrac{K}{K'} - 1\right)\left(MS_i\right)\right]} \tag{4.2}$$

where K is the actual number of days and K' is the number of days generalized.

$$.915 = \frac{3.3917 - .5324}{3.3917 + \left[\left(\dfrac{4}{8} - 1\right)\left(.5324\right)\right]}$$

Facets, EMS, and MS (Steps 1 through 3)

Consider the EMS presented in the middle of Table 4.2. Note that the expected mean square for subjects not only has the variation associated with subjects but also contains the Subject × Day interaction (S × D) source of variation. The coefficient of 4 indicates that subjects' scores are actually summed across four days. The S × D source must also be considered when estimating the variation among subjects, because the days themselves are considered to be random (i.e., representative of the universe of days from which data can be obtained). Thus, the subjects' variance (i.e., Mean Square Subjects) would be *expected* to differ had the researcher chosen some other four days on which to base the estimates. A similar argument is made for the mean square for days, because subjects are considered randomly representative of the universe of potential subjects. In actuality, the alpha or intraclass reliability typically considers both subjects and days *random* rather than *fixed* facets. Therefore, the mean square for subjects (3.3917) can be thought of as consisting of variation associated not only with the variation of subjects but also with how subjects interact with days.

Variance Components and G Study (Steps 4 and 5)

Calculation of G Study statistics utilizes the expected mean squares and calculated mean square values to estimate variance components for each source of variation in the model. In this example, the components of variation include subjects, days, and subjects × days. The variance component ($\hat{\sigma}^2$) for each source of variation is the first term (without the coefficient) in each respective expected mean square. However, note that coefficients are associated with both subjects and days (4 and 10, respectively). In order to isolate and determine the numerical value associated with a particular variance component, the variation contributed by other sources of variation within the expected

Table 4.3   G and D Study Results for Subjects × Days Example 1

Source of Variation	G Study Variance Component $(\hat{\sigma}^2)$	Percent of Variance
Subjects	0.71483	48.0
Days	0.24259	16.3
Subjects × Days	0.53241	35.7
Total	1.48983	100

D Study	
Number of Days	G Coefficient
4	0.843
8	0.915

mean square must first be extracted. An estimate of this contribution, however, is available from other terms in the model. Estimates of the variance components should be calculated from the most complex to the simplest terms in the model. The variance components for each source of variation are presented in Table 4.3. Note that the coefficient for the Subjects × Days expected mean square (see Table 4.2) is 1. Thus, the mean square for this term is also the variance component (0.5324). However, to determine the variance component for Days, one must first subtract the contribution of the Subjects × Days variation from the calculated mean square for Days and then divide this result by 10 to estimate the Days variance component without the coefficient:

$$\text{Day } (\hat{\sigma}^2) = (MS_d - MS_{sd})/s$$
$$\text{Day } (\hat{\sigma}^2) = (2.9583 - 0.5324)/10 \tag{4.3}$$
$$= 2.4259/10$$
$$= 0.24259$$

Similar steps are performed to determine the variance component for the subjects:

$$\text{Subjects } (\hat{\sigma}^2) = (MS_s - MS_{sd})/d$$
$$\text{Subjects } (\hat{\sigma}^2) = (3.3917 - 0.5324)/4 \tag{4.4}$$
$$= 2.8593/4$$
$$= 0.71483$$

Also presented in Table 4.3 are the summary results from the G Study. Note that in a G Study, interest centers on the percentage of variance associated with each source of variation in the model. To determine this percentage, simply sum the variance components for each source of variation and then determine the percentage of this total associated with each variance component. Note that nearly half (48%) of the variation is associated with differences among subjects, while about one-third (35.7%) is associated with the Subjects × Days interaction (i.e., undifferentiated error).

D Study (Step 6)

The essence of a D Study is based on G Study values and results in **G coefficients**, which represent the generalizability of scores across particular universes of interest. In the present example, generalizing to the universe of potential days is of interest. A G coefficient (Brennan, 1977) is the ratio of the universe score variance to the expected universe score variance. It is calculated using Equation 4.5:

$$G = \frac{\text{universe score variance for the object of measurement}}{\text{universe score variance for the object of measurement} + \text{error variance for making comparative decisions among objects of measurement}} \tag{4.5}$$

This is analogous to the calculation from classical test theory:

$$r_{xx'} = \frac{\text{true score variance}}{\text{true score variance} + \text{error score variance}} \tag{4.6}$$

Different variance components will be part of the universe score variance or error variance, depending on the universes of generalization and the facets that are perceived as fixed for the generalizability coefficient. The universe score variance for the object of measurement (typically, but not always, subjects) contains the component of variance for the object of measurement *plus* all other facets that interact with the object of measurement to which one is *not* generalizing. Each variance component (except that of the object of measurement) is divided by the number of levels of the facet used to estimate a G coefficient (i.e., the number of scores to be averaged). Interaction terms among effects which interact with the object of measurement are divided by the multiplicative number of levels for the respective facets. For example, if in another model $i = 3$ and $c = 4$ with no generalization across I or C, then the variance component for $S \times I \times C$ is divided by 12; that for $S \times I$ is divided by 3, and that for $S \times C$ is divided by 4.

The error variance for making comparative decisions is calculated by summing the variance components for all interaction terms associated with the object of measurement and universes of generalization. This is, in effect, an estimate of the error variation when generalizing across universes of interest, because these sources are expected to contribute to measurement error from one level of the facet to another as they interact with subjects. Once again, the variance components are divided by the number of levels of the facet of generalization. Interaction terms are divided as described in the preceding paragraph.

Different definitions of universes to which one generalizes result in changes in the numerator and denominator. Thus, changes occur in the G coefficients. Many different estimates of reliability can be obtained from a single study.

Using the $S \times D$ design, a G coefficient can be calculated across the universe of days. The universe score variance is simply that associated with subjects, i.e., the object

of measurement, sometimes referred to as the face of differentiation (Cardinet, Tourneur, & Allal, 1981). The variance component is 0.71483. The error variance is calculated
as:

$$\hat{\sigma}^2_{sd}/d = \text{Error}\ (\hat{\sigma}^2) \tag{4.7}$$
$$0.53241/4 = 0.13310$$

because the interaction between the object of measurement (subjects) and the facet of
generalization across days is 0.53241 and the number of levels of days is 4. Calculating
the G coefficient results in:

$$G = \hat{\sigma}^2_s/[\hat{\sigma}^2_s + (\hat{\sigma}^2_{sd}/d)]$$
$$G = 0.71483/[0.71483 + (0.53241/4)] \tag{4.8}$$
$$= 0.71483/0.84793$$
$$= .843$$

This is exactly the value obtained with the alpha coefficient earlier. To generalize across
eight days rather than four, the G coefficient is forecast:

$$G = \hat{\sigma}^2_s/\hat{\sigma}^2_s + (\hat{\sigma}^2_{sd}/d')$$

where d' is the number of days generalized.

$$G = 0.71483/[0.71483 + (0.53241/8)]$$
$$= 0.71483/0.781381 \tag{4.9}$$
$$= .915$$

This is the value obtained when using the intraclass correlation coefficient equation to
step-up the previously calculated alpha coefficient.

The Best Protocol (Step 7)

The use of four days results in an acceptable reliability. This procedure does necessitate
using the *average* of three testers per day. The index of reliability is .918, and the SEM
is .440 units. The SEM is calculated using Equation 4.10:

$$\text{SEM} = \sqrt{\hat{\sigma}^2_d/d + \hat{\sigma}^2_{sd}/d}$$
$$\text{SEM} = \sqrt{.24259/4 + .53241/4} \tag{4.10}$$
$$= \sqrt{.19375}$$
$$= .440$$

The benefit of generalizability theory is that the researcher can conduct these same
logical steps when more than two facets (e.g., subjects, days, teachers) are in the design.
Although Brennan (1983) indicates that in almost all cases, the intraclass correlation
coefficient equation does not apply when generalizing over *more* than a single facet,
the logic of such a procedure does generalize.

Table 4.4   Example Data Set 2 and Expected Mean Squares

	D1			D2			D3			D4			
	T1	T2	T3	T1	T2	T3	T1	T2	T3	T1	T2	T3	Total
S1	5	5	5	3	4	5	3	4	2	4	4	4	48
:	5	5	5	3	3	3	2	3	4	0	1	2	36
:	5	5	5	3	4	5	4	4	4	3	3	3	48
:	5	5	5	5	4	3	4	4	4	3	4	2	48
:	3	4	2	2	3	1	0	1	2	1	2	3	24
:	4	4	4	3	2	1	2	2	2	3	4	2	33
:	3	2	1	3	2	1	1	1	1	0	1	2	18
:	1	2	3	1	1	1	2	2	2	2	2	2	21
:	3	4	2	4	4	4	3	2	1	3	3	3	36
10	3	2	1	2	2	2	1	1	1	3	3	3	24
Total	37	38	33	29	29	26	22	24	23	22	27	26	336

Sums: D1 = 108; D2 = 84; D3 = 69; D4 = 75; T1 = 110; T2 = 118; T3 = 108

Calculation of Expected Mean Squares

	R s 10	R d 4	R t 3	Expected Mean Square
S	1	4	3	$12\,\sigma^2 S + 3\,\sigma^2 S{\times}D + 4\,\sigma^2 S{\times}T + \sigma^2 S{\times}D{\times}T$
D	10	1	3	$30\,\sigma^2 D + 3\,\sigma^2 S{\times}D + 10\,\sigma^2 D{\times}T + \sigma^2 S{\times}D{\times}T$
T	10	4	1	$40\,\sigma^2 T + 4\,\sigma^2 S{\times}T + 10\,\sigma^2 D{\times}T + \sigma^2 S{\times}D{\times}T$
S×D	1	1	3	$3\,\sigma^2 S{\times}D + \sigma^2 S{\times}D{\times}T$
S×T	1	4	1	$4\,\sigma^2 S{\times}T + \sigma^2 S{\times}D{\times}T$
D×T	10	1	1	$10\,\sigma^2 D{\times}T + \sigma^2 S{\times}D{\times}T$
S×D×T	1	1	1	$\sigma^2 S{\times}D{\times}T$

Example 2: Volleyball Ratings

Facets, EMS, and MS (Steps 1 through 3)

Example 1 assumed that each of three teachers rated each student during each of four days, but the researcher simply used the average of the three teacher ratings for each day. Note that the data used in example 1 are simply average teacher ratings by day from the data presented in Table 4.4. Interest might now focus on the generalizability of the ratings across both days *and* teachers. In actuality, one might expect different teachers to rate students differently across days. That is, ratings might vary as a function of the day or as a function of the teacher who does the rating. Additionally, it may be

Table 4.5   ANOVA Source Table—Example 2

Source of Variation	Degrees of Freedom	Sum of Squares	Mean Squares
Subjects	9	101.7000	11.3000
Days	3	29.4000	9.8000
Teachers	2	1.4000	0.7000
Subjects × Days	27	44.1000	1.6333
Subjects × Teachers	18	9.6000	0.5333
Days × Teachers	6	2.2000	0.3667
Subjects × Days × Teachers	54	26.8000	0.4963
Total	119	215.2000	

that students (subjects) and days and/or teachers interact to reduce the generalizability of obtained scores. Finally, interest may center on ascertaining the particular measurement protocol that will result in reliable information and still be obtained in the most efficient manner. Generalizability theory analysis will help the researcher answer each of these questions. The example 2 data set and expected mean squares (fully crossed random model) are shown in Table 4.4, the ANOVA source table is shown in Table 4.5, and the BMDP8V and SPSS^X computer commands are shown in Figure 4.2.

Variance Components (Step 4)

The logic followed to determine the variance components for the facets is the same as that with the Subjects × Days model presented in example 1. However, careful inspection of the expected mean squares found in Table 4.4 indicates that there are now *four* sources of variation associated with the subjects, days, and teachers facets. The four sources of variation differ with each facet because of the nature of the interactions among the random facets. Thus, additional steps are needed to isolate the variance component for each facet. Note that if interest lies in isolating the variance component for Subjects, one must subtract the variance associated with the S × D, S × T, and S × D × T components and then divide by 12. However, subtracting the three sources of variance requires three steps before dividing by 12. The steps are:

$$\text{Subjects } (\hat{\sigma}^2) = (MS_s - MS_{sd} - MS_{st} + MS_{sdt})/dt \tag{4.11}$$

Note that the addition of the S × D × T mean square is necessary because subtraction of both the mean squares for S × D and S × T results in extracting the S × D × T variation twice. Thus, the S × D × T mean square is added back to ascertain the

```
                      BMDP8V
PROBLEM TITLE IS 'Example 2 BMDP8V'./
INPUT   VARIABLES ARE 12.
        FORMAT IS '(12F2.0)'./
DESIGN LEVELS ARE 10,4,3.
       NAMES ARE S,D,T.
       RANDOM IS S,D,T.
       MODEL IS 'S,D,T'.
       DEPEND = 1 TO 12.
       PRINT = SDT./
END/
5 5 5 3 4 5 3 4 2 4 4 4
5 5 5 3 3 3 2 3 4 0 1 2
5 5 5 3 4 5 4 4 4 3 3 3
5 5 5 5 4 3 4 4 4 3 4 2
3 4 2 2 3 1 0 1 2 1 2 3
4 4 4 3 2 1 2 2 2 3 4 2
3 2 1 3 2 1 1 1 1 0 1 2
1 2 3 1 1 1 2 2 2 2 2 2
3 4 2 4 4 4 3 2 1 3 3 3
3 2 1 2 2 2 1 1 1 3 3 3
                      SPSSx
TITLE 'Example 2 SPSSx MANOVA'
DATA LIST/V1 TO V12 1-24
MANOVA V1 TO V12/
       WSFACTORS = DAY(4) TEACHER(3)/
       WSDESIGN = DAY, TEACHER, DAY BY TEACHER/
       ANALYSIS(REPEATED) = V1 TO V12/
       DESIGN/
BEGIN DATA
5 5 5 3 4 5 3 4 2 4 4 4
5 5 5 3 3 3 2 3 4 0 1 2
5 5 5 3 4 5 4 4 4 3 3 3
5 5 5 5 4 3 4 4 4 3 4 2
3 4 2 2 3 1 0 1 2 1 2 3
4 4 4 3 2 1 2 2 2 3 4 2
3 2 1 3 2 1 1 1 1 0 1 2
1 2 3 1 1 1 2 2 2 2 2 2
3 4 2 4 4 4 3 2 1 3 3 3
3 2 1 2 2 2 1 1 1 3 3 3
END DATA
FINISH
```

Figure 4.2   Computer Set-Up For Example 2

Table 4.6   G Study Results for Subjects × Days × Teachers Example 2

Source of Variance	Variance Component $(\hat{\sigma}^2)$	Percent of Variance
Subjects	0.80248	40.3
Days	0.28877	14.5
Teachers	0.01658	0.8
Subjects × Days	0.37900	19.0
Subjects × Teachers	0.00925	0.5
Days × Teachers	0.00000	0.0
Subjects × Days × Teachers	0.49630	24.9
Total	1.99238	100.0

Note. Days × Teachers variance component was set to 0.00000 because of negative variance estimate.

proper variance component for Subjects. Similar steps are used for the Days and Teachers facets. When models consist of large numbers of facets, it can become quite cumbersome to subtract and then add back the proper mean squares. But the logic remains the same (i.e., isolation of the particular variance component), which requires knowledge of the expected mean squares. Table 4.6 contains the variance components for example 2. The variance component for Subjects is:

$$\text{Subjects } (\hat{\sigma}^2) = (MS_s - MS_{sd} - MS_{st} + MS_{sdt})/dt$$
$$\text{Subjects } (\hat{\sigma}^2) = (11.3000 - 1.6333 - 0.5333 + 0.4963)/12 \qquad (4.12)$$
$$= 0.80248$$

The variance components presented on the BMDP8V output are *not* always correct. Notice that a negative variance component has been obtained for the D × T facet:

$$\text{D} \times \text{T } (\hat{\sigma}^2) = (MS_{dt} - MS_{sdt})/s$$
$$\text{D} \times \text{T } (\hat{\sigma}^2) = (0.3667 - 0.4963)/10 \qquad (4.13)$$
$$= -0.01296$$

Logic suggests that it is impossible to have a negative variance component, although this can occur because of sampling error. When a negative variance component is obtained, it is set equal to zero. Should the mean square associated with this variance component be utilized in further variance component calculations in the model (as it often will be in multifaceted designs and is demonstrated here with both the D and T EMS), use zero as the mean square rather than the value actually obtained by the computer. This is done because zero is now the best estimate of the actual variance component.

The algorithm used in the BMDP8V package does not adjust for negative variance components, as suggested by Cronbach, Gleser, Nanda, and Rajaratnam (1972). In effect, if the program calculates a negative variance component (a theoretical impossibility but mathematical reality), the BMDP8V program uses the negative variance throughout the remaining calculations. However, once a negative variance component is calculated, assume the mean square for that facet to be zero and use the value of zero throughout further variance component determinations when that particular mean square is required. For example, the variance component for the Day facet is:

$$\text{Day}\ (\hat{\sigma}^2) = (MS_d - MS_{sd} - MS_{dt} + MS_{sdt})/st \tag{4.14}$$

which is obtained from

$$0.28877 = (9.8000 - 1.6333 - 0.0 + 0.4963)/30$$

because 0.0 is the best estimate of the D × T variation (calculated at −0.01296).

G Study (Step 5)

As indicated in the G Study results presented in Table 4.6, the largest percentage of variation is associated with differences among subjects (40.3%). Notice that the Days facet is associated with 14.5% of the total variation, but the variation associated with Teachers is only 0.8%. Variation across days and teachers might be considered sources of potential error. (In actuality, differences in days might *not* be considered a source of error but only differences in teachers. Generalizability theory studies permit differentially defined sources of error.) The results suggest that while variation due to days might negatively impact the generalizability of the results, teacher variation appears to contribute little toward measurement error. Subjects (students) also tend to have variable performance across days (19.0% of the variation). The single remaining large source of variation (S × D × T) indicates that there is still some (24.9%) variation associated with the highest order interaction. This is analogous to the undifferentiated error described earlier with the alpha coefficient. Other facets might be associated with this error (e.g., court position, game). Thus, other facets may be perceived as unexplained, because they were not included in the present model. However, days are associated with a potentially large source of variation while differences in teachers are associated with little variation. Note also the small amount of variation associated with the S × T (0.5%) and D × T (0.0%) sources of variation. These indicate that the ratings assigned by teachers tend to be constant across subjects (S × T) and days (D × T).

D Study and Best Protocol (Steps 6 and 7)

The D Study results are presented in Table 4.7. The first line (with 4 days and 3 teachers) indicates the G coefficient obtained with the present analysis. That is, the estimated

Table 4.7   D Study Results for Subjects $\times$ Days $\times$ Teachers Example 2

Number of Days	Levels for Teachers	G Coefficient
4	3	.852
4	2	.833
4	1	.779
3	3	.813
3	2	.790
3	1	.727
2	3	.745
2	2	.716
1	3	.594
1	1	.476
5	1	.813
5	2	.861

reliability (generalizability) coefficient for the average of 3 teacher ratings across 4 days (a total of 12 measurements) is .852. This value was obtained from

$$G = \hat{\sigma}_s^2/(\hat{\sigma}_s^2 + \hat{\sigma}_{sd}^2/d + \hat{\sigma}_{st}^2/t + \hat{\sigma}_{sdt}^2/dt)$$
$$.852 = 0.80248/(0.80248 + 0.37900/4 + \tag{4.15}$$
$$0.00925/3 + 0.4963/12)$$

In practical terms, it is unlikely that a teacher could conscript two colleagues to help rate each of the players during each of four days. Thus, estimated (forecasted) G coefficients for various measurement protocols are also presented in Table 4.7. As the number of levels of each facet declines, one would expect the generalizability to be reduced. This is observed in the G coefficients presented in Table 4.7. However, note that G coefficients drop more appreciably with a reduction in the number of days than with a reduction in the number of teachers. This is a function of the relatively larger variation associated with Subjects $\times$ Days compared with that associated with Subjects $\times$ Teachers. To achieve sufficient reliability (i.e., $G \geq 0.83$) measurements need to be obtained on at least four days using two different teachers. Note that the estimated generalizability for a single teacher on a single day is only 0.476. Note also that the estimated generalizabilities are 0.813 for five days and one teacher and 0.861 for five days and two teachers. The latter value was obtained by

$$G = \hat{\sigma}_s^2/(\hat{\sigma}_s^2 + \hat{\sigma}_{sd}^2/d' + \hat{\sigma}_{st}^2/t' + \hat{\sigma}_{sdt}^2/d't') \tag{4.16}$$

where d' and t' are the number of days and teachers, respectively, to be generalized.

$$0.861 = 0.80248/(0.80248 + 0.37900/5 + 0.00925/2 + 0.49630/10)$$

Had this generalizability not met a minimally acceptable level, the obtained variance components could have been used to forecast the measurement protocol, which would produce the reliability (generalizability) required.

The index of reliability for ratings by three teachers across each of four days is 0.923. The SEM for the G of 0.852 obtained with four days and three teachers is

$$\begin{aligned} \text{SEM} &= \sqrt{\begin{aligned}(\hat{\sigma}_d^2/d + \hat{\sigma}_t^2/t + \hat{\sigma}_{sd}/d + \hat{\sigma}_{st}^2/t \\ + \hat{\sigma}_{dt}^2/dt + \hat{\sigma}_{sdt}^2/dt)\end{aligned}} \\ \text{SEM} &= \sqrt{\begin{aligned}(0.28877/4 + 0.01658/3 \\ + 0.37900/4 + 0.00925/3 \\ + 0.00000/12 + 0.49630/12)\end{aligned}} \\ &= \sqrt{0.21691} \\ &= 0.466 \end{aligned}$$

(4.17)

These values indicate sufficient reliability for the protocol.

Generalizability Uses in Physical Education and Exercise Science

A number of generalizability theory applications are available in physical education, the exercise sciences, and related content areas. Safrit, Atwater, Baumgartner, and West (1976) introduced generalizability theory to the physical education literature.

Taylor (1979) used a generalizability model to investigate the inter- and intra-rater reliability of the Physical Education Observation Instrument (PEOI). Methods were described for determining G coefficients within observers (repeated measures by the *same* observer) as well as among observers (ratings of the same behavior by *different* observers). Three teachers rated each of three videotaped volleyball teaching episodes on each of two occasions. Twelve different PEOI variables were evaluated. The instrument was found to be reliable (generalizable) for use in rating teacher and student behaviors across raters and occasions. G coefficients exceeded 0.87 for eleven of the twelve variables evaluated.

Stamm and Moore (1980) demonstrated the use of generalizability theory with bowling classes and investigated the generalization across gender, scores (frames), and days of first-ball bowling scores. They obtained G coefficients of 0.93 when generalizing to scores (s = 10), 0.92 when generalizing to days (d = 10) and scores (s = 10), and 0.84 within gender when generalizing to days (d = 10) and scores (s = 10). Godbout and Schutz (1983) presented a variety of generalizability models in ratings of motor performance and investigated the effect of various statistical models on the resultant G coefficients. They illustrated that a fully crossed model (as illustrated in this chapter) provides the greatest flexibility in determining G coefficients.

Boodoo and O'Sullivan (1982) demonstrated the appropriateness of generalizability theory in the development of rating scales for students in nursing clinical settings. Mosher and Schutz (1983) used generalizability analysis in the development and evaluation of an objective means of rating overarm throwing ability. The components of foot placement, body rotation, and arm action were evaluated. High G coefficients were obtained when generalizing to raters (G typically greater than 0.84), to occasions (G typically greater than 0.83), and to both teachers and occasions (G typically greater than 0.76). However, the G coefficients varied as a function of the throwing component assessed.

Generalizability theory has been used by a number of investigators (e.g., Lohman, Pollock, Slaughter, Brandon, & Boileau, 1984; Morrow, Fridye, & Monaghen, 1986; Oppliger, Looney, & Tipton, 1987) to ascertain the percentage of variance and/or effective G coefficients in body fatness measures with facets such as calipers, sites, equations, and testers. Collectively, their analyses indicate that results are quite generalizable across calipers and testers (G coefficients greater than .90) but not as generalizable across equations or sites. Since subcutaneous fatness can be observed to vary as a function of location, lower G coefficients would be expected when generalizing to sites. Percentage of fat equations are based on different sites; thus it would be expected that generalization across equations would also be lower. However, the major source of variation in each of these body fatness studies is people, and generalization across facets of primary interest to educators and clinicians is quite good. As is true in classical test theory, if the major source of variation is people, one can assume a relatively high reliability (i.e., generalizability).

Conclusion

Generalizability theory, an extension of classical test theory, is an appropriate method for determining the reliability of a measurement schedule when measurements are obtained across more than a single facet. Increasing the number of facets in the measurement schedule results in potentially large sources of measurement error. Generalizability theory results in estimates of the impact of the various error sources and helps the researcher develop measurement schedules that control error and increase reliability (generalizability).

Another use for the G Study variance components is for a researcher who has *not* utilized the particular facet within a generalizability study to estimate the effects of this facet on a measurement protocol by using variance component estimates from a variety of different studies. This will help in the development of better measurement protocols without having to personally obtain the relatively large number of measurements required when many facets are involved. Smith (1981) presents suggestions for utilizing such procedures when sample sizes are limited.

The reader interested in further study of generalizability theory techniques is encouraged to review the work of Cronbach, Gleser, Nanda, and Rajaratnam (1963) and Brennan (1983). The purpose of this chapter was to introduce concepts related to univariate generalizability. That is, there is a single score for each person across various facets. Interest might also center on *multivariate generalizability*, in which more than one variable is assessed at each level of the facets. The reader interested in multivariate generalizability should investigate the work of Webb and Shavelson (1981). Wood and

Safrit (1987) provide an example of the use of multivariate generalizability in physical education. Finally, the discussion in this chapter has been related to norm-referenced decisions. For examples related to the use of generalizability theory in criterion-referenced decisions, see the work of Brennan and Kane (1977) and Patterson and Safrit (1987).

References

Bell, J.F. (1985). Generalizability: The software problem. *Journal of Educational Statistics,* *10,* 19–29.

Boodoo, G.M., & O'Sullivan, P. (1982). Obtaining generalizability coefficients for clinical evaluations. *Evaluation & the Health Professions, 5,* 345–358.

Brennan, R.L. (1977). *Generalizability analyses: Principles and procedures* (ACT Testing Bulletin Number 26). Iowa City: American College Testing Program.

Brennan, R.L. (1983). *Elements of generalizability theory.* Iowa City: American College Testing Program.

Brennan, R.L., & Kane, M.T. (1977). An index of dependability for mastery tests. *Journal of Educational Measurement, 14,* 277–289.

Brennan, R.L., & Kane, M.T. (1979). Generalizability theory: A review. *New Directions for Testing and Measurement, 4,* 33–51.

Cardinet, J., Tourneur, Y., & Allal, L. (1976). The symmetry of generalizability theory: Applications to educational measurement. *Journal of Educational Measurement, 13,* 119–135.

Cardinet, J., Tourneur, Y., & Allal, L. (1981). Extension of generalizability theory and its application in educational measurement. *Journal of Educational Measurement, 18,* 183–204.

Crick, J.E., & Brennan, R.L. (1982). *GENOVA: A generalized analysis of variance system computer program* [Computer program]. Dorchester, MA: University of Massachusetts at Boston, Computer Facilities.

Cronbach, L.J., Gleser, G.C., Nanda, H., & Rajaratnam, N. (1972). *The dependability of behavioral measurements: Theory of generalization for scores and profiles.* New York: Wiley.

Cronbach, L.J., Rajaratnam, N., & Gleser, G. (1963). Theory of generalizability: A liberalization of reliability theory. *The British Journal of Statistical Psychology, 16,* 137–163.

Dixon, S.J., & Brown, M.B. (Eds.) (1983). *BMDP biomedical computer programs P-Series.* Berkeley: University of California Press.

Glass, G.V, & Hopkins, K.D. (1984). *Statistical methods in education and psychology* (2nd ed.). Englewood Cliffs, NJ: Prentice-Hall.

Gleser, G., Cronbach, L.J., & Rajaratnam, N. (1965). Generalizability of scores influenced by multiple sources of variance. *Psychometrika, 30,* 395–418.

Godbout, R., & Schutz, R.W. (1983). Generalizability of ratings of motor performance with reference to various observational designs. *Research Quarterly for Exercise and Sport, 54,* 20–27.

Hopkins, K.D. (1976). A simplified method for determining expected mean squares and error terms in the analysis of variance. *Journal of Experimental Education, 45,* 13–18.

Hopkins, K.D. (1983). Estimating reliability and generalizability coefficients in two-facet designs. *Journal of Special Education, 17,* 371–375.

Joe, G.W., & Woodward, J.A. (1976). Some developments in multivariate generalizability. *Psychometrika, 41,* 205–217.

Lohman, T.G., Pollock, M.L., Slaughter, M.H., Brandon, L.J., & Boileau, R.A. (1984). Methodological factors and the prediction of body fat in female athletes. *Medicine and Science in Sports and Exercise, 16,* 92–96.

Morrow, J.R., Jr., Fridye, T., & Monaghen, S.D. (1986). Generalizability of the skinfolds recommended on the AAHPERD Health Related Fitness Test. *Research Quarterly for Exercise and Sport, 57,* 187–195.

Mosher, R.E., & Schutz, R.W. (1983). The development of a test of overarm throwing: An application of generalizability theory. *Canadian Journal of Applied Sport Sciences, 8,* 1–8.

Oppliger, R.A., Looney, M.A., & Tipton, C.M. (1987). Reliability of hydrostatic weighing and skinfold measurements of body composition using a generalizability study. *Human Biology, 59,* 77–96.

Patterson, P., & Safrit, M.J. (1987). *The bias and consistency of two dependability indices based on criterion-referenced generalizability theory.* Manuscript submitted for publication.

Rentz, R.R. (1980). Rules of thumb for estimating reliability coefficients using generalizability theory. *Educational and Psychological Measurement, 40,* 575–592.

Safrit, M.J., Atwater, A.E., Baumgartner, T.A., & West, C. (Eds.) (1976). *Reliability theory,* Washington, DC: American Alliance for Health, Physical Education and Recreation.

SAS user's guide. (1979). Cary, NC: SAS Institute, Inc.

Shout, P.E., & Fleiss, J.L. (1979). Intraclass correlations: Uses in assessing rater reliability. *Psychological Bulletin, 86,* 420–428.

Smith, P.L. (1981). Gaining accuracy in generalizability theory: Using multiple designs. *Journal of Educational Measurement, 51,* 147–154.

SPSS^X User's Guide. (1983). Chicago: SPSS Inc.

Stamm, C.L., & Moore, J.E. (1980). Application of generalizability theory in estimating the reliability of a motor performance test. *Research Quarterly for Exercise and Sport, 51,* 382–388.

Taylor, J.L. (1979). Development of the physical education observation instrument using generalizability study theory. *Research Quarterly, 50,* 468–481.

Webb, N.M., & Shavelson, R.J. (1981). Multivariate generalizability of general educational development ratings. *Journal of Educational Measurement, 18,* 13–22.

Wood, T.M., & Safrit, M.J. (1987). A comparison of three multivariate models for estimating test battery reliability. *Research Quarterly for Exercise and Sport, 58,* 150–159.

Supplementary Readings

Brennan, R.L. (1983). *Elements of generalizability theory.* Iowa City: American College Testing Program.

Crocker, L., & Algina, J. (1986). Generalizability theory. In L. Crocker & J. Algina (Eds.), *Introduction to classical and modern test theory* (pp. 157–191). New York: Holt, Rinehart, and Winston.

Cronbach, L.G., Gleser, G., Nanda, H., & Rajaratnam, N. (1972). *The dependability of behavioral measurements: Theory of generalization for scores and profiles.* New York: Wiley.

Godbout, R., & Schutz, R.W. (1983). Generalizability of ratings of motor performance with reference to various observational designs. *Research Quarterly for Exercise and Sport, 54,* 20–27.

CHAPTER 5

The Use of Validity Generalization in Exercise Science

Patricia Patterson, Ph.D.
San Diego State University

Validity generalization is a method of synthesizing evidence of validity from studies involving the correlation between the same **criterion-predictor** combination. It allows a researcher to determine if the variability in observed validity coefficients across studies is real or due to statistical artifacts.

A common occurrence in exercise science research is the reporting of validity coefficients that vary in size from study to study for the same criterion-predictor combination. For example, validity coefficients for the 12-min run and maximal oxygen uptake have ranged from .27 to .94. This variability in coefficients has meant that researchers must conduct new validation studies for each situation in which the test might be used. The result is a burgeoning body of literature that is often difficult to integrate in a meaningful way. Validity generalization provides the methodology to synthesize all previous work in a quantifiable way to clarify conflicts and formulate theories.

The purpose of this chapter is to outline the impetus for the development of validity generalization, describe the model itself, and provide a tutorial on the implementation of validity generalization in exercise science. The final section of the chapter deals with a discussion of controversies surrounding validity generalization and implications for the future.

Early Methods for Cumulating Findings

An important element of scientific research is the synthesis of findings. Facts are accumulated across studies in order to formulate theories that explain relationships among variables. In the past, the most common methods for cumulating findings have been narratives, vote counting, and cumulating p values.

Several investigators have found flaws in the use of these traditional methods (Glass, 1976, 1977; Glass, McGaw, & Smith, 1981; Hedges & Olkin, 1980; Hunter, Schmidt, & Jackson, 1982). A major drawback is the lack of quantitative information available to examine the strength of the relationship between the independent and dependent variables (Glass, 1977; Hunter, Schmidt, & Jackson, 1982). These problems in the usual literature review procedure led Glass (1976) to propose another method of integrating studies, which he called **meta-analysis**.

Meta-analysis provides a quantitative framework for synthesizing and generalizing the results of many studies of the same hypothesis. The findings of each study are quantified by calculating the *effect size*, which is then averaged across all studies of interest to yield information about the magnitude of treatment outcomes. Study characteristics such as gender, age, and quality of design can be examined to determine if a relationship exists between any of these variables and the dependent variable. Proponents of meta-analysis believe that the quantification this model allows leads to more substantive support in theory development. Thomas and French (1986) wrote an excellent tutorial on meta-analysis in which they provide an in-depth discussion of modifications to Glass's original work and offer a step-by-step guide to carrying out a meta-analysis, complete with an empirical example.

Meta-analysis has been used in a variety of physical education and exercise science settings (Feltz & Landers, 1983; Kavale & Mattson, 1983; Sparling, 1980; Thomas & French, 1985; Tran, Weltman, Glass, & Mood, 1983). For example, it has been employed to examine gender differences in maximal oxygen uptake (Sparling, 1980), the effect of mental practice on motor and cognitive tasks (Feltz & Landers, 1983), the use of perceptual motor training as an intervention technique for exceptional children (Kavale & Mattson, 1983), the effect of exercise on serum lipids (Tran et al., 1983), and gender differences across motor tasks (Thomas & French, 1985).

Validity Generalization

Validity generalization is a quantitative method of combining the results of all previous studies of the validity of a test to establish the generalizability of validity. It was developed by Schmidt, Hunter, and Urry (1976) to resolve the problem of situation specificity in predictive validity studies in the field of personnel psychology. Historically, psychologists have proposed that the variability in validity coefficients for tests used in job selection resulted from the unique nature of each situation. In other words, although the same test might be used to predict performance in similar jobs, the underlying factor of *job structure* was perceived to be different from situation to situation, even though job analysts were often incapable of detecting these differences. Thus, an empirical validity study must be designed for each situation.

Schmidt et al. (1976) provided an alternative explanation to situation specificity. An examination of the literature in the field of personnel psychology revealed that psychologists were guilty of believing in the *law of small numbers*. While the law of large numbers guarantees that large random samples will be representative of the population from which they were drawn, no such guarantee can be applied to small samples. Thus, not only is information gleaned from a small sample more likely to be inaccurate, but the power to detect *true* validity is very low. In addition, unreliability in the criterion will attenuate the validity coefficient. And finally, in a selection situation, range restriction will lower the validity coefficient, since variation in the selected pool of subjects will always be smaller than the variation in the applicant pool of subjects.

These observations led Schmidt et al. (1976) to examine the effect of sample size, criterion unreliability, and range restriction on the variability of observed validity coefficients. Formulas were developed to correct for these artifacts. The corrected validity coefficients were found to be quite stable across jobs. This initial study served as the foundation for the validity generalization model.

Schmidt and Hunter (1977) outlined the theoretical framework of validity generalization. The hypothesis of interest in validity generalization is that the variance of true validities is zero. This hypothesis differentiates validity generalization from the meta-analytic work of Glass (1976). Early meta-analysts accepted the variability in effect size as real and attempted to explain it by correlating effect size with moderating variables. In contrast, Schmidt and Hunter suggested that variability in effect sizes (or validity coefficients, in the case of validity generalization) could be attributed to artifacts in the data. If validity coefficients could be corrected for these artifacts and the variance of the corrected validity coefficient was zero, validity generalization was possible. That is, conducting a new validity study was unnecessary, and the mean corrected validity coefficient could be accepted as the best estimate of true validity.

Conceptually, the test of this hypothesis is straightforward. All validity coefficients of the same predictor-criterion combination are obtained from both published and unpublished studies. The mean and variance of each observed validity coefficient and the error variance of artifacts are calculated. These artifactual sources include criterion reliability, test reliability, range restriction, sample size, criterion contamination and deficiency, computational and typographical errors, factor structure of tests, and factor structure of criterion tests. Usually only the first four artifacts are quantifiable; but although sample size is routinely reported in validity studies, the reliability coefficients often are omitted. Thus, Hunter, Schmidt, and Jackson (1982) have provided methods for estimating these coefficients from assumed frequency distributions. The variances of the quantifiable artifacts are calculated, summed, and subtracted from the observed variance. If the residual variance is zero, the hypothesis is confirmed, providing evidence of validity generalization.

Schmidt and Hunter (1977) also provided a **decision rule** for the case in which the residual variance is not zero. As noted previously, not all artifacts are quantifiable. According to the decision rule, if 75% of the variance can be accounted for by artifacts, the variance of true validities can still be assumed to be zero. Furthermore, a **confidence interval** can be constructed, with the lower bound representing a minimum value of validity. For example, if the lower bound of a 90% interval was .70, there is a 90% probability that a new validity study using the same predictor-criterion combination would yield a validity coefficient of .70 or higher.

Bayesian Statistics as a Framework for Validity Generalization

Test validation in the validity generalization model uses **Bayesian statistics** rather than the more traditional maximum likelihood approach. The advantage of using the Bayesian approach is that it not only employs sample-derived information from the current study but also utilizes relevant information from past research. The information from past validity studies is called the **prior distribution** and is combined with new information to form a **posterior distribution**. The mean of the posterior distribution, in this case the mean of the validity coefficients (prior and new), is taken as the best estimate of test validity. In the context of validity generalization, the prior distribution is the distribution of validity coefficients corrected for quantifiable artifacts. If the variance of the distribution is zero, validity generalization is justified and no new study is necessary. If generalization is not justified, however, a new study should be conducted and added to the prior distribution to expand the model. Thus, even when validity generalization is not possible, the use of Bayesian statistics provides a framework for improved decision-making in the new situation. Because the prior distribution is empirically based, the usual criticisms of the Bayesian approach of "pulling the prior distribution out of a hat" are unfounded (Schmidt & Hunter, 1977).

Examples of the Use of Validity Generalization

The validity generalization model has been used in a variety of personnel selection studies (Pearlman, Schmidt, & Hunter, 1980; Schmidt, Hunter, Pearlman, & Shane, 1979; Schmidt, Gast-Rosenberg, & Hunter, 1980; Hirsh, Northrop, & Schmidt, 1986). Safrit, Costa, and Hooper (1986) modified the validity generalization model to examine **concurrent validity** studies in exercise science. A tutorial for the implementation of validity generalization was presented, along with a small empirical example. The work of Safrit et al. (1986) was extended by conducting a large-scale validity generalization study to ascertain if the validity of distance run tests was generalizable (Safrit, Costa, Hooper, Patterson, & Ehlert, 1988).

Table 5.1 Data from Studies Using Submaximal Bicycle Tests

R_{tc}	N	R_{tt}	R_{cc}
.83[a]	15	.95	
.54[b]	48		
.74[c]	16	.82	.99
.91[d]	44	.85	.96
.76[e]	35		.96

Note. R_{tc} are the observed validity coefficients. R_{tt} are the test reliability coefficients. R_{cc} are the criterion reliability coefficients. N is the sample size.

[a]Patton, Vogel, & Mello, 1982; [b]Oja, Partanen, & Teraslinna, 1970; [c]deVries & Klafs, 1965; [d]Wilmore, Roby, Stanforth, Buono, Constable, Tsao, & Lowdon, 1986; [e]Siconolfi, Cullinane, Carleton, & Thompson, 1982.

An Empirical Example

The following small empirical example, presented in a tutorial format, illustrates the use of validity generalization in exercise science. For a full-fledged validity generalization study, however, Schmidt, Hunter, Pearlman, and Hirsh (1985) recommended 100 to 200 validity coefficients.

The question of interest is whether the validity of submaximal bicycle ergometer tests employing the Åstrand-Rhyming protocol (Åstrand & Rhyming, 1954) can be generalized. The observed validity coefficients vary from study to study, making it appear that validity must be evaluated in each situation. Validity generalization can be employed to ascertain whether these observed differences are real or due to statistical artifacts.

Step 1: For a full-scale study, consider all published and unpublished studies employing a submaximal bicycle test as a field test of aerobic capacity. Each study must be examined carefully for the following information: sample size, validity coefficient (preferably a Pearson product moment correlation coefficient), and test and criterion reliability coefficients. In addition, all pertinent study characteristics should be recorded, including sex, age, fitness level, and any other factors that may seem important.

For the purpose of this example, five studies were selected that used a submaximal bicycle test (*indirect* measure of maximal oxygen uptake) as the predictor and a maximal bicycle ergometer test (*direct* measure of maximal oxygen uptake) as the criterion. Information including sample size, test reliability, and criterion reliability were recorded. Only studies using males were selected for this example. Table 5.1 presents data from the five studies. Not all test and criterion reliability coefficients were reported in each study; therefore, assumed distributions were used, as suggested by Schmidt, Hunter, and Pearlman (1982).

Step 2: Correct the distribution of observed validity coefficients for sampling error by weighting each coefficient by its sample size, using Equation 5.1:

$$\bar{r}_{tc} = \frac{\Sigma r_{tc_i} N_i}{\Sigma N_i} \tag{5.1}$$

where $\bar{r}_{tc}$ = weighted mean of observed validity coefficients, r_{tci} = validity coefficient of ith study, N_i = sample size of ith study, t = test, and c = criterion. The data from Table 5.1 result in $\bar{r}_{tc} = .739$:

$$\bar{r}_{tc} = [.83(15) + .54(48) + .74(16)$$
$$+ .91(44) + .76(35)]/158$$
$$= .739$$

Step 3: Correct the corrected distribution for sampling error to obtain $\bar{\rho}_{TC}$, the fully corrected mean validity. The weighted means for the test and criterion reliabilities must be calculated before making this correction.

Step 3a: Compute $\bar{r}_{tt}$, the weighted mean of the observed test coefficients, using Equation 5.2:

$$\bar{r}_{tt} = \frac{\Sigma r_{tt_i} N_i}{\Sigma N_i} \tag{5.2}$$

where r_{tt_i} = test reliability for the ith study and N_i = sample size for the ith study.

Because the test reliabilities were not available for each study, the following assumed distribution was used:

$$\bar{r}^*_{tt} = \frac{\Sigma r_{tt_i} f_{ti}}{\Sigma f_{ti}} \tag{5.2a}$$

where f_{ti} = frequency of ith test reliability coefficient,

$$\bar{r}^*_{tt} = \frac{.95(1) + .82(1) + .85(1)}{3}$$
$$= .873, \text{ and}$$
$$\sqrt{\bar{r}^*_{tt}} = .934$$

Step 3b: Compute $\bar{r}_{cc}$, the weighted mean of the observed criterion reliability. Substitute r_{cc} for r_{tt} in Equation 5.2a to calculate this value.

$$\bar{r}^*_{cc} = \frac{2(.96) + 1(.99)}{3}$$
$$= .97 \tag{5.2b}$$
$$\sqrt{\bar{r}^*_{cc}} = .984$$

Step 3c: Compute $\bar{\rho}_{TC}$, the fully corrected mean validity, by using Equation 5.3.

$$\bar{\rho}_{TC} = \frac{\bar{r}_{tc}}{\sqrt{\bar{r}_{tt}} \sqrt{\bar{r}_{cc}}} \tag{5.3}$$

Because assumed values were used for the test and/or criterion reliabilities, Equation 5.3 was modified as follows:

$$\bar{\rho}^*_{TC} = \frac{\bar{r}_{tc}}{\sqrt{\bar{r}^*_{tt}} \ \sqrt{\bar{r}^*_{cc}}}$$

$$\bar{\rho}^*_{TC} = \frac{.739}{(.934)\,(.984)}$$

$$= .804$$

(5.3a)

Step 4: The fully corrected distribution is now used to calculate the variance of each quantifiable artifact.

Step 4a: Compute σ^2_{cc}, variance due to criterion reliability differences.

1. Compute r_{tc_i}, the estimated validity coefficient of each study, corrected for criterion unreliability.

$$r_{tc_i} = \sqrt{r_{cc_i}} \ (\bar{\rho}_{TC})$$

(5.4)

where

r_{cc_i} = criterion reliability coefficient for ith study,

$\bar{\rho}_{TC}$ = fully corrected mean validity,

$r_{tc_1} = \sqrt{.99} \ (.804) = .799969899$,

$r_{tc_2} = \sqrt{.96} \ (.804) = .787755901$, and

$r_{tc_3} = \sqrt{.96} \ (.804) = .787755901$

2. Calculate $\Sigma r_{tc_i} f_{c_i}$ and $\Sigma r^2_{tc_i} f_{c_i}$ where

r_{tc_i} = estimated validity corrected
for criterion reliability
in the ith study,

f_{c_i} = frequency of r_{tc_i},

$\Sigma r_{tc_i} f_{c_i} = .799969899(1) + .787755901(2)$

$= 2.375481701$, and

$\Sigma r^2_{tc_i} f_{c_i} = 1.881070558$

3. Compute σ^2_{cc} using Equation 5.5:

$$\sigma^2_{cc} = \frac{\Sigma r^2_{tc_i} f_{c_i}}{\Sigma f_{c_i}} - \left[\frac{\Sigma r_{tc_i} f_{c_i}}{\Sigma f_{c_i}} \right]^2$$

$$= \frac{1.881070558}{3} - \left[\frac{2.37548170}{3} \right]^2$$

(5.5)

$$= .000033152$$

Step 4b: Compute σ_{tt}^2, variance due to test reliability differences.

1. Compute $\bar{\rho}_{cT}$, mean validity corrected only for test unreliability:

$$\bar{\rho}_{cT} = \frac{\bar{r}_{tc}}{\sqrt{\bar{r}_{tt}}} \tag{5.6}$$

where $\bar{r}_{tc}$ is the weighted mean of observed validity coefficients and $\bar{r}_{tt}$ is the weighted mean of observed test reliability coefficients:

$$\bar{\rho}_{cT} = \frac{.739}{.934}$$
$$= .791$$

2. Calculate r_{cT_i}, the estimated validity coefficient of each study corrected for test unreliability:

$$r_{cT_i} = \sqrt{r_{tt_i}}\,(\bar{\rho}_{cT}) \tag{5.7}$$

where r_{tt_i} is the test reliability for the ith study, $\bar{\rho}_{cT}$ is the mean validity corrected for test unreliability,

$$r_{cT_1} = \sqrt{.95}\,(.791) = .770971432,$$
$$r_{cT_2} = \sqrt{.82}\,(.791) = .716280964,\text{ and}$$
$$r_{cT_3} = \sqrt{.85}\,(.791) = .729265966$$

3. Calculate $\Sigma r_{cT_i} f_{t_i}$ and $\Sigma r_{cT_i}^2 f_{t_i}$ where

r_{cT_i} = estimated validity coefficient of each study corrected for test unreliability,

$\quad f_{t_i}$ = frequency of r_{cT_i},
$\Sigma r_{cT_i} f_{t_i}$ = .770971432 (1) + .716280964 (1) + .729265966 (1)
$\qquad\quad = 2.216518362,\text{ and}$
$\Sigma r_{cT_i}^2 f_{t_i}$ = 1.639284217

Compute σ_{tt}^2 using Equation 5.8:

$$\sigma_{tt}^2 = \frac{\Sigma r_{cT_i}^2 f_{t_i}}{\Sigma f_{t_i}} - \left[\frac{\Sigma r_{cT_i} f_{t_i}}{\Sigma f_{t_i}}\right]^2$$
$$= \frac{1.639284217}{3} - \left[\frac{2.216518362}{3}\right]^2 \tag{5.8}$$
$$= .000544334$$

Step 4c: Compute $\sigma_{\bar{s}}^2$ variance due to sampling error.

1. Compute weighted variance for each observed validity coefficient, using Equation 5.9:

$$\sigma_{\bar{s}_i}^2 = \frac{N_i\,(1-r_{tc_i}^2)^2}{N_i - 1} \tag{5.9}$$

where

N_i = sample size of study i,

r_{tc_i} = observed validity coefficient for study i,

$$\sigma_{\bar{s}_1}^2 = \frac{15(1-.83^2)^2}{14} = .103696296,$$

$$\sigma_{\bar{s}_2}^2 = \frac{48(1-.54^2)^2}{47} = .512507806,$$

$$\sigma_{\bar{s}_3}^2 = \frac{16(1-.74^2)^2}{15} = .218310144,$$

$$\sigma_{\bar{s}_4}^2 = \frac{44(1-.91^2)^2}{43} = .03023681, \text{ and}$$

$$\sigma_{\bar{s}_5}^2 = \frac{35(1-.76^2)^2}{34} = .183669458$$

2. Compute $\sigma_{\bar{s}}^2$, the weighted average sampling error, using Equation 5.10:

$$\sigma_{\bar{s}}^2 = \frac{\Sigma\sigma_{\bar{s}_i}^2}{\Sigma N_i}$$

$$= \frac{1.048420514}{158} \tag{5.10}$$

$$= .006635572873$$

Step 4d: Compute σ_{PRED}^2, the predicted variance, using Equation 5.11:

$$\sigma_{\text{PRED}}^2 = \sigma_{\bar{s}}^2 + \sigma_{tt}^2 + \sigma_{cc}^2$$

$$= .006635572873 + .000544334 + \tag{5.11}$$

$$.000033152$$

$$= .007213058$$

Step 5: Compute σ_{TOT}^2, the total observed variance, using Equation 5.12:

$$\sigma_{\text{TOT}}^2 = \frac{\Sigma[N_i(r_{tc_i} - \bar{r}_{tc})^2]}{\Sigma N_i}$$

$$\sigma_{\text{TOT}}^2 = [15(.83 - .739556962)^2 + 48(.54 - .739556962)^2$$

$$+ 16(.74 - .739556962)^2 + 44(.91 - .739556962)^2 \tag{5.12}$$

$$+ 35(.76 - .739556962)^2]/158$$

$$= .021057398$$

Step 6: Compute residual variance, using Equation 5.13:

$$\sigma^2_{res} = \sigma^2_{TOT} - \sigma^2_{PRED}$$
$$\sigma^2_{res} = .021057398 - .007213058 \qquad (5.13)$$
$$= .01384434$$
$$\sigma_{res} = .117661973$$

Step 7: Compute the percentage of variance accounted for by each artifact.

1. Compute the percentage of variance accounted for by criterion reliability differences ($\%\sigma^2_{cc}$) using Equation 5.14:

$$\%\sigma^2_{cc} = \frac{\sigma^2_{cc}}{\sigma^2_{TOT}} \times 100$$

$$\%\sigma^2_{cc} = \frac{.000033152}{.021057398} \times 100 \qquad (5.14)$$

$$= .157436355$$

2. Compute the percentage of variance accounted for by test reliability differences ($\%\sigma^2_{tt}$) using Equation 5.15:

$$\%\sigma^2_{tt} = \frac{\sigma^2_{tt}}{\sigma^2_{TOT}} \times 100$$

$$\%\sigma^2_{tt} = \frac{.000544334}{.021057398} \times 100 \qquad (5.15)$$

$$= 2.585001243$$

3. Compute the percentage of variance accounted for by sampling error ($\%\sigma^2_{s}$) using Equation 5.16:

$$\%\sigma^2_{s} = \frac{\sigma^2_{s}}{\sigma^2_{TOT}} \times 100$$

$$= \frac{.006635572873}{.021057398} \times 100 \qquad (5.16)$$

$$= 31.51183256$$

4. Compute the percentage of variance accounted for by all artifacts, using Equation 5.17:

$$\%\sigma^2 = \frac{\sigma^2_{PRED}}{\sigma^2_{TOTAL}} \times 100$$

$$\%\sigma^2 = \frac{.007213058}{.021057398} \times 100 \qquad (5.17)$$

$$= 34.25427016$$

With the above information, the *null hypothesis* can be tested. According to this hypothesis, the variance of true validities (residual variance) is zero.

Since the residual variance in the example was not zero, the null hypothesis cannot be accepted. When this occurs, examine the percentage of variance accounted for by the artifacts. Validity generalization can still be supported if at least 75% of the variance can be accounted for by the artifacts. If the 75% rule has been met, go to Step 8 to calculate descriptive statistics.

Step 8a: Compute $\bar{\rho}$, the mean true validity, using Equation 5.18:

$$\bar{\rho} = \frac{\bar{r}_{tc}}{\sqrt{\bar{r}_{cc}}} \tag{5.18}$$

Step 8b: Compute σ_ρ, the standard deviation of true validity, using Equation 5.19:

$$\sigma_\rho = \frac{\sigma_{res}}{\sqrt{\bar{r}_{cc}}} \tag{5.19}$$

Step 8c: Compute the lower and upper limits of the 90% confidence interval, using Equation 5.20:

Upper Limit $= \bar{\rho} + 1.28\sigma_\rho$

Lower Limit $= \bar{\rho} - 1.28\sigma_\rho$ $\qquad$ (5.20)

The descriptive information in Step 8 indicates the best estimate of validity (ρ) if a new study were carried out. The confidence interval limits show that 90% of the time validity coefficients involving similar predictor/criterion tests can be expected to fall between the lower and upper bounds.

In the empirical example, the percentage of variance accounted for by the artifacts was 34.25%. Thus, the 75% decision rule was not met. Had this been a full-scale validity generalization study, the conclusion would be that the validity of submaximal bicycle tests does not appear to be generalizable. However, a model is in place for future use. A new validity study should be carried out. This new study will represent new data and should be added to the prior information to form the posterior distribution. The posterior distribution can be used in a subsequent validity generalization study. Bear in mind that a decision based on this small empirical example may not represent the *true* state of validity for submaximal cycle tests. A much larger study should be carried out to determine whether validity can be generalized.

Table 5.2 includes summary information for this small empirical example. Figure 5.1 illustrates a flowchart of the validity generalization model. For an example of a full-scale validity generalization study, see Safrit et al. (1988).

Controversy Surrounding Validity Generalization

Whenever a provocative model is developed and presented as an alternative to a firmly entrenched idea, there inevitably is reaction from the research community. Validity generalization is no exception. Reactions have ranged from the development of different approaches for calculating validity generalization to questions regarding the model's assumptions.

Table 5.2   Summary Information from Validity Generalization

Weighted mean of observed validity coefficients	.739
Fully corrected mean validity	.804
Variance due to criterion reliability differences	.000033
Variance due to test reliability differences	.000544
Variance due to sampling error	.006635
Predicted variance	.007213
Total variance	.021057
Residual variance	.013844
Percent variance accounted for by artifacts	34.25%

Alternative approaches to calculating validity generalization.   Two other methods for calculating validity generalization have been proposed by researchers who have identified potential weaknesses in the Schmidt and Hunter (1977) model. Callender and Osburn (1980) developed an approach they termed *multiplicative*, because it allowed for an interactive effect between the artifacts rather than the additive approach of Schmidt and Hunter. Further work (Callender, Osburn, Greener, & Ashworth, 1982) with computer simulation suggested that the approach of Callender and Osburn was more accurate in estimating the variance of the validity coefficients when sample size, shape of distribution, and the mean and standard deviation of the distribution were varied. This led to considerable debate (Callender & Osburn, 1982; Hunter, Schmidt, & Pearlman, 1982; Schmidt, Hunter, & Pearlman, 1982) regarding the merits of each approach. Later research (Raju & Burke, 1983) has suggested that although slight differences exist in these two approaches, the practical impact is minimal.

Type I and Type II errors.   Several studies (Kemery, Mossholder, & Roth, 1987; Osburn, Callender, Greener, & Ashworth, 1983; Spector & Levine, 1987) have examined **Type I** and **Type II errors** in validity generalization through the use of **Monte Carlo studies**. Osburn et al. found that power was low over all conditions when the sample size in the studies was less than 100. Spector and Levine employed a validity generalization model accounting for sampling error only and examined Type I and Type II errors using the 75% decision rule of Schmidt and his colleagues, an approach they called S&H−75%. Their results indicated that Type I errors for the S&H−75% approach ranged from 0.02 when 100 correlations were employed to 0.20 when 6 to 10 correlations were used. Type II errors were fairly high, except with large sample sizes and greater numbers of correlations. They suggested cautious interpretation of results from small validity generalization studies and recommended using tables developed for estimating the Type I and Type II errors under various conditions. These authors

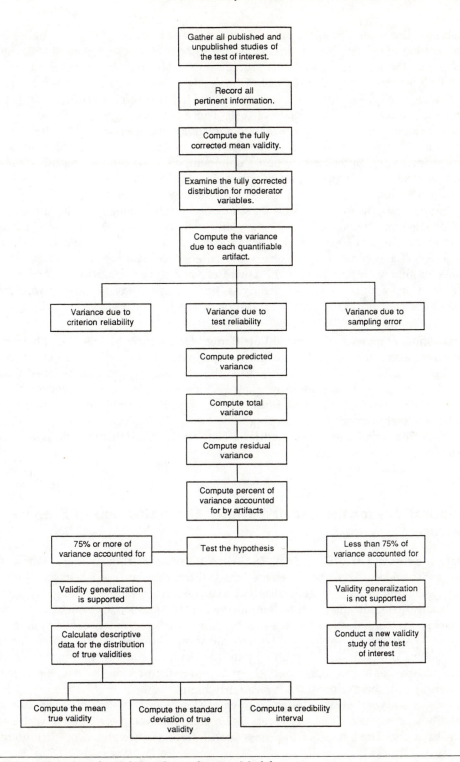

Figure 5.1 Flowchart for Validity Generalization Model

discussed the related problem of the accuracy of the calculation of the variance in the distribution of validity coefficients. They suggested that if the estimate of variance was too small, the need for moderators would be detected too rarely; and if the variance estimate was too high, the presence of moderators would be implicated too often.

Kemery et al. (1987) found that when true validity was zero, the Schmidt and Hunter approach had a Type II error rate of 0.30. These authors suggested the possibility of the coexistence of validity generalization and situational specificity. They believed that some of the variation in validity coefficients was due to the interaction of the job environment (e.g. budgetary support, equipment, collegial support) on the job holder, and that these factors may affect people differentially.

Schmidt, Hunter, Pearlman, and Hirsh (1985) have countered some of the arguments regarding low power by stating that simulation studies underestimate the power of validity generalization, since they can only include quantifiable artifacts. Empirical studies, on the other hand, will always include nonquantifiable artifacts, such as typographical and computational errors and criterion contamination and bias; thus *real* power is higher. In addition, if the power of validity generalization is low, what alternative procedures are there? Clearly, a small single study of validity would have even lower power. It appears that this area merits further research.

Assumptions of the model. Some authors (James, Demaree, & Mulaik, 1986) have raised questions about the assumption of normally distributed errors and the effect that violating this assumption has on computing the variance. James et al. believed that this problem could be taken care of by using Fisher's *z* transformation; however, Schmidt et al. (1985) disagreed and have not used the transformation since they have found it to be positively biased. Other investigators (Burke, 1984; Callender et al., 1982) have found similar results and suggest that a skewed distribution has little effect on the estimation of the variance.

Implications for the Use of Validity Generalization in Exercise Science

Only one study to date (Safrit et al., 1988) has utilized the validity generalization model in exercise science. This study examined the validity of distance-run tests and illustrated the application of validity generalization to a concurrent validity setting.

Validity generalization can be employed in any situation in which several small sample correlational studies exist using the same predictor/criterion combination. The use of Bayesian statistics in validity generalization allows researchers to cumulate information from past studies and integrate conflicting results. If the hypothesis of situational specificity can be rejected, theories and constructs can be developed and relationships can be explored.

There are several areas of research in exercise science in which many small sample validity studies exist. The body composition area, for example, is replete with studies that have correlated skinfold thickness with hydrostatic weighing, or circumferences and girths with hydrostatic weighing. Validity generalization studies would allow integration of an enormous body of research to ascertain the generalizability of the findings and estimate the *true* mean validity. The effects of age, gender, fitness level, and other variables on these relationships also could be clarified. The sport psychology field might also benefit from validity generalization. The psychobiological models for predicting success on athletic teams could employ validity generalization to integrate the literature. In this setting, when athletes actually are selected from a larger pool of athletes, the effects of range restriction should be included. Exercise physiologists might wish to examine the generalizability of various submaximal bicycle protocols as predictors of maximal oxygen uptake. Another possibility is the variability in step test results when correlated with measures of maximal oxygen uptake. And finally, studies of the relationship of perceived exertion and workload could be examined across a variety of settings. These are just a few of the many questions that could be answered with validity generalization. If situational specificity can be rejected, knowledge in an area can be integrated and theory development can move forward. If validity generalization cannot be substantiated, a model is in place for additional research.

Conclusion

Just as an examination of the statistical assumptions of meta-analysis has led to modification in its use, so may validity generalization become refined as researchers examine the effects of variations in the artifacts and explore ways to improve the accuracy of variance estimates. However, the basic tenets of validity generalization have withstood 10 years of scrutiny by personnel psychologists, and it remains one of the most powerful advancements in the study of validity. Validity generalization holds considerable promise as a tool for exercise scientists to use in integrating knowledge in the area of criterion-related validity.

Study Questions

1. What is the purpose of validity generalization?
2. What prompted the development of validity generalization?
3. What is the major difference between meta-analysis and validity generalization?
4. List the eight artifacts that may cause validity coefficients to vary. Which artifacts are considered quantifiable?
5. Why did Schmidt and Hunter develop a 75% rule?
6. How is a Bayesian approach different from traditional hypothesis testing?
7. What problems may arise when validity generalization is based on a small number of validity coefficients?
8. What is the recommended number of validity coefficients for a full-scale validity generalization study?

9. An exercise scientist wished to determine if validity generalization was possible for step test results when correlated with maximal oxygen uptake. The following data were collected:

R_{tc}	N	R_{tt}	R_{cc}
.45	30	.65	.90
.70	25	.80	.95
.85	28	.72	.91
.60	20	.85	.94
.59	35	.68	.89

Now answer these questions:

    a. Is validity generalization supported? Why or why not?
    b. What is the mean observed validity coefficient?
    c. What is the fully corrected mean validity?
    d. What is the variance due to:
      criterion reliability differences?
      test reliability differences?
      sampling error?
    e. What is the percentage of variance accounted for by:
      criterion reliability differences?
      test reliability differences?
      sampling error?
    f. What is the mean true validity?
    g. What is the standard deviation of true validity?
    h. Construct a 90% confidence interval.

Answers to Study Questions

1. The purpose of validity generalization is to determine if the variability in observed validity coefficients is real or due to artifacts.
2. Personnel psychologists noted that validity coefficients varied considerably from situation to situation, even though the same test was used as the predictor.
3. Meta-analysts accept variability in effect sizes as real and explain it by correlating effect size with moderator variables. Validity generalization attempts to correct variability in validity coefficients and hypothesizes that the variance of true validity is zero.
4. Criterion reliability, test reliability, range restriction, sample size, criterion contamination and deficiency, computational and typographical errors, factor structure of tests, and factor structure of criterion tests. The first four artifacts are quantifiable.
5. Because not all artifacts are quantifiable, if 75% of the variance can be accounted for by the artifacts, validity generalization can still be assumed.

6. Bayesian statistics incorporates relevant information from past research to form a prior distribution, which is used to test a hypothesis.
7. The variance estimates may be inaccurate. Both Type I and Type II errors are more likely to occur.
8. 100–200
9. a. Yes. 80.54% of the variance is accounted for by the artifacts.
   b. .634
   c. .777
   d. criterion = .0000878
      test = .001025
      sampling error = .0136
   e. criterion = .4805%
      test = 5.61%
      sampling error = 74.44%
   f. .6627
   g. .0624
   h. .583–.743

References

Åstrand, P.O., & Rhyming, I. (1954). A nomogram for calculation of aerobic capacity (physical fitness) from pulse rate during submaximal work. *Journal of Applied Physiology, 7,* 218–221.

Burke, M.J. (1984). Validity generalization: A review and critique of the correlation model. *Personnel Psychology, 37,* 93–115.

Callender, J.C., & Osburn, H.G. (1980). Development and test of a new model for validity generalization. *Journal of Applied Psychology, 65,* 543–558.

Callender, J.C., & Osburn, H.G. (1982). Another view of progress in validity generalization: Reply to Schmidt, Hunter, and Pearlman. *Journal of Applied Psychology, 67,* 846–852.

Callender, J.C., Osburn, H.G., Greener, J.M., & Ashworth, S. (1982). Multiplicative validity generalization model: Accuracy of estimates as a function of sample size, mean and variance, and shape of distribution of true validities. *Journal of Applied Psychology, 67,* 859–867.

deVries, H.A., & Klafs, C.E. (1965). Prediction of maximal oxygen intake from submaximal tests. *Journal of Sports Medicine and Physical Fitness, 5,* 207–214.

Feltz, P.L., & Landers, D.M. (1983). The effects of mental practice on motor skill learning and performance: A meta-analysis. *Journal of Sports Psychology, 5,* 25–57.

Glass, G.V. (1976). Primary, secondary, and meta-analysis of research. *The Educational Researcher, 10,* 3–8.

Glass, G.V. (1977). Integrating findings: The meta-analysis of research. *Review of Research in Education, 5,* 351–379.

Glass, G.V., McGaw, B., & Smith, M.L. (1981). *Meta-analysis in social research.* Beverly Hills, CA: Sage.

Hedges, L.V., & Olkin, I. (1980). Vote-counting methods in research synthesis. *Psychological Bulletin, 88,* 359–369.

Hirsh, H.R., Northrop, L.C., & Schmidt, F.L. (1986). Validity generalization results for law enforcement occupations. *Personnel Psychology, 39,* 399–420.

Hunter, J.E., Schmidt, F.L., & Jackson, G.B. (1982). *Meta-analysis: Cumulating research findings across studies.* Beverly Hills, CA: Sage.

Hunter, J.E., Schmidt, F.L., & Pearlman, K. (1982). History and accuracy of validity generalization equations: A response to the Callender and Osburn reply. *Journal of Applied Psychology, 67,* 853–858.

James, L.R., Demaree, R.G., & Mulaik, S.A. (1986). A note on validity generalization procedures. *Journal of Applied Psychology, 71,* 440–450.

Kavale, K., & Mattson, P.D. (1983). One jumped off the balance beam: Meta-analysis of perceptual training. *Journal of Learning Disabilities, 16,* 165–173.

Kemery, E.R., Mossholder, K.W., & Roth, L. (1987). The power of the Schmidt and Hunter additive model of validity generalization. *Journal of Applied Psychology, 72,* 30–37.

Oja, P., Partanen, T., & Teraslinna, P. (1970). The validity of three indirect methods of measuring oxygen uptake and physical fitness. *Journal of Sports Medicine and Physical Fitness, 10,* 67–71.

Osburn, H.G., Callender, J.C., Greener, J.M., & Ashworth, S. (1983). Statistical power of tests of situational specificity hypotheses in validity generalization studies: A cautionary note. *Journal of Applied Psychology, 68,* 115–122.

Patton, J.F., Vogel, J.A., & Mello, R.P. (1982). Evaluation of a maximal predictive cycle ergometer test. *European Journal of Applied Physiology, 49,* 131–140.

Pearlman, K., Schmidt, F.L., & Hunter, J.E. (1980). Validity generalization results for tests used to predict job proficiency and training success in clerical occupations. *Journal of Applied Psychology, 65,* 373–406.

Raju, N.S., & Burke, M.J. (1983). Two new procedures for studying validity generalization. *Journal of Applied Psychology, 68,* 382–395.

Safrit, M.J., Costa, M.G., & Hooper, L.M. (1986). The validity generalization model: An approach to the analysis of validity studies in physical education. *Research Quarterly for Exercise and Sport, 57,* 288–297.

Safrit, M.J., Costa, M.G., Hooper, L.M., Patterson, P., & Ehlert, S.A. (in press). The validity generalization of distance run tests. *Canadian Journal of Sport Sciences.*

Schmidt, F.L., Gast-Rosenberg, I., & Hunter, J.E. (1980). Validity generalization results for computer programmers. *Journal of Applied Psychology, 65,* 643–661.

Schmidt, F.L., & Hunter, J.E. (1977). Development of a general solution to the problem of validity generalization. *Journal of Applied Psychology, 62,* 529–540.

Schmidt, F.L., Hunter, J.E., & Pearlman, K. (1982). Progress in validity generalization: Comments on Callender and Osburn and further developments. *Journal of Applied Psychology, 67,* 835–845.

Schmidt, F.L., Hunter, J.E., Pearlman, K., & Hirsh, H. (1985). Forty questions about validity generalization and meta-analysis. *Personnel Psychology, 38,* 697–798.

Schmidt, F.L., Hunter, J.E., Pearlman, K., & Shane, G.S. (1979). Further tests of the Schmidt-Hunter Bayesian validity generalization procedure. *Personnel Psychology, 32*, 257–281.

Schmidt, F.L., Hunter, J.E., & Urry, V.W. (1976). Statistical power in criterion-related validation studies. *Journal of Applied Psychology, 61*, 473–485.

Siconolfi, S.F., Cullinane, E.M., Carleton, R.A., & Thompson, P.D. (1982). Assessing $\dot{V}O_{2max}$ in epidemiologic studies: Modification of the Åstrand-Rhyming test. *Medicine and Science in Sports and Exercise, 14*(5), 335–338.

Sparling, P.B. (1980). A meta-analysis of studies comparing maximal oxygen uptake in men and women. *Research Quarterly for Exercise and Sport, 51*, 542–552.

Spector, P.E., & Levine, E.L. (1987). Meta-analysis for integrating study outcomes: A Monte Carlo study of its susceptibility to Type I and Type II errors. *Journal of Applied Psychology, 72*, 3–9.

Thomas, J.R., & French, K.E. (1985). Gender differences across age in motor performance: A meta-analysis. *Psychological Bulletin, 98*(2), 260–282.

Thomas, J.R., & French, K.E. (1986). The use of meta-analysis in exercise and sport: A tutorial. *Research Quarterly for Exercise and Sport, 57*, 196–204.

Tran, Z.V., Weltman, A., Glass, G.V., & Mood, D.P. (1983). The effects of exercise on blood lipids and lipoproteins: A meta-analysis of studies. *Medicine and Science in Sports and Exercise, 15*, 393-402.

Wilmore, J.H., Roby, F.B., Stanforth, P.R., Buono, M.J., Constable, S.H., Tsao, Y., & Lowdon, B.J. (1986). Ratings of perceived exertion, heart rate, and power output in predicting maximal oxygen uptake during submaximal cycle ergometry. *The Physician and Sportsmedicine, 14*, 133–144.

Supplementary Readings

Guion, R.M. (1987). Changing views for personnel selection research. *Personnel Psychology, 40*, 199–213.

McDaniel, M.A., Hirsh, H.R., Schmidt, F.L., Raju, N.S., & Hunter, J.E. (1986). Interpreting the results of meta-analytic research: A comment on Schmitt, Gooding, Noe, and Kirsch (1984). *Personnel Psychology, 39*, 141–148.

Schmitt, N., & Noe, R.A. (1986). On shifting standards for conclusions regarding validity generalization. *Personnel Psychology, 39*, 849–851.

Criterion-Referenced Measurement

An alternative approach to measurement in physical education and the exercise sciences is criterion-referenced measurement (CRM). Section III contains two chapters that describe the test characteristics of CRM and give examples. Chapter 6, by Margaret J. Safrit, treats validity as it applies to criterion-referenced tests. The validity of a domain-referenced test is differentiated from that of a mastery test. The focus of Chapter 7, by Marilyn A. Looney, is reliability in a CRM context. Reliability indices are described and the underlying assumptions of each are delineated, along with strengths and weaknesses of these procedures. Looney's scholarly treatise of CRM reliability includes a detailed overview of familiar indices as well as estimation procedures not yet used in our field.

Criterion-Referenced Measurement: Validity

Margaret J. Safrit
University of Wisconsin, Madison

Before the 1970s, many psychomotor tests were developed as norm-referenced tests. Then another approach to measurement began receiving emphasis in the world of education. This approach, known as criterion-referenced measurement, focuses on the examinee's ability to display a well-defined criterion behavior. Performance on a test is not compared with that of other examinees, as is characteristic of the norm-referenced approach. A **criterion-referenced test** is defined as:

> . . .one that is deliberately constructed so as to yield measurements that are directly interpretable in terms of specified performance standards. The performance standards are usually specified by defining some domain of tasks that the student should perform. Representative samples of tasks from this domain are organized into a test. Measurements are taken and are used to make a statement about the performance of each individual relative to that domain. (Glaser & Nitko, 1971, p. 653)

The key element of this definition is that performance on the test is tied to a criterion behavior. The set of criterion behaviors is referred to as the domain of behaviors, and the test is a sample from this domain.

The purpose of this chapter is to examine test validity in the context of criterion-referenced measurement. In general, validity has the same meaning in all measurement theories. It is defined as the soundness of the interpretation of the test:

> The concept [of validity] refers to the appropriateness, meaningfulness, and usefulness of the specific inferences made from test scores. . . . Although evidence may be accumulated in many ways, validity always refers to the degree to which that evidence supports the inferences that are made from the scores. The inferences regarding specific uses of a test are validated, not the test itself. (American Psychological Association, 1985, p. 9)

However, the precise definition of validity varies depending on the conceptual framework of the model. When a criterion-referenced test is developed, two approaches to test validation are most frequently used: domain-referenced validity and decision accuracy.

Domain-Referenced Validity

When a test is used to identify the percentage of a domain of tasks an examinee can achieve, the appropriate approach to validation is **domain-referenced validity**. It is similar in many respects to content validity. No standard of performance is set for the examinee. Domain-referenced validity is the extent to which a test measures the objectives identified within the domain. The domain encompasses all possible objectives for the content area of interest. The objectives should not be sampled randomly from the domain, because the end result may not be representative of the domain. Rather, the categories of objectives within the domain should be weighted according to their importance, and the test should reflect this weighting.

When criterion-referenced test theory was in the early stage of development, the domain of content was expected to be narrow enough in scope to encompass a set of objectives that could be measured in its entirety. It was possible to generate questions for each objective and include all questions in a single test form. Every operation in the domain could thus be defined and measured precisely. But many potential domains could not be identified with such precision. Therefore, researchers proposed the concept of *amplified objectives*, which lays down precise rules for the specifications of test items but acknowledges that including items for all objectives in the domain is not feasible. It is appropriate to use the amplified-objectives protocol in specifying representative motor tasks or components of a motor task.

As in content validity, a table of specifications is essential to determining domain-referenced validity. The categories of objectives are listed as well as the individual objectives. The number of tasks or trials within each category is a function of the weighting of each category. The process of evaluating domain-referenced validity is primarily subjective. A pool of judges and measurement specialists is often used to assess the representativeness of items and item bias.

In testing motor behavior, domain-referenced validity would be appropriate for assessing the developmental stages of motor tasks such as walking, running, and hopping. Each of these tasks might be associated with an objective and consist of measurable subcomponents of the task. The test user may be interested in the extent to which a child displays mature behavior on the task. These types of assessment procedures are especially effective in diagnosing weaknesses and correcting performance.

Developing Written Tests

When preparing a written test, an important aspect of domain-referenced validity is whether the content areas are relevant to the test user's goals. Should an area be emphasized more, deemphasized, added, or eliminated? In a test of the effects of physical activity, a substantial number of items might be included on the acute effects of physical activity. One might question whether the degree of emphasis on this content area is warranted. Some users might feel the acute effects of exercise should not be emphasized; others might disagree. The relative importance of various areas of content might differ markedly across school districts, depending on the curricular objectives of the physical education program. Including a substantial number of test items on the short-term and long-term effects of physical activity might be desirable in a program where physical fitness is an important part of the curriculum. In a program stressing skill development, emphasizing exercise physiology might be unacceptable.

The following steps are recommended for reviewing a published test to determine its domain-referenced validity:

1. Answer the test items and score your responses.
2. Review the publisher's statement on domain-referenced validity.
3. Examine the table of specifications.
4. Assess the appropriateness of the placement of items in the domain categories.
5. Examine the domain and respond to the following four questions:
   a. Are important elements of the domain omitted?
   b. Are unimportant elements of the domain erroneously included?
   c. Are any categories included in the domain weighted improperly?
   (Weighting is reflected in the number of items included in a category.)
   d. Are all elements of the test content-relevant?

The following steps should be taken to demonstrate domain-referenced validity when you have developed the test yourself:

1. Develop a table of specifications for the test. Determine the number of items that should be written for each cell of the table. Write the appropriate number of items for each cell.
2. Place the test items in test form.
3. Take the test and score your responses. Take this step even if the test is your own.

4. Select 25% of the test items and reexamine the appropriateness of their placement in the content categories of the table of specifications. Revise the items, if necessary. If more than 5% (of the 25% selected) of the items were placed inappropriately, reexamine the placement of the remaining 75% of the items.
5. Determine whether the content categories should be altered in any way. Look for possible additions, deletions, increased emphasis, and decreased emphasis.

Often a test is developed by writing items as each one comes to mind, until enough items have been written to fill the testing period. Such an approach may lead to haphazard results. The test may be weighted heavily in one or two categories and slighted in others. It behooves the test developer to begin by preparing a table of specifications, deciding in advance the number of items for each category based on its relative importance. Then when the item-writing process is begun, it has greater purpose. The test developer can also have greater confidence that the test will be valid.

Logical Validity

The above procedures must be modified somewhat to determine the validity of sports skills tests. In many cases, only one skill is being measured. In this case, the test should identify and assess the most important components of the skill. Sport specialists and measurement experts should assess the representativeness of the components. The test should also be reviewed for appropriateness regarding gender, age, skill level, and so forth.

The general procedure to be followed in constructing a skills test is to define good performance in executing the skill, construct a test that measures the important components of skill in the definition, and score the test so that the best score represents a performance that approximates the definition of good performance.

Because **logical validity** is the degree to which the components of skill measured by a test correspond with those required to perform the skill adequately, the identification of important components of a skill is important. Although it is appropriate to measure specific skills when students are learning a sport, skills tests should not mistakenly be thought to measure playing ability. To measure playing ability, a battery of tests is often used. One of the first steps in validating a test battery of this type is to use logical validity. In this context, logical validity involves the definition of the important skills comprising playing ability. Tests are then selected to measure each of the skills identified as important. Of course, each individual test must have logical validity as well.

An important interpretive point should be considered in any discussion of domain-referenced and logical validity. Both refer to the validity of the test; however, most test users are ultimately interested in the validity of test scores, i.e., the validity of the intended *use* of the test. As Messick (1975) noted:

The major problem . . . is [that validity is] focused upon test forms rather than test scores, upon instruments rather than measurements. Inferences in educational and psychological measurement are made from scores, and scores are a function of

Table 6.1 Procedure for Establishing the Congruence Between Fitness Specialists and Test Battery Subtests

Subtest	Ratings — Fitness specialist								Mean	Median	Range
	1	2	3	4	5	6	7	8			
Distance Run	5	5	5	4	4	5	5	5	4.75	5	2
Sit-and-Reach	4	4	5	4	4	4	5	5	4.38	4	2
Sum of Skinfolds	3	4	3	3	4	4	4	4	3.63	4	2
Sit-ups	5	5	4	4	5	4	5	5	4.63	5	2
Discrepancy between rating and median summed by judge	1	0	3	3	1	1	1	1			

subject responses. . . . Content coverage is an important consideration in test construction and interpretation, to be sure, but it in itself does not provide validity. (pp. 960–961)

It is possible to quantify domain-referenced validity to some extent, although all such procedures retain a substantial element of subjectivity. Hambleton (1984) describes a procedure for evaluating item-objective congruence which could be applied in a motor behavior test setting. The major question to be answered is whether the psychomotor test matches the objective or competency. For example, in developing a battery of tests for physical fitness, the overall validity of the test is established by demonstrating that the subtests represent the most important components of fitness. This could be assessed by asking a group of fitness specialists to rate each component according to the extent to which it represents a designated component of fitness.

Table 6.1 provides an example of this procedure. A group of 8 fitness specialists were asked to rate the representativeness of each subtest as a measure of a specific component of fitness. A 5-point rating scale was devised for this purpose. An acceptable subtest was one that received a mean rating of 3.5 or higher. The subtests were the four tests in the Health-Related Physical Fitness Test (American Alliance for Health, Physical Education, Recreation & Dance, 1980). The components of health-related fitness were identified and defined, along with the tests used to measure each component. Note that in Table 6.1 the representativeness of all four subtests was assessed as acceptable by the raters.

In addition to the mean of the ratings, the median is also calculated. The number of individual ratings that deviate from the median rating is then calculated for each rater. In this case, the discrepancies between the ratings and the medians exceeded 1 in only two instances. The success of this procedure rests on selecting a well-qualified pool of raters and training them to use the rating scale properly. The disadvantages are the usual ones. Raters have a tendency to rate all items or tasks high. Also, this procedure does not provide for the identification of components that were not included but should have been.

This approach also could be used to test sports skills. Instead of the subtests in the above example, list components of the skill and ask experts in the sport to rate the importance of each component.

Decision Accuracy

Establishing the domain-referenced validity of a test is the primary approach to validating a test that will be used to assess the percentage of a domain the examinee can achieve. However, the more predominant use of criterion-referenced measurement in physical education has been to classify examinees as *masters* or *nonmasters*. This approach is known as **mastery testing** and is based on the *binomial error model*. Dichotomous scores are used, with a score of 1 representing mastery and a score of 0, nonmastery. To classify examinees in this way, a cutoff score must be identified. Those scoring at or above the cutoff are classified as masters; those scoring below the cutoff, as nonmasters.

Errors of classification can be made in a mastery test setting. When an examinee is actually a master but is classified as a nonmaster based on a test score, this is known as a **false negative classification**. A **false positive classification** is made when a nonmaster is erroneously classified as a master. Loss ratios, which assess the relative seriousness of the consequences, can be specified for the misclassifications. If, for example, a false positive classification is considered more serious than a false negative classification, the former error can be assigned a higher weighting than the latter.

Validity in the context of a mastery test can be defined more precisely as the accuracy of classifications. This is referred to as *decision accuracy*. In and of itself, decision accuracy does not provide sufficient evidence of the validity of a mastery test. Satisfactory domain-referenced validity must be established before determining other validity methods. The knowledge that a test classifies examinees accurately is of little value if it is not a valid indicator of the domain being measured.

The procedures for validating a test include both judgmental and empirical approaches, although it is impossible to avoid the judgmental element entirely in either approach. Berk (1986) categorized the methods used to set performance standards, i.e., to determine the most valid standards. He identified three categories: judgmental, judgmental-empirical, and empirical-judgmental. In the first category, the validity of the cutoff score is determined by one or more judges. For example, several teachers who are knowledgeable about the ability levels of students could assign each student to mastery or nonmastery status on each item or task based on their perceptions of each student's performance. The judgmental-empirical category is primarily judgmental, but performance data are made available to guide the judgments. If the teachers in the previous example used data from the students' official records to help assign their

True State

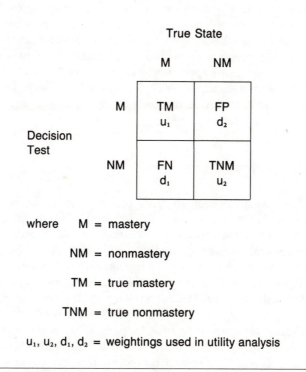

where   M = mastery

NM = nonmastery

TM = true mastery

TNM = true nonmastery

u_1, u_2, d_1, d_2 = weightings used in utility analysis

Figure 6.1   Contingency Table for Decision Validity

classifications, they would have used a judgmental-empirical method. The third category, empirical-judgmental, is primarily data-based, with judgments being made in some instances. Three empirical-judgmental approaches are described in this chapter. These are the *criterion test*, *criterion groups*, and *borderline groups*.

Estimating Decision Accuracy

One of the more desirable procedures for the empirical validation of a cutoff score is to use a comparison of statistical procedures (Berk, 1976). All decision accuracy models utilize a contingency table, as shown in Figure 6.1. At the top of the table, the true state is shown. This is the actual status of the examinee on the attribute being measured. It is assumed that it is possible to classify the examinees as true masters or true nonmasters, with no errors in the classifications. To the left of the table, the predicted state is identified. The predicted state is determined using the test of interest. The examinee is classified as a master or a nonmaster by the test; however, some of these classifications are known to be in error. When the classifications made using the predictor test match the predictions in the true state, the test is highly valid. Note in Figure 6.1 that these are the cells represented by TM (true mastery) and TNM (true nonmastery). Validity can be determined by summing the proportions in the main diagonal (TM and TNM), yielding c, the classification of outcome probabilities. The remaining cells represent errors of classification. The label *FP* represents examinees who are falsely classified as masters. The label *FN* represents those falsely classified as nonmasters.

A major problem in using this approach to criterion-referenced test validation is that the true state of the examinee can never be determined precisely. Therefore, the major quest of test developers is to devise methods of closely approximating the true state. Several approaches have been explored.

Use of a Criterion Test

The criterion test approach has been applied in an exercise science setting by Washburn and Safrit (1982). In this study, the model was used for the empirical validation of a cutoff score on a physical performance test used for job selection. Specifically, the physically demanding job of the wildland firefighter was cited. The physical demands of this job as related to the energy cost of doing the work have been determined through direct field measurements of firefighting tasks and have been shown to average 22.5 ml $O_2 \cdot kg^{-1} \cdot min^{-1}$ (Sharkey, 1977). Given the intermittent nature of firefighting tasks, it is assumed that a physically fit individual could sustain work rates of not more than 50% of his maximum capacity over an 8-hr period. Therefore, a maximum aerobic capacity of at least 45 ml $O_2 \cdot kg^{-1} \cdot min^{-1}$ would be required. This criterion has been adopted by the U.S. Forest Service and represents the true value for the cutoff score on the criterion test. Because of the drawbacks inherent in the direct measurement of maximal aerobic capacity, particularly for large groups, a more practical test is needed in the actual job selection. In the Washburn and Safrit study, the use of a submaximal step test of aerobic capacity as a decision test was investigated.

Six steps are recommended when a criterion test model is used. These are described below, using a hypothetical data set.

1. Establish a true value for the cutoff score on the criterion.
2. Identify a test as a practical decision test. The remaining task is to identify the appropriate cutoff.
3. Administer both the criterion test and the decision test to the same group of subjects. The sample should include at least 100 examinees in both the true mastery and true nonmastery cells.
4. Select cutoff scores on the decision test for investigation. In this example, three cutoff scores were selected, as shown in Table 6.2.
5. Apply analytic procedures. The cutoff score consistently selected across analyses is considered the optimal cutoff score on the decision test for the sample. This combination of procedures was recommended by Berk (1976). In Table 6.2, an example is presented using a small number of subjects. The small number is used merely for convenience and would not be considered adequate in a full-fledged

Table 6.2   Mastery/Nonmastery Scores Using Three Cutoff Scores on Decision Test

Examinee	Criterion Test	1st Cutoff Score - DT[a]	2nd Cutoff Score - DT	3rd Cutoff Score - DT
1	1	1	1	1
2	0	1	1	0
3	0	0	0	0
4	1	1	1	1
5	1	1	1	1
6	1	0	0	1
7	0	1	1	0
8	1	1	1	1
9	0	0	0	0
10	1	1	1	1
11	0	1	0	0
12	0	1	0	1
13	0	0	0	0
14	1	1	1	1
15	1	1	1	1
16	1	0	1	1
17	1	1	1	1
18	1	1	1	1
19	0	0	0	0
20	1	0	0	0

[a]Decision test

study. The criterion test scores have been converted to 0/1 scores. This cutoff score is never altered, since classifications based on this score represent the true state. The decision test score can be varied until the proportions of true masters and true nonmasters have been maximized. In the example in Table 6.2, three cutoff scores were used to classify examinees.

The three analytical procedures are carried out using the first cutoff score on the decision test, as shown in the contingency table in Table 6.3. The first procedure is the calculation of c, identified earlier as the classification of outcome probabilities. This value is determined by simply adding the proportions in the main diagonal (cells A + D in Table 6.3) as shown in Table 6.4.

The second analysis is the calculation of the phi (ϕ) coefficient, a correlational approach. The phi coefficient can also be calculated using the number of examinees in the cells of the contingency table rather than the proportions. An example of this variation is shown in Table 6.5. The third analysis is a utility analysis. Rather than assigning equal weights to each possible classification, as is done in the calculation of the phi coefficient, the utility analysis allows judgments to be made regarding the

Table 6.3   Contingency Table Using 1st Cutoff Score on Decision Test

		Criterion Test	
		M	NM
		A[c]	B
	M	(9)[a] .45[b]	(4) .20
Decision Test			
	NM	C (3) .15	D (4) .20

[a]Number of examinees.

[b]Proportion of examinees.

[c]Letter used to identify cell.

relative weight assigned to each classification. In this example, one combination of weights was considered. A weight of -1 was given to the false negative classifications and -2 to the false positive ones. A weight of $+2$ was given to the true master classifications and $+1$ to the true nonmastery ones. Thus, classifying examinees either erroneously as masters or correctly as masters was viewed as most important.

Table 6.4   Results of Empirical Analysis of Data Using 1st Cutoff Score

Classification of outcome probabilities:

$$c = .45 + .20 = \boxed{.65}$$

Correlational approach:

$$\phi_{uc} = \frac{.45 - .39}{\sqrt{.60(1-.60)\ .65(1-.65)}}$$

$$= \frac{.06}{\sqrt{(.24)(.2275)}} = \boxed{.2568}$$

Utility analysis:

$$\text{Disutility (D)} = [(.15)(-1)] + [(.20)(-2)] = -.55$$
$$\text{Utility (U)} = [(.45)(2)] + [(.20)(1)] = 1.10$$
$$\text{Maximal utility } (\gamma) = (-.55 + 1.10) \times (20) = 13$$

where $d_1 = -1$, $d_2 = -2$, $u_1 = 2$, and $u_2 = 1$.

Table 6.5 Calculating Phi From the Number of Examinees Rather Than the Proportion in Each Cell

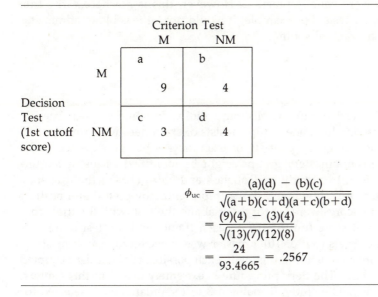

$$\phi_{uc} = \frac{(a)(d) - (b)(c)}{\sqrt{(a+b)(c+d)(a+c)(b+d)}}$$

$$= \frac{(9)(4) - (3)(4)}{\sqrt{(13)(7)(12)(8)}}$$

$$= \frac{24}{93.4665} = .2567$$

Calculations using the second and third cutoff points are not included in this chapter; however, the reader can go through these calculations if desired. The summary information for all three decision-test cutoff points is given in Table 6.6. The third cutoff score is clearly superior. It yields the highest c coefficient, the highest phi coefficient, and the highest maximal utility.

6. Cross-validate the results. The optimal cutoff score selected on the first sample should be tested on other similar samples. A valid cutoff score will be optimal across all samples tested.

Berk (1986) did not discuss the criterion test method in his category scheme, but he identified a similar method labeled *norm-referenced criterion*. He was critical of this

Table 6.6 Summary of Results Across Cutoff Scores

Cutoff Scores	Coefficients				
	c	ϕ_{uc}	D	U	γ
1st	.65	.2568	−.55	1.10	13
2nd	.80	.5833	−.30	1.30	20
3rd	.90	.7916	−.15	1.45	26

method for several reasons, but primarily because a standarized test was used as the criterion. He correctly noted that the criterion test in this case could be used as the mastery test, since both were equally practical. However, this is not necessarily true in all studies using criterion tests. For example, it would not be feasible to administer a maximal stress test in a practical setting.

Criterion Groups

Often no criterion test is available in establishing validity. In some cases a criterion group approach can be used, where one group consists of examinees who are expected to master a task and another group consists of examinees who are expected to be nonmasters. Such mastery-nonmastery groups might be identified as instructed-un-instructed or pretest-posttest. In a study by Douglass and Safrit (1983), the true state of mastery and nonmastery on a bowling task was represented by pretest and posttest group membership. Cutoff scores were set for the trial and the test, with the trial score represented by the first-ball score (out of 10) on each frame, and the test score represented by the number of trials (out of 10) a master was expected to exhibit mastery.

This creates a much more complex situation, with each possible trial standard coupled to each possible test standard. The Berk procedure is extremely useful in this context. In the Douglass and Safrit (1983) study, 3 trial and 3 test standards were selected for each of two groups, one consisting of males and one of females. This resulted in 9 possible combinations for each gender. The Berk procedure was then used to select the best trial-test standard combination for each group.

If the criterion groups are truly different in terms of mastery-nonmastery, this is a useful procedure. However, substantially different groups may be difficult to identify in physical education and exercise science. Note, for example, Figure 6.2. This figure represents the distributions of men's and women's scores. Although they were intended to help set the best standard in the Douglass and Safrit study, there is considerable overlap in the two distributions.

Only when the distributions overlap minimally, as in Figure 6.3, can a valid cutoff score be identified. The pretest group in a physical education setting would have to consist of examinees unfamiliar with the activity to be taught.

Borderline Groups

An alternate strategy is to ask a group of judges (usually teachers) to identify individuals whose skills are borderline, i.e., neither masters nor nonmasters. Administer the mastery test to these examinees, and use the median test score for this group as the cutoff score. Berk (1986) is critical of this method, because judges frequently have difficulty placing individuals in the borderline group, sometimes because they do not have sufficient information to make an appropriate classification. The advantage of this method is that it is simple to use in a school setting, where teachers can assess the ability levels of students with some degree of accuracy.

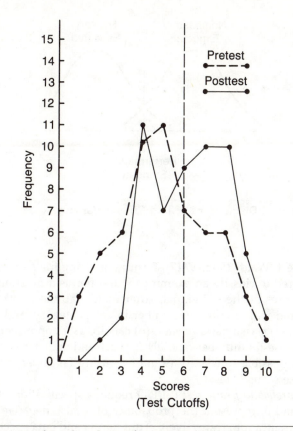

Figure 6.2   Distributions of Bowling Scores for Men and Women

Sequential Testing

Other alternatives to setting a performance standard have been explored in physical education and exercise science. When a mastery test is administered, the appropriate length of the test is determined by taking into account four parameters: (a) probability of false positive classifications, (b) probability of false negative classifications, (c) minimum level of skill for mastery classification, and (d) maximum level of skill for non-mastery classification. When these four parameters are taken into account, a fixed-length test will often require too many trials to be feasible in a practical test setting.

Instead of using a fixed-length test with a performance standard to identify masters and nonmasters, the number of trials can be allowed to vary according to the successes and failures of the examinees, instead of administering the same number of trials to each examinee. Furthermore, the misclassification errors can be held to a minimum. This can be done by using a **sequential testing method**, in particular the sequential

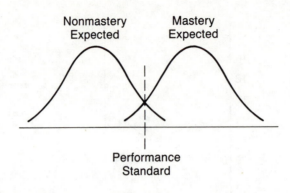

Nonmastery
Expected

Mastery
Expected

Performance
Standard

Figure 6.3   Hypothetical Distributions of Two Criterion Groups

probability ratio test (Wald, 1945, 1947). By administering trials sequentially, the number of trials required to classify an examinee will differ as a function of the pattern of successes and failures of the individual. After each trial, the number of successes or failures is compared with a criterion number in each category, and then one of three decisions is made: (a) classify as a master, (b) classify as a nonmaster, or (c) administer another trial. Because the number of trials for each individual has not been predetermined, it is often possible to classify examinees using far fewer trials than would be needed for the fixed-length test.

The *sequential probability ratio test* (SPRT) requires specification of four parameters. The first two, α and β, represent the probability of a false negative classification and a false positive classification, respectively. Thus, alpha and beta specify tolerance limits for errors of misclassification. They can be equal or unequal and must range between 0 and 1. The minimum probability of success for mastery classification is theta 0, and theta 1 represents the maximum probability of success for nonmastery. These values also must range between 0 and 1, with the restriction that theta 0 > theta 1. Generally, theta 0 is set equal to the cutoff score for a criterion-referenced mastery test. The test user controls the precision of classification by setting each of the four parameters.

A sample scoresheet is depicted in Figure 6.4. Once the parameters have been set, a computer-generated scoresheet can be printed. In the first column, this form includes the number of successful trials needed to be classified as a nonmaster. This number changes as the total number of trials (successes and failures) increases. The third column gives the number of successful trials needed to be classified as a master. In this case, the nonmastery decision is made when the number of successful trials is smaller than the minimum number of successes. The fifth column is used by the scorer to record cumulatively the number of successful trials performed by the examinee. In this example, the examinee was successful on the first trial and a score of 1 is recorded at the top of the fifth column. On the second trial, the examinee was again successful and given 1 point. The score is cumulative; thus, the second trial score, $1 + 1 = 2$, is recorded in column 5. Following an unsuccessful performance on the third trial, a

NM	-	TR#	-	M	#TR	SUC
		1			1	1
		2			2	2
		3			3	2
0	-	4			4	3
		5	-	5	5	4
1	-	6			6	5
2	-	7	-	6	7	6
		8	-	7	8	

Figure 6.4 Sample Scoresheet for Sequential Test

0 was given and the score was recorded as 2, and so on. Refer to Safrit, Wood, Ehlert, Hooper, and Patterson (1985) for an example of the application of this method to a test of motor skill.

Item Response Theory

Item response theory (IRT) has been the focus of considerable research during the last decade. IRT, also known as *latent trait theory*, is viewed as a means of improving the efficiency and accuracy of a test. It is considered superior to many other approaches to measurement. It consists of a family of mathematical models and, because of the computational complexity involved in estimating parameters, requires the use of a computer. One of the most notable advantages of IRT models is that examinees' ability can be estimated on the basis of their performance on a set of tasks, using the same metric as the task-difficulty parameter. IRT is described in detail in chapter 10. It is mentioned briefly here because of its usefulness in setting a cutoff score on a mastery test.

Consider, for example, using as a mastery test a test consisting of repeated trials of a task. Several cutoff scores could be identified to form equivalent sets of dichotomous data. An IRT model could be applied to each data set. The cutoff score representing the distribution with the smallest number of misfit values, the most precise parameter estimates, and the most test information would be the best performance standard for the test under the conditions it was given. Two IRT models were applied to motor-behavior data in a study by Costa, Safrit, and Cohen (1987). Performance standards were varied to identify the best test setting.

Conclusion

When a test user is interested in comparing test scores to a performance standard representing a criterion behavior, the validity of the *standard* must be considered as well as the validity of the *test*. Test validity can be established by forming a table of specifications and examining the content of items within the cells of the table. If the test items adequately represent the domain of behavior being measured, this provides evidence of domain-referenced validity. Quantitative procedures are recommended when validating a performance standard, although a degree of arbitrariness in setting standards cannot be avoided. Item response theory provides a methodology that allows the test developer to set more accurate standards, by identifying the point on an ability scale that maximally discriminates between masters and nonmasters.

The more traditional research on the validity of criterion-referenced tests has waned in recent years, for at least two reasons. First, the majority of test theorists have focused on item response theory as a more accurate and efficient approach to testing. Second, political and legal considerations associated wih mastery testing have led to a redirection of the research effort. Nonetheless, the practical use of mastery tests has *increased*, if anything, in physical education and exercise science. For example, as physical fitness tests are being revised, many of the new versions include criterion-referenced standards in the accompanying test manual (cf., American Health and Fitness Foundation, 1986). Thus, the importance of identifying valid standards based on scientific evidence remains a key element in the development of a mastery test.

References

American Alliance for Health, Physical Education, Recreation and Dance. (1980). *The Health-Related Physical Fitness Test*. Reston, VA: Author.

American Health and Fitness Foundation. (1986). *FYT program manual*. Austin, TX: Author.

American Psychological Association. (1985). *Standards for educational and psychological tests*. Washington, DC: Author.

Berk, R.A. (1976). Determination of optimal cutting scores in criterion-referenced measurement. *Journal of Experimental Education, 45,* 4–9.

Berk, R.A. (1986). A consumer's guide to setting performance standards on criterion preferred tests. *Review of Educational Research, 56,* 137–172.

Costa, M.G., Safrit, M.J., & Cohen, A.J. (1987). *The appropriateness of two item response theory models for measurement of motor behavior*. Manuscript submitted for publication.

Douglass, J.A., & Safrit, M.J. (1983). An empirical approach to the validation of a criterion referenced measure of motor performance. *Journal of Human Movement Studies, 9,* 57–69.

Glaser, R., & Nitko, A.J. (1971). Measurement in learning and instruction. In R.L. Thorndike (Ed.), *Educational measurement* (2nd ed.) (pp. 625–670). Washington, DC: American Council on Education.

Hambleton, R.K. (1984). Validating the test scores. In R.A. Berk (Ed.), *A guide to criterion-referenced test construction* (pp. 199–230). Baltimore: Johns Hopkins University Press.

Messick, S.A. (1975). The standard problem: Meaning and values in measurement and evaluation. *American Psychologist, 30,* 955–966.

Safrit, M.J., Wood, T.M., Ehlert, S.A., Hooper, L.M., & Patterson, P. (1985). The application of sequential probability ratio testing to a test of motor skill. *Research Quarterly for Exercise and Sport, 56,* 58–65.

Sharkey, B.J. (1977). *Fitness and work capacity* (Publication FS-315). Washington, DC: U.S. Department of Agriculture.

Wald, A. (1945). Sequential method of sampling for deciding between two courses of action. *Journal of the American Statistical Association, 40,* 277–306.

Wald, A. (1947). *Sequential analysis.* New York: Wiley.

Washburn, R.A., & Safrit, M.J. (1982). Physical performance tests in job selection: A model for empirical validation. *Research Quarterly for Exercise and Sport, 53,* 267–270.

Supplementary Readings

Berk, R.A. (1980). A framework for methodological advances in criterion-referenced testing. *Applied Psychological Measurement, 4,* 563–573.

Berk, R.A. (1986). A consumer's guide to setting performance standards on criterion-referenced tests. *Review of Educational Research, 56,* 137–172.

Bloom, B.S. (1987). A response to Slavin's mastery learning reconsidered. *Review of Educational Research, 57,* 507–508.

Hambleton, R.K. (1980). Test score validity and standard setting methods. In R.A. Berk (Ed.), *Criterion-referenced measurement: The state of the art* (pp. 80–123). Baltimore: Johns Hopkins University Press.

Safrit, M.J., Baumgartner, T.A., Jackson, A.S., & Stamm, C.L. (1980). Issues in setting motor performance standards. *Quest, 32,* 152–162.

Slavin, R.E. (1987). Mastery learning reconsidered. *Review of Educational Research, 57,* 175–213.

CHAPTER 7

Criterion-Referenced Measurement: Reliability

Marilyn A. Looney
Northern Illinois University

The application of criterion-referenced tests in the psychomotor domain has been the focus of several researchers and practitioners (Brownlie et al., 1985; Douglass & Safrit, 1983; Safrit & Stamm, 1980; Safrit, Stamm, & Douglass, 1981; Shifflett & Schuman, 1982; Washburn & Safrit, 1982). Two popular applications of criterion-referenced tests are measuring psychomotor proficiency and screening job applicants. In the first situation, a criterion-referenced test is used to determine which students have mastered a domain of sport skills. If the purpose of the test is to exempt students from a physical education class, examinees classified as masters are given credit for a course and are not required to take the class. In the second application, criteria established for motor tasks are used to screen a pool of job applicants. Those who meet minimum standards can proceed to the next stage of the evaluation or interview process.

In both applications, criterion-referenced tests are not designed to discriminate among the examinees' abilities. No attempt is made to select test items that will produce maximum variability among the examinees' scores. Norm-referenced reliability estimates indicate the degree of consistency in replicating scores and in placing examinees in the same relative order from one test administration to another. Thus, greater variability among examinees' scores results in higher reliability coefficients. Criterion-referenced reliability is concerned with consistently replicating an examinee's domain (or true) score independent of other examinees' performance. Evaluation is not based on comparing an individual's score to the group's performance. As a result, the statistical techniques used to establish reliability for norm-referenced tests are not appropriate for criterion-referenced tests.

The reliability indices for criterion-referenced tests can be categorized into three areas: **threshold loss agreement** indices, **squared-error loss agreement** indices, and **domain score estimation** statistics. The categorization of these indices is based on the type of decision to be made with the scores (Berk, 1984).

Domain score estimation statistics do not utilize cutoff scores and the assignment of mastery or nonmastery status in their calculation. They estimate the reliability of the examinee's score (proportion correct or completed successfully) in the item domain. These statistics fall into one of two categories: estimates of standard error of a proportion that are computed and interpreted separately for each examinee, and estimates of standard error of measurement that represent the average of individual-specific errors of measurement. When an estimate of standard error is available, confidence intervals can be specified for each examinee's domain score (Berk, 1984; Hambleton, Swaminathan, Algina, & Coulson, 1978). A more detailed description of these statistics is provided by Berk (1984).

When a cutoff score is used to distinguish between masters and nonmasters, error in classification can be viewed from one of two perspectives. In the first perspective, misclassifications to mastery or nonmastery status based on scores far above or below the cutoff score are considered to be more serious than misclassifications based on scores close to the cutoff value. Reliability indices that describe the squared deviations of individual scores from the cutoff score are called *squared-error loss agreement indices*. Livingston (1972) and Brennan and Kane (1977a, 1977b) have developed two of these indices, which are described in two review papers (Berk, 1984; Hambleton et al., 1978).

The second perspective, or way of viewing misclassification error, is that all errors are assumed to be equally serious. It does not matter how far above or below the cutoff a domain score falls. In other words, the error associated with a domain score that lies far above the cutoff but results in a false classification as a nonmaster is the same as the error associated with a domain score that lies slightly above the cutoff but also results in a false classification as a nonmaster. Reliability indices that incorporate this perspective of error are called *threshold loss agreement indices* (Berk, 1984; Hambleton et al., 1978). This chapter focuses on three of these indices (proportion of agreement, coefficient kappa, modified kappa), because they are more appropriate for determining reliability or consistency in assignment to mastery-nonmastery status from one time to another.

Proportion of Agreement (*P*)

The *proportion of agreement index* is defined as the proportion of decisions consistently made across test occasions. When Hambleton and Novick (1973) first proposed this method of reliability, they defined it as being "the proportion of times that the same decision would be made with two parallel instruments" (p. 168). The use of two parallel instruments implies that (a) the expected observed scores for the two sets of measurements are equal and (b) the observed score variances are equal (Lord & Novick, 1968). The way in which parallel measurements are obtained differs for written and psychomotor tests. Within the written context, two different tests that measure the same content are administered; in the psychomotor context, the same test is administered twice to the same group of examinees. Regardless of how parallel measurements are obtained, the proportion of agreement can be used to describe decision-making consistency.

The most common procedure for determining reliability is to administer a test to a group of individuals on one day. Based on the individuals' test scores, each person is assigned to master or nonmaster status. On another day, the group is administered the same test and again assigned to master or nonmaster status. The proportion of the group that was classified as masters on Day 1 and Day 2 plus the proportion that was classified as nonmasters on both days equals the proportion of agreement. This will be illustrated by an example.

Shifflett and Schuman (1982) developed a criterion-referenced archery test where 12 arrows are shot at a standard target from a distance of 20 yd. Target scores of 1 and 3 are assigned an arrow score of 0 and target scores 5, 7, and 9 are assigned an arrow score of 1. The sum of the 12 arrow scores equals the test score (0–12), where 5 is the mastery cutoff value. Hypothetical data depicting the test-retest performance of an instructed group of college students are presented in Table 7.1. Of the 30 individuals tested, 26 were classified as masters on the initial test. Suppose that the same test was administered to the group of students again under identical conditions. The proportion of agreement can be computed to determine the reliability of classification decisions over time. Table 7.2 presents a 2 × 2 contingency table depicting the hypothetical test-retest situation illustrated in Table 7.1. Note that the proportion of agreement (.83) is the sum of the proportions on the main diagonal of the contingency table (Step A, in Table 7.2).

The values of P may range from 0 to $+1$, but the general interpretable range is .50 $\leq P \leq 1.00$ (Huynh, 1979). A P value below .50 is attributed to chance agreement when no information is available concerning the contingency table. When information is available, the lower limit (proportion of chance agreement) can be determined by a procedure that is described later, in the discussion of coefficient kappa. This procedure was used to determine the lower limit for the data depicted in Table 7.1. P values that fall below .69 are attributed to chance agreement (Step B, Table 7.2).

The proportion of agreement describes overall decision consistency that is not adjusted for chance agreement. It is affected by two factors: the accuracy of the test and the mastery and nonmastery composition of the group (Subkoviak, 1984). As the proportion of nonmasters or masters in the group approaches zero, the probability of consistently classifying individuals by chance alone increases. The example in Table 7.2 shows that 86% of the examinees were classified as masters on Day 1; therefore, it is not surprising that the proportion of agreement (.83) is high.

Subkoviak (1984) has demonstrated that proportion of agreement is sensitive to the position of the cutoff score in the score distribution. For a given set of test-retest data

Table 7.1   Hypothetical Archery Test-Retest Scores (N=30)

Subject Number	Initial Score	Retest Score	Subject Number	Initial Score	Retest Score
1	10	9	16	7	6
2	10	10	17	7	6
3	9	10	18	7	4
4	9	9	19	6	8
5	9	9	20	6	7
6	8	9	21	6	6
7	8	8	22	6	4
8	8	8	23	5	7
9	8	7	24	5	5
10	8	7	25	5	4
11	7	8	26	5	4
12	7	7	27	4	6
13	7	7	28	4	4
14	7	6	29	3	4
15	7	6	30	3	3

Note. Individuals are classified as masters if their scores are greater than or equal to five.

that follow a unimodal distribution, the proportion of agreement calculated for various cutoff scores will vary. When the cutoff is near the mean of the score distribution, P is lower than when the cutoff is in the tails of the distribution. As noted earlier, P is influenced by the mastery and nonmastery composition of the group. P is fairly large when there is a large percentage of masters or nonmasters comprising the group. This large percentage occurs when the cutoff score falls in either tail of the score distribution.

Proportion of agreement is also affected by test length. As the number of trials (items) increases, P increases (Berk, 1984; Safrit, Stamm, & Douglass, 1981). P also increases as the dispersion of the test scores increases (Berk, 1984).

Since proportion of agreement is easy to compute and interpret, it has great potential for use with teacher-made tests where sample sizes are small ($N = 30$). For motor tasks, small sample estimates have been found to be unbiased estimates of large sample ($N = 100$) values (Safrit et al., 1981). Using SAT data, Subkoviak (1978) also found unbiased estimates of P, but with relatively large standard errors.

Reliability Indices Corrected for Chance Agreement

Sometimes it may be more desirable to use an index that describes the test's contribution to making consistent mastery classifications independent of the mastery and nonmastery composition of the group tested. As a result, an index should be reported that has

Table 7.2   Decision-Consistency Indices for Hypothetical Archery Data

		Day 2		$P_{i.}$	$P_{.i}$
		Master	Nonmaster		
Day 1	Master	.73 (22)	.13 (4)	.86	.77
	Nonmaster	.04 (1)	.10 (3)	.14	.23
	$P_{.j}$	.77	.23		
	$P_{j.}$	.86	.14		

Note. Cell frequencies are placed in parentheses.

A. $\hat{P} = \sum_{i=1}^{2} P_{ii} = .73 + .10 = .83$

B. $\sum_{i=1}^{2} P_{i.}P_{.i} = (.77)(.86) + (.23)(.14) = .69$

C. $\hat{k} = \dfrac{.83 - .69}{1 - .69} = .45$

D. $\sum_{i=1}^{2} \min(P_{i.}, P_{.i}) = .77 + .14 = .91$

E. $\max k = \dfrac{.91 - .69}{1 - .69} = .71$

F. $\sum_{i=1}^{2}(P_{i.} - P_{.i})^2 = (.86 - .77)^2 + (.14 - .23)^2 = .02$

G. $M = 1 - \dfrac{.02}{2(1 - .69)} = .97$

H. $\hat{k}/(\max k) = \dfrac{.45}{.71} = .63$

I. $\hat{k}_q = \dfrac{.83 - .50}{1 - .50} = .66$

been corrected for chance agreement. Several of these indices have been developed to describe observer agreement (Cohen, 1960; Flanders, 1967; Frick & Semmel, 1978, Garrett, 1972; Light, 1971; Scott, 1955). Only one of these, Cohen's kappa, has been recommended as an index of consistency for mastery and nonmastery decisions (Swaminathan, Hambleton, & Algina, 1974).

Coefficient Kappa (*k*)

Coefficient kappa is an index of agreement that was initially used to assess agreement between observers. Three assumptions must be met: (a) objects to be categorized are independent of each other; (b) observers are independent; and (c) the assignment categories are independent and mutually exclusive. Kappa is defined as:

$$
k = \frac{\sum_{i=1}^{q} P_{ii} - \sum_{i=1}^{q} P_{i.} P_{.i}}{1 - \sum_{i=1}^{q} P_{i.} P_{.i}} . \tag{7.1}
$$

where $\Sigma_{i=1}^{q}$ is the proportion of observed agreement and $\Sigma_{i=1}^{q} P_{i.} P_{.i}$ is the proportion of chance agreement (Cohen, 1960). The terms of Equation 7.1 are cell and marginal proportions of a $q \times q$ contingency table. Although the general case has been presented, the configuration for mastery and nonmastery classifications is a 2×2 contingency table.

The proportion of chance agreement is affected by the composition of the group (Livingston & Wingerksy, 1979). For example, if in 100 students there are 90 masters and 10 nonmasters, the probability of selecting (or classifying) a student as a master is .9 on Trial 1. On Trial 2 the probability of classifying a student as a master is also .9. However, the *joint* probability, i.e., classifying a student as a master on both occasions, is .81 ($.9^2$). The proportion of chance agreement is the sum of the joint probabilities for classifying students as masters and nonmasters ($.9^2 + .1^2$). When the proportion of nonmasters or masters is high, kappa will be attenuated, because the estimate of chance agreement is also high. As a result, Brennan and Prediger (1981) have argued that using kappa is only appropriate when the proportions are considered to be fixed or are determined before classification of examinees. This implies that an examiner knows the sizes of marginal proportions before each trial begins. In this situation the cutoff score is considered to be a relative or adjustable standard for the testing situation. In other words, the cutoff score is determined by the score distribution if only a specified proportion of examinees can be classified as masters or nonmasters (Berk, 1984). Consider the situation where each year a fire department administers a battery of psychomotor tests to prospective firefighters. Because the number of available positions may vary from year to year, the cutoff may be manipulated based on the actual score distributions to allow a predetermined percentage of applicants to be classified as masters or nonmasters (pass/fail). A cutoff score determined in this manner will diminish the validity of mastery and nonmastery classifications (Looney, 1987).

The computation of kappa is illustrated in Table 7.2 (Steps A–C). The proportion of consistent classifications to mastery and nonmastery status from one day to another after the influence of chance agreement has been removed is .45. Kappa is, as expected, smaller than the proportion of agreement (.83).

It is only under certain conditions that kappa's values can range from -1 to $+1$. Little attention is paid to the lower limit of kappa, because any value less than zero implies inconsistent decision-making at an unrealistic extreme. For a negative value to occur, the proportion of observed agreement must be less than the proportion of chance agreement. This would be a rare but possible situation for reliability studies; thus, a general range for interpretation is $.00 \leq k \leq 1.00$. However, the upper limit of kappa (max k) can equal $+1$ only when all of the marginal proportions are symmetrical (Cohen, 1960). The marginal proportions in Table 7.2 are asymmetrical, because the proportion assigned to each category on Day 1 is not the same for Day 2. When the marginal proportions for a given category are not equal, the upper limit is less than 1 but greater than or equal to 0 (Collis, 1985). Also, kappa is less than the product-moment correlation for the dichotomous case (phi coefficient) when the marginal proportions are asymmetric. Otherwise, kappa equals phi for a 2×2 contingency table (Cohen, 1960).

Coefficient kappa's response to score dispersion and test length appears to be similar to the proportion of agreement. As test length and score variability increase, kappa increases (Safrit et al., 1981; Subkoviak, 1984). However, coefficient kappa's sensitivity to placement of the cutoff score in the distribution is the inverse of proportion of agreement. For a unimodal score distribution, kappa will have larger values when the cutoff score is near the mean of the score distribution (Berk, 1984; Subkoviak, 1976, 1984).

For motor task data, small sample ($N = 30$) estimates of kappa have been shown to provide substantial overestimates of large sample values (Safrit et al., 1981) and to be unpredictable when trial criteria and test criteria were manipulated (Safrit & Stamm, 1980).

It is known that the sampling distribution of kappa approximates normality when the sample size is greater than 100 (Cohen, 1960). However, the equations appearing in the literature to approximate large sample variance have been misleading (Cohen, 1960, 1968; Everitt, 1968). They provide an overestimate because they are based on "contradictory assumptions of fixed marginal totals and binomial variation of cell frequencies" (Fleiss, Cohen, & Everitt, 1969, p. 323). Everitt (1968) derived an equation to compute the exact large-sample variance of kappa, but it is very tedious to use.

Fleiss, Cohen, and Everitt (1969) proposed a correct approximation to the variance of kappa based on a multinomial sampling model, where only N is fixed. It is defined as:

$$\hat{\sigma}_\kappa^2 = \frac{1}{N(1 - P_c)^4} \left\{ \sum_{i=1}^{q} P_{ii} \left[(1 - P_c) - (P_{.i} + P_{i.})(1 - P_o) \right]^2 \right.$$

$$\left. + (1 - P_o)^2 \sum_{i \neq j}^{qq} P_{ij} (P_{.i} + P_{j.})^2 - (P_o P_c - 2P_c + P_o)^2 \right\} \quad (7.2)$$

where N is sample size, P_c is $\Sigma_{i=1}^{q} P_{i.} P_{.i}$, and P_o is $\Sigma_{i=1}^{q} P_{ii}$. Fleiss and Cicchetti (1978) confirmed Equation 7.2 for $N \geq 16q^2$, where q is the number of classification categories. However, the design of the Monte Carlo study included only contingency tables where q equaled 3, 4, and 5.

With an estimate of large sample variance for kappa, a confidence interval for the true or population value of kappa can be constructed. It would be beneficial to establish confidence intervals in numerous physical education settings. For example, this procedure can be used in examining the consistency of observers' ratings. Consider an example where 100 students are videotaped while performing an overarm throw. After three instructors independently classify the students as masters and nonmasters on two separate occasions, kappa coefficients and confidence intervals are computed for each instructor. The instructor with the largest kappa value and confidence band that did not overlap confidence bands of the other instructors would be identified as being more consistent in classifying students from one trial to the next. This interpretation, however, should be tempered by the magnitude of the confidence band. If the interval is very large, the estimate of kappa is not precise. To increase the precision of the estimate, a larger sample size would be required to reduce sampling error.

Neither the standard error of kappa nor a confidence interval was determined for the example in Table 7.2 because the sample size ($N = 30$) was too small. When confidence intervals can be constructed, interpretation may be misleading if the upper limit of kappa is not identified. If marginal proportions are not symmetrical, the maximum value of kappa permitted by the marginal proportions is defined as (Cohen, 1960):

$$\max k = \frac{\sum_{i=1}^{q} \min(P_{i.}, P_{.i}) - \sum_{i=1}^{q} P_{i.}P_{.i}}{1 - \sum_{i=1}^{q} P_{i.}P_{.i}} \tag{7.3}$$

where

$$\sum_{i=1}^{q} \min(P_{i.}, P_{.i}) = \begin{cases} P_{i.}, \text{ if } P_{i.} \le P_{.i} \\ P_{.i}, \text{ if } P_{.i} \le P_{i.} \end{cases}$$

In addition to an index of asymmetry, max k, Collis (1985) has proposed M as an index of marginal symmetry. This value approaches 1 as the marginal proportions approach symmetry. It describes the "proportion of potential agreement-above-chance that would remain under perfect marginal symmetry, conditional on the observed marginal dispersion" (Collis, p. 58).

$$M = \frac{1 - \sum_{i=1}^{q} (P_{i.} - P_{.i})^2}{2(1 - \sum_{i=1}^{q} P_{i.}P_{.i})} \tag{7.4}$$

Another index that has received some attention estimates item-by-item agreement adjusted for marginal asymmetry (Collis, 1985) or the "proportion of marginally permitted agreement beyond chance" (Brennan & Prediger, 1981, p. 691). This value is the ratio of kappa to max k. Because it will equal kappa when the marginals are symmetrical, it has an upper limit of 1.

Whenever marginal asymmetry exists, at least one of the three indices [max k, M, or $\hat{k}/(\max k)$] should be reported along with kappa. These values have been calculated for the example and are presented in Table 7.2 (max k in Steps B, D, E; M in Steps B,

F, G; $\hat{k}/(\max k)$ in Steps C, E, H). The maximum value that kappa can attain is .71. This indicates that part of the disagreement or inconsistency is due to marginal discrepancies. The value of M (.97) also supports the claim that marginal discrepancies exist but that the proportions are close to symmetry. M is sensitive to whether the proportions are symmetrical but not sensitive to whether the proportions are close to .50. Max k is more sensitive to the magnitude of the marginal proportions, which is one reason it differs from M. The interpretation of $\hat{k}/(\max k)$ is that 63% of the marginally permitted agreements beyond chance occurred. With this additional information, a kappa value of .45 should not be judged too harshly.

Modified Kappa (k_q)

Brennan and Prediger (1981) have suggested that the definition of chance agreement may be too large when the proportion of masters in the group is not .50. In a typical reliability study the investigator does not predetermine how many individuals may be classified as masters. Thus, defining chance agreement by the natural composition of masters and nonmasters in a group is not appropriate. An example will illustrate this point.

Assume that a group of teachers has attended a training workshop on how to administer a gross motor test to elementary school students. Toward the end of the workshop they are tested on two occasions to see if they can administer and score the test consistently. In this situation there should be a large percentage ($>80\%$) of teachers classified as masters if the training was effective. Because the proportion of masters is large, the proportion of chance agreement will also be large, resulting in a small kappa value. Brennan and Prediger (1981) suggest that the proportion of chance agreement should be determined by the probability of being assigned to one of q categories. In this context the marginals are not *fixed* by group composition but are *free*. For the typical master and nonmaster classification scheme, proportion of chance agreement is 1/2, or .50. When the marginal proportions are considered free to vary, the equation for kappa (7.1) can be modified to equal:

$$k_q = \frac{\sum_{i=1}^{q} P_{ii} - 1/q}{1 - 1/q} \tag{7.5}$$

where q equals the number of classification categories. The interpretation of k_q is the same as kappa. The only difference is that chance agreement has been defined differently. When the proportion of masters equals .50, kappa will equal the modified kappa. Otherwise, modified kappa will be greater than kappa. Its upper limit will always be 1 because marginal proportions ($1/q$) are always symmetrical.

Modified kappa may be artificially large when no examinees are assigned to some categories. As the number of categories increases, modified kappa increases. For example, holding the proportion of observed agreement constant and changing the number of assignment categories from 2 to 4 reduces the definition of chance agreement from .50 to .25, resulting in a larger modified kappa. Using $1/q$ as the proportion of chance agreement is based on the assumption that the examiner will not restrict the range of category assignment for each test administration. If some classification categories are never used, the proportion of chance agreement is usually higher than $1/q$ (Brennan & Prediger, 1981). Thus, categories should be collapsed before determining $1/q$ to adjust for the nonfunctional categories that exist (Brennan & Prediger, 1981; Lawlis & Lu, 1972). Because individuals typically are classified as masters or nonmasters, the proportion of chance agreement is .50. Modified kappa determined for the data in Table 7.2 (Steps A, I) is .66.

Single-Test Administration Estimates of P, k, and k_q

In the previous section, reliability was described from a test-retest perspective, i.e., a group of individuals was tested twice using the same test or parallel forms. Sometimes it is not possible to administer a test twice. When this is the case, the investigator may choose one of several methods that require only one test administration. However, estimates of P and k generated from single administration methods do not reflect all influences of instability that occur across repeated testings.

Two methods have been developed to estimate both P and k (Huynh, 1976; Subkoviak, 1976) and one that estimates only P (Marshall & Haertel, 1976). Since the advantages and disadvantages of these methods are fairly similar and Huynh's method is the most mathematically elegant, it is discussed in detail in this chapter. Subkoviak (1984) provides a review of the other two methods.

Huynh's method simulates scores on the retest given scores on the initial test. As a result, a joint probability distribution is generated that specifies the probability of scoring X on the first test and Y on the retest. This method is based on the assumption that the observed scores follow a beta-binomial distribution. This distribution occurs when the true scores are distributed as a beta distribution and the distribution of test scores after repeated testing for a fixed individual is binomial (Subkoviak, 1984; Peng & Subkoviak, 1980; Huynh, 1976). The binomial distribution is tenable if (a) the test items are scored 0 or 1, (b) the items are statistically independent, and (c) the items have equal difficulty (Subkoviak, 1984).

To use the Huynh method, there must be more than one item on the test. With this information, $\hat{\mu}$, $\hat{\sigma}^2$, Kuder-Richardson 21 coefficient (see chapter 12), and parameters of the beta distribution $(\hat{\alpha}, \hat{\beta})$ can be determined. Subsequent computations to form the joint distribution table are very tedious and require the use of a computer. For the data in Table 7.1 the Huynh estimates of P (P_H) and k (k_H) are .80 and .08, respectively. In an effort to help the practitioner, Huynh (1978) has provided tabled values of P_H and k_H for short tests containing between five and ten items with various cutoff scores. The tables also include asymptotic standard errors of P_H and k_H. These tables are reprinted in Subkoviak (1980).

Small sample standard errors of P_H and k_H can be determined when the beta-binomial assumptions are met by multiplying asymptotic standard error by the constant $(1 + 1/m^{3/4})$ (Huynh, 1981). This adjustment is adequate for sample sizes as small as 25.

Huynh's P_H (Safrit & Stamm, 1980; Subkoviak, 1978) and k_H (Huynh, 1976) increase as the number of items increases. There is some question as to whether small sample estimates of P_H overestimate or underestimate large sample estimates. One study (Safrit & Stamm, 1980) found small sample estimates ($N = 30$) of psychomotor data to overestimate large sample estimates ($N = 100$). On the other hand, Subkoviak (1978) found small sample estimates of P_H for SAT data to underestimate large sample estimates ($N = 300$) when 10 test items were examined.

Additionally, Huynh's P_H underestimates the test-retest coefficient for psychomotor (Safrit & Stamm, 1980) and cognitive data (Huynh & Saunders, 1980). Huynh's kappa is also an underestimate of the test-retest index; however, kappa is more biased than P_H. This bias is more pronounced when the proportion of chance agreement approaches 1. Smaller sampling variability associated with Huynh's estimates of P and kappa may occur, because the data are expected to conform to the beta-binomial model. Alternatively, the test-retest estimates are not contingent on assumptions made about the score distributions. These estimates also incorporate sources of systematic or random error that are encountered in repeated testings. Thus, test-retest estimates will have larger sampling errors than estimates based on the beta-binomial model (Huynh & Saunders, 1980).

Huynh (1976) proposed an *arcsin normal approximation method* that assumes the joint distribution of test-retest scores is approximately normal. This assumption may be reasonable if (a) the number of test items is greater than eight and (b) the mean test score divided by the number of test items ($\hat{\mu}/n$) is between .15 and .85 (Huynh, 1976). This method requires normalization of the data by an arcsin transformation, the computation of a normal deviate (z) corresponding to the cutoff score, and the use of a bivariate normal distribution table. Peng and Subkoviak (1980) have shown that the arcsin transformation is not required to provide good estimates of P and kappa. Their simple normal approximation method incorporates all of the steps used by Huynh's approximation method except the arcsin transformation. For 125 simulated cases, the simple normal approximation yielded smaller errors than the arcsin normal estimates, but both approximation methods tended to underestimate estimates generated by the exact method. Additionally, the estimates were better when the score distribution was unimodal than when it was U-shaped. For more information on the Peng-Subkoviak method, refer to Subkoviak (1980) or Peng and Subkoviak (1980). This method was used to estimate P and kappa for the hypothetical data, but only the estimates are provided in Table 7.3. The approximation of proportion of agreement (.81) was very close to the test-retest estimate (.83); however, the approximation for kappa (.13) was considerably less than .45. If defining chance agreement as $1/q$ can be justified, then a modified kappa can be determined by substituting P_H into Equation 7.5. This estimate (.62) is smaller but very close to the test-retest estimate (.66).

Guidelines for Selecting Index of Reliability

In selecting an index of reliability the practitioner must first determine how the test scores will be used or interpreted. If the distance of the domain score from the cutoff

Table 7.3 Summary of Reliability Estimates for Hypothetical Data

Method	$\hat{P}$	$\hat{k}$	$\hat{k}_q$
Test-Retest	.83	.45	.66
Huynh (1976)	.80	.08	.60
Peng-Subkoviak (1980)	.81	.13	.62

Note. Summary statistics required to compute Huynh's estimates or Peng and Subkoviak's estimates are: $\hat{\mu} = 6.7$, $\hat{\alpha}^2 = 3.528$, $\hat{\sigma}_{21} = .176$, $\hat{\sigma} = 31.37$, $\hat{\beta} = 24.81$.

score is of no interest when classifying individuals as masters or nonmasters, threshold loss agreement indices would be appropriate descriptors of reliability. Otherwise, one of the indices described briefly at the beginning of this chapter should be selected.

If threshold loss agreement indices are appropriate, the next decision is whether to calculate an index based on test-retest or single-test administration methods. If the reliability estimate is expected to reflect variations in performance that occur from one day to the next, the test-retest method should be used. When administering a retest is not practical, a single-test administration method may be used; but it should not be interpreted as a test-retest coefficient, even though data are simulated for the retest.

Before determining reliability, the location of a valid cutoff score in the score distribution should be identified. If it lies in the tails of the distribution, the proportion of agreement will have higher relative values and kappa will have lower relative values than when the cutoff score is in the middle of the score distribution. Additionally, if the examinees to be tested are likely to have a large percentage of masters or nonmasters, a large P and small kappa is expected.

Perhaps the most important decision is to determine if the marginal proportions of a contingency table are considered *fixed* or *free to vary*. If the proportion of individuals to be classified as masters is determined before classification begins, then kappa is the only appropriate index (Berk, 1984; Brennan & Prediger, 1981). Confidence limits and an index of symmetry or asymmetry should be reported along with kappa to enhance the interpretation.

When the proportion of masters is not restricted, then proportion agreement (Berk, 1984) and modified kappa are appropriate indices to use (Brennan & Prediger, 1981). It is probably best to report both indices, because they reflect different types of consistency. Proportion of agreement describes overall consistency, which is influenced by group composition and test consistency. Alternatively, modified kappa is adjusted for chance agreement independent of group composition of masters and nonmasters. It indicates only test consistency. If the proportion of masters is .50, then modified kappa and kappa are equal.

These recommendations have implications for the use of single-test administration methods. The Huynh method (1976) has been recommended as the best of the three procedures (Subkoviak, 1980). Although it requires tedious computations, a simple normal approximation (Peng & Subkoviak, 1980) exists that is simpler to compute. The use of Huynh's procedure to estimate kappa is appropriate only when marginals are considered fixed; estimates of proportion of agreement and modified kappa should be used when marginal proportions are free to vary.

Conclusion

Since Hambleton and Novick (1973) first proposed using proportion of agreement as a threshold loss agreement index, other indices and methodologies have been presented. These indices (k, k_q) make adjustments for chance agreement while the alternate methodologies require only a single test administration.

Previous studies in which the characteristics of P and kappa have been investigated primarily used cognitive data. More studies should be undertaken using a variety of psychomotor data to investigate the influence of item difficulty. There is some evidence to indicate that heterogeneity of item difficulty does not affect estimates of P and kappa that are based on the beta-binomial model (Huynh & Saunders, 1980). This needs to be explored further for psychomotor data with small samples, particularly, because two studies have reported conflicting results concerning the bias of small sample estimates (Safrit, Stamm, & Douglas, 1981; Subkoviak, 1978).

The ability to estimate a reliability index from a single test administration is appealing. From a psychomotor perspective, however, the use of Huynh's (1976) and Peng-Subkoviak's (1980) approximation methods may not be appropriate, because at least 8 test items are required. Some psychomotor tests are based on fewer than 8 items (trials); thus, the small-sample bias for psychomotor tests with 3 to 10 items should be explored.

The modified kappa coefficient proposed by Brennan and Prediger (1981) is an attractive alternative to kappa. The argument for using modified kappa appears to be sound; however, its characteristics and properties relative to the merits of P and kappa have not been described. More specifically, the small and large sampling distributions of modified kappa should be determined for both cognitive and psychomotor data. In addition, modified kappa's sensitivity to the cutoff score location in the score distribution is not known.

Although several issues still need to be addressed concerning threshold loss agreement indices, sufficient information exists to guide the practitioner's selection and use of the most appropriate index.

References

Berk, R.A. (1984). Selecting the index of reliability. In R.A. Berk (Ed.), *A guide to criterion-referenced test construction* (pp. 231–266). Baltimore: Johns Hopkins University Press.

Brennan, R.L., & Kane, M.T. (1977a). An index of dependability for mastery tests. *Journal of Educational Measurement, 14,* 277–289.

Brennan, R.L., & Kane, M.T. (1977b). Signal/noise ratios for domain-referenced tests. *Psychometrika, 42,* 609–625; Errata (1978), *43,* 289.

Brennan, R.L., & Prediger, D.J. (1981). Coefficient kappa: Some uses, misuses, and alternatives. *Educational and Psychological Measurement, 41,* 687–699.

Brownlie, L., Brown, S., Diewert, G., Good, P., Holman, G., Laue, G., & Bannister, E. (1985). Cost effective selection of fire fighter recruits. *Medicine and Science in Sports and Exercise, 17,* 661–666.

Cohen, J. (1960). Coefficient of agreement for nominal scales. *Educational and Psychological Measurement, 20,* 37–46.

Cohen, J. (1968). Weighted kappa: Nominal scale agreement with provision for scaled disagreement or partial credit. *Psychological Bulletin, 70,* 213–220.

Collis, G.M. (1985). Kappa, measures of marginal symmetry and intraclass correlations. *Educational and Psychological Measurement, 45,* 55–62.

Douglass, J.A., & Safrit, M.J. (1983). An empirical approach to the validation of a criterion referenced measure of motor performance. *Journal of Human Movement Studies, 9,* 57–69.

Everitt, B.S. (1968). Moments of the statistics kappa and weighted kappa. *The British Journal of Mathematical and Statistical Psychology, 21,* 97–103.

Flanders, N.A. (1967). Estimating reliability. In E.J. Amidon & J.B. Hough (Eds.), *Interaction analysis: Theory, research, and application* (pp. 161–166). Reading, MA: Addison-Wesley.

Fleiss, J.L., & Cicchetti, D.V. (1978). Inference about weighted kappa in the non-null case. *Applied Psychological Measurement, 2,* 113–117.

Fleiss, J.L., Cohen, J., & Everitt, B.S. (1969). Large sample standard errors of kappa and weighted kappa. *Psychological Bulletin, 72,* 323–327.

Frick, T., & Semmel, M.I. (1978). Observer agreement and reliabilities of classroom observational measures. *Review of Educational Research, 48,* 157–184.

Garrett, C.S. (1972). *Modification of the Scott coefficient as an observer agreement estimate for marginal form observation scale data* (Occasional Paper #6). Bloomington: Indiana University, Center for Innovation in Teaching the Handicapped.

Hambleton, R.K., & Novick, M.R. (1973). Toward an integration of theory and method for criterion-referenced tests. *Journal of Educational Measurement, 10,* 159–170.

Hambleton, R., Swaminathan, H., Algina, J., & Coulson, D. (1978). Criterion-referenced testing and measurement: A review of technical issues and developments. *Review of Educational Research, 48,* 1–47.

Huynh, H. (1976). On the reliability of decisions in domain-referenced testing. *Journal of Educational Measurement, 13,* 253–264.

Huynh, H. (1978). Computation and inference for two reliability indices in mastery testing based on the beta-binomial model (Research Memorandum 78-1). *Publication Series in Mastery Testing,* Columbia, SC: University of South Carolina, College of Education.

Huynh, H. (1979). Statistical inference for two reliability indices in mastery testing based on the beta-binominal model. *Journal of Educational Statistics, 4,* 231–246.

Huynh, H. (1981). Adequacy of asymptotic normal theory in estimating reliability for mastery tests based on the beta-binominal model. *Journal of Educational Statistics, 6,* 257–266.

Huynh, H., & Saunders, J.C. (1980). Accuracy of two procedures for estimating reliability of mastery tests. *Journal of Educational Measurement, 17,* 351–358.

Lawlis, G.F., & Lu, E. (1972). Judgment of counseling process: Reliability, agreement, and error. *Psychological Bulletin, 78,* 17–20.

Light, R.J. (1971). Measures of response agreement for qualitative data: Some generalizations and alternatives. *Psychological Bulletin, 76,* 365–377.

Livingston, S.A. (1972). Criterion-referenced applications of classical test theory. *Journal of Educational Measurement, 9,* 13–26.

Livingston, S.A., & Wingersky, M.S. (1979). Assessing the reliability of tests used to make pass/fail decisions. *Journal of Educational Measurement, 16,* 247–260.

Looney, M.A. (1987). Threshold loss agreement indices for criterion-referenced measures: A review of applications and interpretations. *Research Quarterly for Exercise and Sport, 58,* 360–368.

Lord, F.M., & Novick, M.R. (1968). *Statistical theories of mental test scores.* Menlo Park, CA: Addison-Wesley.

Marshall, J.L., & Hartel, E.H., (1976). *The mean split-half coefficient of agreement: A single administration index of reliability of mastery tests.* Unpublished manuscript, University of Wisconsin, Madison.

Peng, C-Y.J., & Subkoviak, M.J. (1980). A note on Huynh's normal approximation procedure for estimating criterion-referenced reliability. *Journal of Educational Measurement, 17,* 359–368.

Safrit, M.J., & Stamm, C.L. (1980). Reliability estimates for criterion-referenced measures in the psychomotor domain. *Research Quarterly for Exercise and Sport, 51,* 359–368.

Safrit, M.J., Stamm, C.L., & Douglass, J.A. (1981). The consistency of mastery classifications for a criterion referenced test of motor behavior: The effect of varying sample size. *Journal of Human Movement Studies, 7,* 131–143.

Scott, W.A. (1955). Reliability of content analysis: The case of nominal scale coding. *Public Opinion Quarterly, 19,* 321–325.

Shifflett, B., & Schuman, B.J. (1982). A criterion-referenced test for archery. *Research Quarterly for Exercise and Sport, 53,* 330–335.

Subkoviak, M.J. (1976). Estimating reliability from a single administration of criterion-referenced test. *Journal of Educational Measurement, 13,* 265–276.

Subkoviak, M.J. (1978). Empirical investigation of procedures for estimating reliability for mastery tests. *Journal of Educational Measurement, 15,* 111–116.

Subkoviak, M.J. (1980). Decision-consistency approaches. In R. A. Berk (Ed.), *Criterion-referenced measurement: The state of the art* (pp. 129–185). Baltimore: Johns Hopkins University Press.

Subkoviak, M.J. (1984). Estimating the reliability of mastery-nonmastery classifications. In R.A. Berk (Ed.), *A guide to criterion-referenced test construction* (pp. 267–291). Baltimore: John Hopkins University Press.

Swaminathan, H., Hambleton, R., & Algina, J. (1974). Reliability of criterion-referenced tests: A decision-theoretic formulation. *Journal of Educational Measurement, 11,* 263–267.

Washburn, R.A., & Safrit, M.J. (1982). Physical performance tests in job selection: A model for empirical validation. *Research Quarterly for Exercise and Sport, 53,* 267–270.

Supplementary Readings

Bintig, A. (1980). The efficiency of various estimations of reliability of rating scales. *Educational and Psychological Measurement, 40,* 619–643.

Froman, T.W., & Llabre, M. (1985). The equivalence of kappa and del. *Perceptual Motor Skills, 60,* 3–9.

Huynh, H., & Saunders, J.C. (1980). *Solutions for some technical problems in domain-referenced mastery testing.* Columbia, SC: University of South Carolina, College of Education.

Kraemer, H.C. (1980). Extension of the kappa coefficient. *Biometrics, 36,* 207–216.

Subkoviak, M.J. (1988). A practitioner's guide to computation and interpretation of reliability indices for mastery tests. *Journal of Educational Measurement, 25,* 47–55.

Advanced Measurement and Statistics

Like many areas of study, the study and practice of measurement reflects the evolution of technology and methodology in other fields. For example, in the past two decades advances in computer technology have contributed to a burgeoning application of multivariate statistical methodology and scaling models to measurement problems. A number of these applications are described in this section.

The first two chapters present multivariate statistical methodology commonly employed in the measurement of psychomotor behavior. In chapter 8, Jim Disch provides a conceptual overview of factor analysis, multiple discriminant analysis, and canonical correlation, focusing on the use of these methodologies in the exploration of construct validity. Regression analysis is highlighted in chapter 9. Andrew Jackson renders a lucid description of regression analysis, focusing on the use of regression in gathering evidence for criterion-related validity.

Exploration of new methods and models for enhancing understanding of measurement problems is the focus of chapters 10 and 11. A persistent problem in measurement concerns the analysis of change. In chapter 10, Robert Schutz addresses the salient issues faced in measuring change. Although recommended statistical procedures for analyzing change in the research process are outlined, Schutz concludes that, despite a vast body of literature and several new computational techniques, measurement of change remains an enigma in the field of measurement. In contrast, Judith Spray examines new approaches to solving measurement problems in the psychomotor domain, emphasizing the application of item response theory. Spray's insightful chapter may well point to a new era of measurement research in the psychomotor domain.

CHAPTER 8

Selected Multivariate Statistical Techniques

James Disch
Rice University

To understand the complex nature of human performance, the behavioral researcher must be able to develop and examine sound theories. Kerlinger (1973) stated that the basic aim of science is theory. He offered the following definition:

> A theory is a set of interrelated constructs (concepts), definitions, and propositions that presents a systematic view of phenomena by specifying relations among variables, with the purpose of explaining and predicting the phenomenon. (p. 11)

Examination of this definition suggests that theories are multivariate in nature. They are derived from a set of measurable constructs that are interrelated in an organized fashion and that can be tested empirically. Popper (1965) stated that the genuine test of a theory is its resistance to refutation. Good scientific theory forbids more than it accepts. This is consistent with the basic tenet of *null hypothesis testing* and further indicates the complex nature of behavioral theory. Popper felt that testability was the element that differentiated scientific theory from other "metaphysical" types. He concurred with Kerlinger that problems of pure knowledge are problems of explanation. To be satisfactory, explanations must be causal in nature. They are formed by sets of statements that describe both the state of affairs to be explained and the explanatory statements themselves. Satisfactory explanations mean improving testability. This in turn means proceeding to theories of richer context. To enrich these theories, more effort must be taken in the development of theoretical schema and more sophisticated modes of analysis must be employed to test these propositions. Both of these factors require not only multivariate thinking but also multivariate research tools.

Multivariate Analysis and Construct Validity

The way **construct validity** evolved is an example of how multivariate analysis can be used to examine theoretically challenging questions. According to Cronbach (1957), before 1955 the only theory dealing with test validation was related to content and criterion areas. There was no recognized way of determining whether a proposed test was sound unless a concrete criterion could be measured or content validity could be established. The application of factor analytic methodology to theory-based psychological models provided a heuristically powerful means of attacking this problem.

Fleishman (1963, 1964) pioneered factor analytic methodology in the area of motor ability testing that was later extended by Harris and Liba (1965), Jackson (1971), and others. These researchers applied appropriate multivariate models to research questions that had been previously examined in a piecemeal fashion. Their work provided foundational theories that were testable. They moved us beyond Student's t-test to Hotelling's T^2. MANOVAs replaced serial ANOVAs. Questions once answered by the application of the tests of Scheffé and Tukey are now examined by partial, sequential, and step down Fs. Researchers are now able to examine complex patterns or paths. They can look at the optimal combination of variables to construct both predictor and criterion sets of variables. Many somewhat different but partially correlated aspects of an organism's behavior can be integrated into a mathematically complex but logically pleasing structure. This is the nature of multivariate analysis.

The Multivariate Nature of Behavioral Research

Amick and Walberg (1975) posed the question, "Why is behavioral research inherently multivariate?" (p. 1). They answer this question by stating that individual differences among people affect behavior. Behavior is further modified by external conditions, both physical and psychological. Differences also result from an interaction between backgrounds and variations of conditions. Stated another way, different people react differently to different stimuli and the same people react differently to the same stimuli on various occasions. This means that a number of factors (conditions, relations) must be considered when examining human behavior.

Harris (1975) stated that the term *multivariate statistics* refers to assorted descriptive and inferential techniques that allow for the analysis of data sets involving multiple variables. *Multiple regression analysis* is a specific technique that allows for the examination of the association between one unmodified variable (criterion) and one modified variable (a linear composite of a set of predictors). This is an example of a multivariate tool that is used for questions of criterion-related validity. Harris further stated that

> . . . the research question should dictate the appropriate statistical analysis, rather than letting the ready availability of a statistical technique generate a search for research paradigms which fit the assumptions of the technique. (p. 3)

Bock (1975) reemphasized this point by stating that the multivariate character of behavioral data has an especially strong bearing on tests of significance. We can no longer compute significance levels separately for each of a multiple number of response variables. We must examine the structural relations among dependent variables. And these explanations must be driven by theory, not data. One drawback of correlational research is the indefinite causal nature of the relationships explored. It can be shown that one set of data can be analyzed to yield several different plausible explanations. In order for the results to be valid, they must be founded in a theory-driven model that is **robust** to falsification.

Amick and Walberg (1975) further stated that multivariate analysis is simply a means of conducting research—a tool. Computers provide us with the medium to analyze large data sets into hierarchical models, but they offer no insight into the "whys" and "hows" of the theoretical paradigm. As Cronbach (1957) warned, the temptation to study the techniques themselves should be resisted. We must logically derive practical research questions and apply the appropriate multivariate technique in an effort to untangle the complex interrelationships that exist in behavioral data.

The Scope of This Chapter

Multivariate analysis is a very general term that encompasses a number of statistical techniques. Technically speaking a two-way ANOVA is a multivariate technique, because it involves one dependent variable and two independent variables. However, ANOVAs are seldom linked with traditional multivariate techniques. Multiple regression (R) (discussed in chapter 9) is a widely used statistical tool that fits the multivariate mode; but because of its versatility and its popularity, R is usually considered separately from the other correlational tools that fall into the multivariate camp. The techniques discussed in this chapter are three of the most widely used and versatile of the traditional multivariate techniques. They are also the ones of greatest benefit to the measurement specialist because of their application to problems of construct and criterion-related validity.

Before a technique can be selected, the researcher must pose several questions:

- What is the specific research question to be answered?
- What are the variables necessary to answer this question?

• What is the appropriate measurement model to answer the question?

As previously discussed, the research question should be based in a well-conceived theory that has been developed through observation, an exhaustive literature search, and the synthesis of previous studies. This will allow the researcher to determine the number and type of variables necessary to thoroughly explore the research question. The number and type (measurement scale) of independent and dependent variables will in turn determine the appropriate statistical model.

If the research question dictates one continuously scaled dependent variable with a number ($n \geq 2$) of independent variables (either categorical or continuous), then the appropriate model is R. But if the dependent variable is categorical, the researcher must use a **multiple discriminant analysis** (MDA). This technique is covered in this chapter. MDA is utilized primarily to examine problems of construct validity. If a number of dependent variables are related to a number of independent variables, then **canonical correlation analysis** (CCA) is the appropriate model. Although CCA can be thought of as a logical extension of R, it can be applied to both criterion and construct validity problems. The nature of CCA allows the researcher to examine the structure of two multifaceted domains: a predictor set and a criterion set.

A third technique to be explored in this chapter is **factor analysis** (FA). This technique allows the researcher to examine the theoretical constructs of a number of variables with no delineation of dependent or independent measures. Many behavioral domains have no concrete criteria, and the mathematical elegance of FA allows the measurement specialist to cluster variables that are logically related to one another into common factors (i.e., **dimensions**, which identify the unobserved but statistically developed constructs of a theoretical domain).

The Purpose of This Chapter

Statistical methodology is simply the researcher's tool for accomplishing a goal—to examine the research question or theory. It is the purpose of this chapter to provide a conceptual look at the three multivariate techniques previously mentioned. No attempt is made to examine the complex mathematics of the methodology, although some statistical equations are presented to enhance the conceptual presentation. Because the practical difference that distinguishes multivariate models from others is in the need for matrix manipulations, some matrix notation is also presented. A more complete, yet readable presentation of matrix information is presented by Pedhazur (1982). An example of the application of techniques is presented, with the emphasis on interpreting the various salient summary statistics. Finally, the chapter discusses the use and interpretation of the models.

Factor Analysis

Factor analysis (FA) is a multivariate correlation technique that does not require the distinction between independent and dependent variables. FA can be conducted in either an exploratory fashion or a confirmatory mode. It will be presented first because of the elegant way it partitions the variance of the variables. Knowledge of this technique will hopefully lead to more thorough understanding of the techniques that follow.

The purpose of factor analysis is to identify common patterns of variation among a set of theoretically related variables (k). These common sources of variation are called factors (p), and the object is to obtain a parsimonious number of factors ($p < k$) that can be related logically to the variables. The variables represent selected measures sampled from some general area termed a **domain**. The factors are said to represent various dimensions within the domain.

Most construct validity studies have involved exploratory FA methodologies. **Confirmatory factor analysis** (CFA) approaches recently have been used because of the development of computer programs such as **LISREL** (Jöreskog & Sörbom, 1986). The approaches could be compared with the choices of the experimentalist using ANOVA. *Exploratory* FA is similar to the post hoc analysis of group differences, whereas *confirmatory* FA is analogous to the planned comparisons approach. Regardless of the approach chosen, the problems of the factor analyst are many.

Conducting a Factor Analytic Study

The next section provides a step-by-step procedure to be used for an exploratory problem. Specific information on confirmatory problems follows.

Step 1: Identify theoretical dimensions and marker variables. The first problem is to identify the theoretical dimensions within the domain examined. This should be accomplished through a thorough search of the literature, both experimental and nonexperimental. Consultation with experts can aid the factor analyst in establishing the theoretical model.

Once the theoretical model has been established, variables are selected to measure the theoretical constructs or factors within the model. These variables are called **marker variables**, and they are extremely important in the exploration of the configuration of the factors, termed the **factor structure**. Approximately the same number of variables should be selected to mark each factor, so that if the proposed factor structure is established each factor will be represented by the same number of markers.

It should be pointed out that the development of the model and the selection of the marker variables limit the results of the study. In other words, factors that are not hypothesized will not be identified. Also, if variables that are theorized to mark a given dimension do not, then the dimension will not be identified. For this reason it is often said that "you only get out of a factor analysis what you put into it." Before discussing more of the methodology associated with factor analysis, a brief explanation of the theoretical manner in which factor analytic techniques partition variance is necessary. The factor analyst is able to partition the variance for each variable into the following components:

Variance Component	*Definition*
Total Variance (S_t^2)	$h^2 + b^2 + e^2 = h^2 + u^2 = 1$

Reliable Variance (S_r^2) $h^2 + b^2 = 1 - e^2$
Common Variance (S_c^2) $h^2 = 1 - u^2$
Unique Variance (S_u^2) $u^2 = b^2 + e^2 = 1 - h^2$
Specific Variance (S_s^2) $b^2 = u^2 - e^2$
Error Variance (S_e^2) $e^2 = 1 - (h^2 + b^2)$

The S_t^2 is a sum of common (h^2) and unique (u^2) portions, and always equals one. The S_r^2 is determined by the sum of the common (h^2) and specific portions (b^2). It is not directly measurable by factor models and must be estimated by external methods. The S_c^2 is measured by h^2, which is equal to the sum of the squared factor loadings for a variable in an orthogonal solution (an orthogonal solution creates factors that are uncorrelated). It is this common portion of variance that the researcher wishes to maximize; it is called the communality estimate. The S_u^2 represents both random error (e^2) and lack of fit, as measured by S_s^2. This is analogous to $1-R^2$ in multiple regression analysis.

Step 2: Collect data and analyze correlation matrix. After the theoretical model is established and the marker variables are selected, the data are collected and analyzed. Correlations among all variables are computed, and the correlation matrix becomes the basis for determining the structure of the factors.

Step 3: Determining the initial factor structure. The intercorrelation matrix is factor analyzed using one or more factoring methods. The problem for the factor analyst becomes one of determining which variables are associated with which factors and to what extent. Statistically this is accomplished by decomposing the correlation matrix among the variables into its latent roots, called *eigenvalues*. This is mathematically complex, and a number of decisions have to be made to determine the exact manner in which this is done. Practically speaking, the $k \times k$ correlation matrix is transformed into a $k \times p$ factor matrix. The p factors identify the common sources of variation and are named in relation to the variables associated with them. The association or relationship between a variable and a factor is called a **factor loading**. Factor loadings can be interpreted as the correlation between a variable and a factor. Through this relationship, the variables that are most highly related to a factor are said to *mark* this factor. By examining the nature of the variables that mark a factor, a name is given to that factor. For example if 50-m, 100-m, and 200-m dashes were found to load on the same factor, this dimension could be named *speed* or *sprinting speed*.

The factors within a factor structure can also be labeled according to the number and configuration of the factor loadings. If more than two variables load on a factor, the factor is called a *common* or *group factor*. If a large number of variables load on a factor it is called a *general factor*. If only two variables load, then the factor is called a *doublet*, and if only one variable is substantially associated with a factor it is called a *specific factor*. From an intuitive standpoint, common factors form the focus of interpretation. Ideally a common factor will be extracted to identify each of the theoretical dimensions in the domain. Sometimes hypothesized factors are represented by doublets, because one or more of the theoretical marker variables do not function as theorized. Specific factors arise from a number of causes. Sometimes a variable that is hypothesized to mark a given factor does not relate to that factor. Also, a variable that has a *primary loading* (its highest loading) on one factor could have a *secondary loading* on another, creating a specific factor. Due to the specific analytical technique selected, factors could be identified that have no substantial loadings. These are called *null factors*. Null factors and specific factors contribute little to the explanation of the structure and usually are deleted from the interpretation.

The next point to consider is the term *substantial loading*. Since factor loadings can be interpreted as correlation coefficients, they are dependent on sample size. Therefore, the standard error of the correlation coefficient (SE_r) can be used as the basis for determining a substantial loading. Usually the magnitude is set at two or three times the SE_r to correspond with the .05 or .01 levels of significance. Another approach is to set a practical level a priori. This means that the researcher is looking for loadings that are of practical value. These values conventionally are set at .30 or .40. It is also appropriate to simply interpret the highest loading for each variable.

Step 4: Determining simple structure and the pattern of factors. This leads to the next methodological point, termed *simple structure*. It is the goal of the factor analyst to establish a factor matrix that adheres to the criterion of simple structure. Simple structure describes a factor matrix in which all or nearly all the variables have substantial loadings on one factor only. Simple structure makes interpretation much easier, but it creates a number of other problems that factor analysts must face. Unlike the experimentalists, who choose ANOVAs to analyze data, or the researchers who use multiple regression where there is only one technique to choose from, the factor analyst must make several analytical decisions. For example, there are a number of methods that can be used to decompose the intercorrelation matrix into a factor matrix. They are differentiated by the manner in which they treat the variability of the variables and the way in which the factor space is manipulated. Principal components and image analysis are techniques that are not technically factor analysis models but accomplish the same purpose. *Alpha* and *canonical factor* analysis are two factor analytic methods that manipulate the variables in different ways. The specific differences among the techniques are primarily mathematical in nature. From a conceptual standpoint, some yield a conservative estimate of factors and others yield a more liberal number. When doing an exploratory factor analysis, it usually is accepted that at least one conservative (e.g., Alpha) and one liberal (e.g., canonical) method be chosen.

Step 5: The question of rotation. Another question related to interpretation is whether the factors should be forced into an uncorrelated structure (orthogonal) or allowed to assume their natural geometric space (oblique). This is accomplished by subjecting the factor patterns of the variables to statistical rotation. Rotations are based on a number of mathematical qualities. The most popular orthogonal rotation is called the *varimax* criterion (Kaiser, 1958). It maximizes the common variance among the factors and is quite useful in determining simple structure. Oblique rotations tend to complicate the interpretation, because factors are allowed to be correlated with one another. However, this allows for a more realistic look at the theoretical structure, because the researcher can examine the relationships among factors.

Step 6: Interpreting the results of the factor analysis. Once the rotated factor structures have been determined, the researcher can relate these results to the hypothesized factor model. To do this the researcher should take the following steps.

a. Examine the rotated factor structure of the selected models. Note the variables that are substantially related to the factors that are identified.

b. Look for common factors across models and rotations. They may not be extracted in the same order in each model. They will be identified by the similarity of the loadings. There are statistical methods of determining the congruence of the factors, but they are beyond the scope of this text. For a thorough discussion of congruency tests, see Rummel (1970).

c. Name the factors in relation to the hypothetical dimensions of the theoretical model. In other words, if the markers of a dimension load on a given factor, that factor is identified and should be named accordingly.

d. Attend to unhypothesized findings, such as specific factors, unhypothesized factors, or hypothesized factors that were not identified. The researcher should examine the reliability of the data, the correlations between oblique factors, and the total amount of variance of the variables accounted for by the factors. Other logical explanations should also be considered.

It should be pointed out that some factor programs print out unrotated factor matrices and that oblique solutions yield both factor structure and factor pattern matrices. It is the loadings of the rotated factor structures that should be interpreted in all orthogonal solutions and in most oblique solutions. For proper interpretation of the oblique solutions, consult the manual for the specific statistical package.

Before presenting an example, a few concluding comments are necessary. FA is as much an art as a science. It is an extremely powerful tool, but it basically is a self-describing technique. In order to be useful for determining construct validity, extreme care must be taken in developing a complete theoretical model; variable selection, factor models, rotation, sample size, and sample composition must all be considered.

There are a number of excellent exploratory factor analytic studies in the domain of human performance. The original work by Fleishman (1954) was later reanalyzed by Harris and Liba (1965) to provide the foundation for the exploration of domains within the general framework of human performance. Jackson and Frankiewicz (1975) and Ismail and Young (1977) present excellent examples of the factor analytic work in our field.

Factor Analysis Example

An excellent study conducted by Hopkins (1977) was selected as the example for this section. Hopkins examined the factor structure of the domain of basketball skills tests. Through a review of the literature he hypothesized the following five dimensions: shooting, passing, jumping, movement without the ball, and movement with the ball. Tests were selected to mark these five dimensions and were administered to 70 male junior and senior high school students. The data were analyzed using four models and two rotations. The full rotated orthogonal solution for the Alpha factoring procedure is presented in Table 8.1. All substantial and nonsubstantial loadings are included to show how each variable relates to each factor. The negative signs associated with various factor loadings represent an inverse relationship between a factor and a variable

Table 8.1   Alpha Factor Analysis, Rotated Orthogonal Solution: Hopkins' Data

| | Factor Loadings | | | |
| | Rotated Factors | | | |
Experimental Tests	1	2	3	4
Front Shot	.024	−.317	.218	.576
Side Shot	.017	−.379	.373	.563
Under Shot	.095	.047	.235	.516
Foul Shot	.044	−.137	.040	.635
Zig Zag Run	−.214	.808	−.006	−.093
Shuttle Run	−.598	.596	−.284	−.105
40-ft Dash	−.670	.395	−.177	.052
Side Step	.356	−.683	.159	.112
Dodge Run	−.474	.715	−.219	−.164
Vertical Jump	.791	−.209	.051	.045
Jump-Reach	.926	−.125	.147	.140
Free Jump	.885	−.184	.076	.251
Standing Broad Jump	.767	−.321	.114	−.026
Wall Pass	.109	−.101	.770	.150
Overarm Pass	.041	−.200	.444	.255
Push Pass	.167	−.501	.341	.157
Speed Pass	−.249	.300	−.609	−.310
Obstacle Dribble	−.357	.532	−.515	−.277
Zig Zag Dribble	−.223	.754	−.242	−.299
Dribble	−.295	.599	−.355	−.329
Dribble Blitz	−.286	.539	−.318	−.468

or an artifact of the rotation procedure. For interpretive purposes, the signs for any row or column of the solution may be inflected without changing the meaning of the relationships. To summarize the results, all of the common factors and their associated substantial loadings are presented in Table 8.2. The variables are clustered according to the factors on which they loaded.

Four common factors were identified in a majority of the eight solutions. Relating the factors to his theoretical model, Hopkins was able to identify robust factors for shooting, passing, and jumping. The variables selected to measure the remaining two movement factors loaded on one general factor. Therefore, the factor structure did not differentiate between movement with or without the ball. Reliability estimates for the variables were not provided; however, lower bound estimates could be derived from the orthogonal solution. By summing the squared factor loading for each variable in a given solution across factors, h^2 (the communality estimate) was computed. The h^2 value can be interpreted as a lower bound reliability estimate. Also, the h^2 in a given solution can be summed and divided by the number of variables to provide a proportion of the total variance in the variable space accounted for by the factor structure. Hopkins

Table 8.2   Common Factors and Factor Loadings Obtained by the Eight Solutions: Hopkins' Basketball Data

| | Factor Loadings | | | | | | | |
| | Orthogonal Solutions | | | | Oblique Solutions | | | |
Factors/Tests	PC[a]	Alpha	C[b]	Image	PC[a]	Alpha	C[b]	Image
Factor I								
Vertical Jump	.787	.791	.794	.816	.815	.821	.784	.873
Jump-Reach	.923	.926	.888	.891	.982	.985	.849	.948
Free Jump	.894	.885	.866	.866	.948	.935	.843	.914
Standing Broad Jump	.772	.767	.774	.782	.755	.753	.506	.776
Factor II								
Zig Zag Run	.828	.808	.781	.822	.917	.882		.877
Shuttle Run	.618	.596	.573	.616	.515	.476		.478
40-ft Dash	.411	.395	.387	.415				
Side Step	.657	.683	.599	.638	.637	.664		.587
Dodge Run	.731	.715	.680	.720	.685	.654		.635
Obstacle Dribble	.540	.532	.548	.522	.409	.387		.360
Zig Zag Dribble	.749	.754	.758	.721	.737	.739		.678
Dribble	.624	.599	.662	.611	.552	.511		.514
Dribble Blitz	.529	.539	.539	.498	.424	.434		.367
Factor III								
Wall Pass	.750	.770			.838	.864		.727
Overarm Pass	.437	.444			.438	.446	.620	.629
Push Pass								.397
Speed Pass	.641	.609		.406	.637	.599		.530
Factor IV								
Front Shot	.611	.576			.576	.537		.717
Side Shot	.569	.563		.408	.481	.473		.431
Under Shot	.491	.516			.472	.504		.420
Foul Shot	.616	.635			.654	.672		.472

[a]PC = Principal Components.

[b]C = Canonical.

concluded that the hypothesized factor structure was substantiated. The fact that two of the hypothesized factors grouped together meant that the domain was essentially a four-dimensional model. By examining the magnitude of the factor loadings, he concluded that a complete, concise test battery to measure basketball skills could consist of the jump and reach, dribble, speed pass, and front shot. This is an example of how an exploratory factor analysis can be conducted to examine the dimensionality of a domain of human performance.

Confirmatory methods allow for a more heuristically powerful test of the hypothesized factor structure. Rather than letting the number of factors and the relationships between factors and variables be determined by the matrix manipulations of the methods and rotations selected, the confirmatory approach suggests a specific number of factors with a definite loading pattern. Factors can be hypothesized to be oblique or orthogonal. The data are analyzed in relation to this specific model and essentially a *goodness of fit* test is conducted to determine if the theoretical model can be refuted. One of the two main purposes of the program LISREL (Jöreskog & Sörbom, 1986) is to examine measurement models of this nature. LISREL methodology provides the researcher with powerful tools, not only for examining the construct validity of a specific factor structure, but also for estimating the multivariate reliability of a battery of tests. To provide an example of the LISREL methodology, the Hopkins basketball data were analyzed using a confirmatory approach.

To examine the basketball skills data from a confirmatory approach, four dimensions were hypothesized: shooting, jumping, passing, and dribbling. The variables associated with factor 2 of the exploratory solution, i.e., the variables that did not involve basketball, were deleted from this analysis. The marker variables that had been selected by Hopkins were chosen to identify the four theoretical factors. It was hypothesized that these factors would be oblique, that is, they were correlated and the data were then analyzed using a confirmatory approach. The results of the confirmatory analysis are presented in Table 8.3. Note by examining the factor loadings in Table 8.3 that all of the marker variables did load substantially on the hypothesized factors. The lowest factor loading was found to be .533 between the overarm pass and the passing dimension. This provides some degree of confirmation of the factor structure. The theta delta values represent the amount of *residual* variance, i.e., variance not identified by the factor structure. From a factor analytical standpoint this could be thought of as $1-h^2$. Because there are no trivial loadings on the other factors, this value normally would be higher than the residual variance in an exploratory factor analysis. The Phi matrix provides the correlations between the hypothesized dimensions. It can be seen that several factors correlate quite highly. It is possible that in a given factor analysis study, if the data were analyzed from an exploratory standpoint, factors this highly correlated would collapse into a single dimension and therefore provide a different solution than hypothesized. This is a brief example of a confirmatory factor analysis. For a more thorough explanation of the use of LISREL methodology see Jöreskog and Sörbom (1986).

Canonical Correlation

Canonical correlation (CCA) can be thought of as an extension of multiple regression with more than one dependent variable. It combines the features of regression analysis and factor analysis to create a more flexible technique for examining the relationships between two variable sets. Whereas factor analysis makes no distinction between predictor and criterion variables and multiple regression limits the researcher to a single criterion measure, CCA allows for multiple variables in the criterion set as well as the predictor set. This is easily expressed in terms of the supermatrix shown in Figure 8.1,

Table 8.3 Confirmatory Factory Analysis: Hopkins' Basketball Skills Data

Tests	Factor Loadings				
	Shooting	Jumping	Passing	Dribbling	Theta Delta
Front Shot	0.693	0.000	0.000	0.000	.520
Side Shot	0.807	0.000	0.000	0.000	.348
Under Shot	0.460	0.000	0.000	0.000	.789
Foul Shot	0.534	0.000	0.000	0.000	.715
Vertical Jump	0.000	0.829	0.000	0.000	.313
Jump-Reach	0.000	0.958	0.000	0.000	.082
Free Jump	0.000	0.938	0.000	0.000	.120
Standing Broad Jump	0.000	0.797	0.000	0.000	.365
Wall Pass	0.000	0.000	0.657	0.000	.568
Overarm Pass	0.000	0.000	0.533	0.000	.715
Push Pass	0.000	0.000	0.585	0.000	.657
Speed Pass	0.000	0.000	−0.809	0.000	.345
Obstacle Dribble	0.000	0.000	0.000	0.865	.252
Zig Zag Dribble	0.000	0.000	0.000	0.850	.278
Dribble	0.000	0.000	0.000	0.888	.211
Dribble Blitz	0.000	0.000	0.000	0.857	.265

Factors	Correlations (Phi)			
	Shooting	Jumping	Passing	Dribbling
Shooting	1.000			
Jumping	0.308	1.000		
Passing	0.775	0.462	1.000	
Dribbling	−0.758	−0.555	−0.837	1.000

where R_{11} represents the correlation matrix of q criterion variables, R_{22} represents the correlation of the p predictors, and R_{12} (and R_{21}) is the intercorrelation matrix between predictor and criterion spaces. In the multiple regression case, the R_{22} matrix is a single criterion measure and the R_{12} matrix is a vector of validity coefficients. By using canonical analysis the researcher can more completely define the criterion space.

Similar to R, CCA can be said to define two variables; however, both are modified. These unobserved modified variables maximize the relationship between the weighted sets of the unmodified variables. In other words, canonical correlation is the maximum relationship between a linear function of two vector variables. The number of canonical correlations that can be obtained from a set of data is determined by the number of variables in p or q, whichever is less. Each canonical correlation is uncorrelated with the others that have been obtained. Since there is more than one criterion measure, there will be weighting coefficients (cs and ds, respectively) for both the predictor

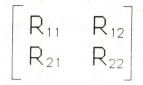

Figure 8.1   Super Matrix for Canonical Correlation Analysis

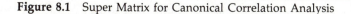

variables (xs for set p) and criterion variables (ys for set q). These are called *canonical weights* or coefficients and can be represented as follows:

$$X = c_1x_1 + c_2x_2 + \ldots + c_nx_n \tag{8.1}$$

$$Y = d_1y_1 + d_2y_2 + \ldots + d_my_m \tag{8.2}$$

$$R_c = r_{XY} \tag{8.3}$$

(Note: this notation assumes that the variables X and Y are in standard score form.)

Each canonical correlation maximizes the relationship between each pair of canonical variates. In CCA the correlation matrix is manipulated to display the structure of the relationship across domains of measurement. This reduces the dimensionality of the test space (essentially the R_{12} matrix) and allows for a more parsimonious representation of the data. Essentially, R_c represents the extent one predictor vector variable maps entities with respect to a criterion vector variable. CCA has several advantages over R. First, the burden of artificially forming a composite criterion is eliminated. Second, the variables do not have to conform to the predictor-criterion relationship; any two sets of variables may be studied. Finally, the distinct advantage of CCA is that successive correlations can be examined that are uncorrelated with the first set. This is superior to arbitrarily weighting criterion variables of R or computing separate R values for each criterion measure.

Conducting a Canonical Correlation Analysis

As with R, the researcher is concerned with the magnitude of the relationship between the criterion variable set and the predictor variable set. This is determined by the decomposition of the R_{12} submatrix.

Step 1: Determining canonical correlations and canonical weights. There will be as many R_c values calculated as there are variables in the smallest variable set. However, only significant R_c values should be reported. These are reported by conventional CCA programs (SPSS and SAS). The square of the R_c represents the shared variance between the vector variables. This value can be quite high, but only represents a small portion of the variance of the original variables. The magnitude of the standardized canonical weights represents the contribution of each variable to its canonical variate. Examination of the R_c values and the standardized weights form the initial phase of the analysis.

Step 2: Analysis of the canonical structure. Once the significant variates have been established and the standardized weights derived, then the *canonical structure* should be examined. This is analogous to interpreting the factor structure in factor analysis research. In order to do this a set of coefficients (similar to factor loadings) must be derived. The mathematical technique for calculating these coefficients is presented and discussed by Cooley and Lohnes (1979) and Marascuilo and Levin (1983). From a conceptual standpoint these coefficients represent the correlations between a variable in one space and the variate representing that space (**canonical loading**) or the correlation between a variable in one space and the variate from the other space (**canonical index**). The examination and interpretation of these coefficients allow the researcher to describe the significant variates.

Step 3: Redundancy analysis. The next step is to examine the amount of variance of the original variables extracted by the significant canonical factors. Stewart and Love (1968) provide a statistic called the **redundancy coefficient** (R_d) for this purpose. There is a mathematical weakness of R_d that causes it to overestimate the actual variance. This limitation is discussed by Jackson (1982). For the purposes of this chapter, R_d is discussed as an appropriate upper bound estimate of the variance of the original variables accounted for by the canonical structure. The R_d is not a symmetrical statistic. That is, the redundant variance of set x given y is not equal to that of y given x: ($R_{dx.y} \neq R_{dy.x}$).

It is worthwhile to note that the application of canonical correlation analysis to complex research questions is still in a somewhat experimental stage. As with any multivariate technique, the results of CCA must be mathematically sound and interpretable to the user.

Canonical Correlation Example

An example of canonical correlation in the area of human movement is the relationship between volleyball skills tests and basic ability tests.[1] A set of four skills tests (criteria) and five motor performance tests (predictors) were administered to a group of female high school volleyball players. The correlation matrix is presented in Table 8.4. The R_{11} matrix is a 4×4 matrix of the criterion variables; the R_{22} matrix is a 5×5 matrix of the motor performance measures. The R_{12} matrix is a 4×5 matrix that represents the overlap between the test spaces. An r of .29 was needed to be significant at $p < .05$. Inspection of the matrices reveals that three of the six intercorrelations among the criterion variables were significant, all ten of the correlations among the predictor

[1]Unpublished data provided by the author.

Table 8.4   Correlation Matrix: Volleyball Skills Tests and Motor Performance Variables

Variables	S	P	A	V	VJ	TH	AR	20	BBT
					Correlations				
Skills Space									
Serve (S)	1.00	−.03	.23	.53	.26	.22	−.36	−.21	.55
Pass (P)	−.03	1.00	.19	.31	.60	.30	−.27	−.29	.28
Spike (A)	.23	.19	1.00	.51	.34	.44	−.44	−.48	.26
Volley (V)	.53	.31	.51	1.00	.59	.47	−.66	−.48	.49
Performance Space									
Vertical Jump (VJ)	.26	.60	.34	.59	1.00	.77	−.70	−.74	.46
Triple Hop (TH)	.22	.30	.44	.47	.77	1.00	−.79	−.85	.47
Agility Run (AR)	−.36	−.27	−.44	−.66	−.70	−.79	1.00	.80	−.49
20-yd Dash (20)	−.21	−.29	−.48	−.48	−.74	−.85	.80	1.00	−.38
Basketball Throw (BBT)	.55	.28	.26	.49	.46	.47	−.49	−.38	1.00

variables were significant, and 14 of the 20 correlations in the R_{12} matrix were significant.

The canonical correlations were then calculated. These values, along with the standardized canonical weights, are presented in Table 8.5. Three significant R_c values were found ($p < .05$). The magnitudes of the R_c values indicated that the first pair of canonical variates were highly correlated ($R_c = .809$), and the second and third sets of variates were correlated to moderate degrees (.508 and .423, respectively). Inspection of the magnitude of the standardized weights indicated that the first canonical factor was best represented by the volley and pass in the skills space and the vertical jump in the performance space. The fact that the loadings were negative is simply an artifact of the mathematical manipulation of the variable space. Since they represent vector variables, the signs can be inflected across all variables and thus do not affect the interpretation of the variate. Therefore, high vertical jump performances would be associated with high volley and pass scores.

The weights that best represent the second variate space are pass and spike with vertical jump and agility run; variate space three is best represented by the serve and spike with basketball throw. To describe the variates more thoroughly, the canonical structure was examined (see Table 8.6).

Variate I resembles a general skills-performance factor with substantial loadings ($>|.55|$) on all variables except the spike. The highest loadings were .86 for the volley and .88 for the vertical jump. Note that the negative signs are now in the direction that would be expected (all positive, except for the two timed tests). Inspection of the canonical indices indicated that the structure was consistent across variate spaces, because the volley was most highly related to the performance variate and the vertical jump was most closely related to the skills variate.

Table 8.5 Standardized Canonical Weights and Canonical Correlations

	Standardized Weights		
Variables	Variate 1	Variate 2	Variate 3
Skills Space			
Serve	−0.275	0.240	0.973
Pass	−0.536	−0.787	0.035
Spike	0.112	0.512	−0.583
Volley	−0.601	0.267	−0.407
Performance Space			
Vertical Jump	−0.930	−1.348	−0.099
Triple Hop	0.493	0.058	−0.486
Agility Run	0.476	−0.833	0.039
20-Yd Dash	−0.223	−0.555	0.434
Basketball Throw	−0.346	0.330	0.913
	Canonical Correlation Results		
R_c	.809	.508	.423
Alpha level	.0001	.017	.049

Interpretation of Variate II is not as simple, because Variate I was a general variate. Remember that canonical variates are derived under the constraint that they are orthogonal. Therefore, the relationships of the variable on the second variate can be thought of as residualized values. Although all the skills variables had loadings above .40, the pass had the highest loading of .61. This can be linked with a high loading of .54 for the agility run in the performance space. This is logical, because the passing test involved a shuffling movement from one spot on the court to another. The pattern of the indices was the same as the loadings; however, the drop in magnitude indicated that the strength of this association was not as great.

Examination of the loadings on Variate III indicated no logical pattern of variation. The serve and spike best represented the skills spaces, but in different directions. The triple hop and 20-yd dash had the highest loadings in the performance space. The low values of the indices (.26 was the highest index) suggest that only a trivial amount of overlap occurred on this variate.

The final step is the redundancy analysis. These values, along with the total battery redundancies, are also presented in Table 8.6. As can be seen, the magnitudes of these redundancies are substantially lower than the respective R_c values. This indicates that, although there is a high degree of relationship between the first set of canonical variates ($R_c = .809$), only 31.7% of the total variance of the skills variables is accounted for by the performance measures. Only 27% of the performance measures variance is associated with that of the skills tests. Even though the second and third R_c values are

Table 8.6 Structure Coefficients and Redundancy Values

| | Structure Coefficients | | | | | |
| | Canonical Loadings | | | Canonical Indices | | |
Variables	V_1[a]	V_2	V_3	V_1	V_2	V_3
Skills Space						
Serve	.55	−.52	−.62	.45	.26	.26
Pass	.69	.61	.23	−.56	−.31	−.10
Spike	.36	−.55	.56	−.29	.29	−.24
Volley	.86	−.41	.18	−.69	.21	−.07
Performance Space						
Vertical Jump	.88	.16	.40	−.71	.08	−.16
Triple Hop	.57	−.30	.54	.47	.15	−.22
Agility Run	−.73	.54	−.39	−.59	−.28	.17
20-yd Dash	−.56	.40	−.60	−.45	−.20	.26
Basketball Throw	.69	−.36	−.46	.57	.18	.19
	Redundancy Analysis					
Rd_{xy}[b]	.317	.036	.042	$Rd_x \cdot y = .395$ Total Battery		
Rd_{yx}	.270	.072	.033	$Rd_y \cdot x = .375$ Redundancy		

[a] Variates.

[b] x represents skills tests, y represents motor performance tests.

significant, the redundancies for these factors are small—especially in view of these redundancy values being upper bound estimates of common variance. The total redundancy of the skills battery given the motor performance tests is .395. This means that the three significant canonical variates account for less than 40% of the variance of the four skills tests.

It is for this reason that CCA should be used cautiously and should be linked closely to a strong theoretical model. Although heuristically powerful, canonical correlation requires a thorough understanding before it can be readily applied to research problems in our field. Recently Wood and Safrit (1984, 1987) outlined and tested a model based on canonical correlation analysis for estimating the multivariate reliability of a motor performance test battery and subsequently applied the method estimating the test-retest reliability of the AAHPERD *Health-Related Physical Fitness Test* (AAHPERD, 1980). Cureton, Boileau, and Lohman (1975) and Disch (1977) have also applied CCA to research questions in the area of human performance. Many more studies must be attempted before the actual utility of this multivariate technique for human performance researchers can be fully evaluated.

Discriminant Analysis

Discriminant analysis is a procedure for estimating group membership. This is accomplished by estimating the position of an individual on a line that best separates the groups. The estimate used is a linear function of a subject's measures on the variables included in the analysis. The maximum number of discriminant functions associated with a study is $(g - 1)$ or m, whichever is less (g = number of groups, m = variables). Multiple discriminant analysis (MDA) is advantageous, because it reduces the dimensionality of the predictor space without a substantial loss of information. Also, multiple discriminant scores may satisfy the assumption of a multivariate normal distribution better than the original tests (because of the *Central Limit Theorem*).

Relationship to Multiple Correlation

Conceptually, MDA may be contrasted with R. Essentially, regression analysis answers the question "Who will perform best in a group?", whereas discriminant analysis determines "Which group is an individual most like?". That is, in prediction (regression) the researcher is interested in the order of a group of individuals according to their ability to perform some set criterion. In classification (discriminant analysis) the question is not *how well* an individual will perform, but in *which group* an individual would best perform. Group membership becomes the criterion, and because it is a categorical measure the purpose of discriminant analysis differs from regression techniques.

Geometrically speaking, MDA represents individuals as points in a multidimensional space. The swarm of points associated with the groups defines the classes. In order for the MDA to function, the means of the g groups on the swarm of points must be significantly different. An individual's original scores can be transformed into a discriminant score by matrix multiplication of the vector of original scores by a vector of discriminant weights. These weights represent the contributions of each variable to the classification procedure. In practice, they are analogous to the weighting coefficients in regression analysis.

A salient point about MDA is that it takes into account the variability of the group means on the m variables, variation of individuals about group means, and the interrelationships among the variables. Statistically MDA can be shown to be a special case of regression analysis. Whereas canonical correlation was a modification of multiple regression with more than one dependent variable, MDA is a multiple regression on a categorical dependent variable. In fact, when the dependent variable is dichotomous, MDA can be run on standard regression computer programs, and the statistics of interest can be derived from the regression printout.[2] Whether two or more groups are contrasted, MDA programs should be used to provide the researchers with the information they need. These programs are written to provide all the information needed for MDA.

---

[2]It should be pointed out that this is not suggested because the weighting coefficients probably will differ if regression programs rather than discriminant programs are used, because of different computing algorithms. Although the amount of variance accounted for will be the same, the values in the MDA program are more appropriate.

Interpreting a Discriminant Analysis

As noted previously, MDA distinguishes among groups. These groups are usually *natural groups* that have some preformed characterisic or construct. If MDA can identify significant variability among the groups, then it can be said that the group can be differentiated on the construct.

Step 1: Examination of descriptive group statistics and the discriminant function. The first statistics to examine are the group means and standard deviations. Essentially, a significant discriminant function indicates that the groups are different on the vector of means.

To test this, a discriminant function is calculated in a manner similar to the way a regression equation is derived. A weighted linear composite variable is formed, using the weights that maximize the differences among groups. They are used along with the original variables to create discriminant scores that are similar to predicted scores in multiple regression. The standardized discriminant weights are similar to regression beta weights, and they are examined to determine which variables contribute most to creating the discriminant function.

There are a number of tests for significance of the discriminant function, but if a two-group problem is analyzed with a regression program, only the F-test for significance of the R is needed. The R^2 reflects the amount of variability in group membership accounted for by the independent variables. For this generalized discriminant solution, the F-test is a multivariate extension of the traditional F-test. The overall F-test is examined by comparing a matrix of mean square between values to the appropriate matrix of mean square within values. The rank of this matrix is determined by the number of independent variables. MDA programs provide various other significance tests that can all be examined for statistical significance in a similar manner.

Step 2: Examination of the structure of the discriminant function. Next, structure coefficients similar to those calculated in CCA should be computed to help clarify the composition of the discriminant function. These are interpreted as correlations between the variables and the discriminant function, and they are calculated by multiplying a row vector of standardized discriminant weights by the correlation matrix of the original predictor variables. This produces a column vector of structure coefficients.[3]

Step 3: Subject classification. The last step is to classify the subjects according to their discriminant scores. Several approaches for classification are described by Marascuilo and Levin (1983). Regardless of the approach used, these predicted group scores are compared with actual group membership.

In the ideal case, all the subjects who actually belonged in a given group would be predicted (or classified) into that group. In a realistic case, misclassifications occur, and often these cases are the ones that are most interesting to interpret.

---

[3]Discriminant programs often calculate these by using the pooled within-groups correlation matrix. Although they will differ in magnitude, they will reflect the same pattern of variation.

Table 8.7   Raw Track Data

Subj. #	Event	Weights (pounds)	Vertical Jump (inches)	Five Bounds (inches)	30-yd Dash (seconds)
01	1	180	23	435	4.8
02	1	138	14	365	5.5
03	1	140	18	373	5.0
04	1	250	13	280	5.7
05	1	150	14	358	5.0
06	1	135	12	352	5.7
07	1	152	23	460	4.4
08	1	176	19	368	4.8
09	0	150	18	407	4.8
10	0	163	22	486	4.2
11	0	135	25	515	4.5
12	0	133	22	511	4.3
13	0	125	21	403	4.5
14	0	143	19	429	4.2
15	0	123	23	425	4.0
16	0	123	21	514	4.0

Multiple Discriminant Analysis Example

In this example, an actual data set is provided and an MDA on the data is performed. The raw data are presented in Table 8.7. It should be noted that in order to create classification tables, the raw data (not the correlation matrix) must be used. The data for this example were taken from a data set on female high school track performers.[4] Sixteen cases were selected for this analysis: 8 throwers and 8 sprinter-jumpers. The data were analyzed using the SPSS program DISCRIMINANT (Nie, Hull, Jenkins, Steinbrenner, & Bent, 1982), with the throwers coded as *1*s and the sprinter-jumpers coded as *0*s on the variable *event*. The correlations between variables, along with the group means, are presented in Table 8.8.

   Also presented in Table 8.8 are the univariate F values and significance levels reported in the program. (No attempt was made to control the pairwise error rate.) The data were then analyzed using a multiple discriminant function. A significant discriminant function ($p < .05$) was derived based on a Wilke's Lambda of .405 (chi square = 10.86). The resulting canonical correlation between predictor variables and group membership (actually just a multiple R) was .772. The standardized discriminant function coefficients, along with the discriminant structure coefficients, are presented in Table

[4]Thanks is given to Dr. Phil Henson, Mike Lacourse, and Paul Turner of Indiana University for providing these data.

Table 8.8   Correlations and Group Means With Associated Univariate *F*-values and Significance Levels

		Correlations						Between
Variables	Weight	Vertical Jump	Five Bounds	30-yd Dash	Event	Group 1 Mean	Group 0 Mean	Group *F* (*p* level)
Weight (pounds)	1.00					165	137	3.8(.07)
Vertical Jump (inches)	−.32	1.00				17.0	21.4	6.3(.02)
Five Bounds (inches)	−.53	.87	1.00			374	461	11.2(.005)
30-yd Dash (seconds)	.48	−.83	−.81	1.00		5.11	4.3	17.1(.001)
Event	.46	−.55	−.67	.74	1.00	—	—	—

8.9. By inspection of these values it can be seen that the function is best described by the 30-yd dash. All the performance variables are positively associated with group membership (when method of scoring is taken into account), whereas weight is negatively associated with group membership.

The classification table is presented in Table 8.10. Based on the results of this study, 14 of the 16 subjects could be classified properly using this discriminant function. The performance characteristics of the two misclassified subjects (numbers 7 and 9, Table 8.7) should be examined to see if they would fit better into the other group or possibly become multi-event performers.

It should be noted that when the subjects are being classified into more than two groups, the interpretation is a little more difficult. More than one significant discriminant

Table 8.9   Standardized Discriminant Weights and Structure Coefficients

Variables	Standardized Discriminant Weights	Structure Coefficients
Weight	.077	−.431
Vertical Jump	.581	.533
Five Bounds	−.488	.736
30-yd Dash	1.021	−.911

Note.—Structure Coefficients are based on the pooled within groups correlation matrix.

Table 8.10   Classification Table: Track Data

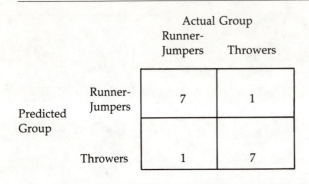

| | | Actual Group | |
		Runner-Jumpers	Throwers
Predicted Group	Runner-Jumpers	7	1
	Throwers	1	7

function could be derived. For illustrative purposes, consider the location of centroids for a hypothetical three-group discriminant analysis presented in Figure 8.2. For a three-group case with more than two variables, two distinct discriminant functions could be calculated. Each function is orthogonal to the other. Classifications are then based on placing individuals in an n dimensional space, where n equals the number of significant discriminant functions. For this example, assume a group of distance runners (DR) were added to the throwers (TH) and sprinter-jumpers (S-J). Assume that function one is defined as a body-structure function and that function two is best represented by speed

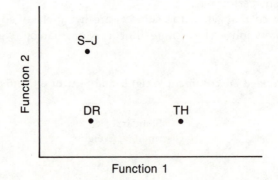

Figure 8.2   Three-Group Discriminant Example

variables. As can be seen by inspection of the figure, the groups are separated differently by the distinct functions. Function one separates the throwers from the other two groups, whereas function two pulls out the sprinter-jumpers. When both functions are considered simultaneously, all three groups are found to occupy distinct geometric locations. This is a real virtue of discriminant analysis. It should be noted that if more than two groups are involved, a regression program will not work. Discriminant analysis programs must be used for analyses of this type.

Conclusion

The three models discussed in this chapter are probably the most widely used multivariate techniques for the analysis of human performance data. They can provide information to untangle complex relationships among variable sets. The three techniques are intertwined in a number of ways. It was shown that MDA and CCA can be considered special cases of R (more correctly, R and MDA are special cases of CCA). Factor analysis does not distinguish among predictors and criterion variables, although it partitions the data much like CCA. The keys to using multivariate techniques properly are to develop the theoretical model thoroughly and then select the proper technique. Multivariate analyses can be very useful tools for the human performance researcher when used appropriately. They are very important in the structuring and examination of theory.

References

American Alliance for Health, Physical Education, Recreation and Dance. (1980). *Health-related physical fitness manual*. Washington, DC: Author.

Amick, D.J., & Walberg, H.J. (1975). *Introductory multivariate analysis*. Berkeley: McCutchan.

Bock, R.D. (1975). *Multivariate statistical methods in behavioral research*. New York: McGraw-Hill.

Cooley, W.W., & Lohnes, P.R. (1979). *Multivariate data analysis*. New York: Wiley.

Cronbach, L.J. (1957). The two disciplines of scientific psychology. *The American Psychologist, 12*, 671–684.

Cureton, K.J., Boileau, R.A., & Lohman, T.G. (1975). Relationship between body composition measures and AAHPER test performances in young boys. *Research Quarterly, 46*, 218–229.

Disch, J.G. (1977, February). *A canonical analysis of the relationships between anthropometric measures and motor performance tests in female volleyball players*. Paper presented at the Southern District Convention of AAHPER, Atlanta.

Disch, J.G. (1979). A factor analysis of selected tests for speed of body movement. *Journal of Human Movement Studies, 5,* 141–151.

Fleishman, E.A. (1954). Dimensional analysis of psychomotor ability. *Journal of Experimental Psychology, 48,* 437–454.

Fleishman, E.A. (1963). *The dimensions of physical fitness: A factor analysis of speed, flexibility, balance, and coordination tests.* New Haven: Yale University.

Fleishman, E.A. (1964). *The structure and measurement of physical fitness.* Englewood Cliffs, NJ: Prentice-Hall.

Harris, C.W., & Liba, M.R. (1965). Components, image and factor analysis of tests of intellect and of motor performance (Cooperative Research Project Number 5-192-64). Madison: University of Wisconsin.

Harris, R.J. (1975). *A primer of multivariate statistics.* New York: Academic Press.

Hopkins, D.R. (1977). Factor analysis of selected basketball skills tests. *Research Quarterly, 48,* 535–540.

Ismail, A.H., & Young, R.J. (1977). Effect of chronic exercises on the multivariate relationships between selected biochemical and personality variables. *Multivariate Behavioral Research, 12,* 49–67.

Jackson, A.S. (1971). Factor analysis of selected muscular strength and motor performance tests. *Research Quarterly, 42,* 164–172.

Jackson, A.S., & Frankiewicz, R.G. (1975). Factorial expressions of muscular stength. *Research Quarterly, 46,* 206–217.

Jackson, A.W. (1982). Canonical correlation: Additional aspects. In J.G. Disch & J.R. Morrow, Jr. (Eds.), *Practical computer applications of multivariate statistics for researchers in HPERD* (pp. 68–75). Houston: University of Houston.

Jöreskog, K.G., & Sörbom, D. (1986). *LISREL: Analysis of linear structural relationships by the method of maximum likelihood: Users guide, Version VI.* Mooresville, IN: Scientific Software, Inc.

Kaiser, H.F. (1958). The varimax criterion for analytic rotation in factor analysis. *Psychometrika, 23,* 187–200.

Kerlinger, F.N. (1973). *Foundations of behavioral research* (2nd ed.). New York: Holt, Rinehart and Winston.

Marascuilo, L.A., & Levin, J.R. (1983). *Multivariate statistics in the social sciences: A researcher's guide.* Monterey, CA: Brooks/Cole.

Nie, N.H., Hull, C.H., Jenkins, J.G., Steinbrenner, K., & Bent, D.H. (1982). *Statistical package for the social sciences* (2nd ed.). New York: McGraw-Hill.

Pedhazur, E.J. (1982). *Multiple regression in behavioral research: Explanation and prediction.* New York: Holt, Rinehart and Winston.

Popper, K.R. (1965). *Conjectures and refutations: The growth of scientific knowledge.* New York: Harper & Row.

Popper, K.R. (1979). *Objective knowledge: An evolutionary approach.* Oxford, U.K.: Clarendon Press.

Rummel, R.J. (1970). *Applied factor analysis.* Evanston, IL: Northwestern University.

Stewart, D.K., & Love, W.A. (1968). A general canonical correlation index. *Psychological Bulletin, 70,* 160–163.

Wood, T.M., & Safrit, M.J. (1984). A model for estimating the reliability of psychomotor test batteries. *Research Quarterly for Exercise and Sport, 55,* 53–63.

Wood, T.M., & Safrit, M.J. (1987). A comparison of three multivariate models for estimating test battery reliability. *Research Quarterly for Exercise & Sport, 58,* 150–159.

CHAPTER 9

Application of Regression Analysis to Exercise Science

Andrew S. Jackson
University of Houston

The terms correlation, regression, and prediction are so closely related in statistics that they are often used interchangeably. **Correlation** refers to the relationship between two variables. When two variables are correlated, it becomes possible to make a prediction. **Regression** is the statistical model used to predict performance on one variable from another.

Regression analysis is a general method used in many different disciplines, ranging in diversity from political science to engineering. It has become a popular method in exercise science. An example is the prediction of percent body fat from anthropometric measurements. The most accurate method of measuring percent body fat is by an underwater weighing technique, which is accurate but expensive in terms of time and need for trained testers. It has been shown that the combination of weight and height

Note. A special thanks is extended to Matt Mahar for his critical review and suggestions in this manuscript.

is correlated with hydrostatically determined percent body fat; however, the correlation between hydrostatically determined percent body fat and skinfold measurements is higher and is a more accurate method of estimating body composition. For this type of research, regression analysis is used to establish the statistical (criterion-related) validity of the field test(s). Since the correlation between these anthropometric variables and hydrostatically determined percent body fat is less than a perfect 1.0, the field methods introduce prediction errors. Regression is the statistical method that not only develops the prediction equation but also quantifies the accuracy of the prediction. The **standard error of estimate** (SE_{est}) is the statistic used to quantify the accuracy of a prediction equation.[1]

Regression analysis is somewhat cumbersome to do by hand, but with mainframe and microcomputers the analysis is relatively simple. The purpose of this chapter is to provide the theory behind simple linear regression analysis and reinforce the theory with exercise examples. Examples include the prediction of body composition from anthropometric variables and estimating $\dot{V}O_2$ from a cycle ergometer and jogging. This topic is an excellent example of the ongoing application of regression analysis. In 1951, Brozek and Keys published the first body composition prediction equation, and this type of research continues today. The logic and data analyses methods of body composition prediction are fully presented in other sources (Jackson, 1984; Jackson & Pollock, 1985; Lohman, 1981).

Equations of a Linear Relationship

In order to predict scores on one variable from another, one must have knowledge of the relationship between the two sets of scores. Many of the relationships are linear and can be represented by a straight line drawn on a graph. The general form of the equation is:

$$Y = bX + c \tag{9.1}$$

where b is a constant and termed the **regression slope** of the line. The slope is the rate at which Y changes with change on X. The constant c is called the **regression intercept** and is the point at which the line crosses the vertical axis. It is the value of Y that corresponds to an X of 0. The slope and intercept can be illustrated with common examples of converting the power output of exercise modes to oxygen uptake ($\dot{V}O_2$). Standard linear equations are used to convert cycle ergometer power output and jogging pace to $\dot{V}O_2$.

---

[1]It is also commonly called the *standard error of prediction*.

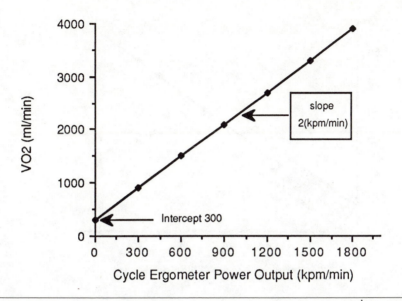

Figure 9.1   The linear relation between cycle ergometer power output and $\dot{V}O_2$ ml·min^{-1}. The equation is: $\dot{V}O_2$ (ml·min^{-1}) = 2(kpm·min^{-1}) + 300.

Example 1: Estimating $\dot{V}O_2$ From a Cycle Ergometer

The power output of a cycle ergometer is typically quantified in kilogram or kilopond meters per minute (kpm·min^{-1}).[2] Both terms have been used; for consistency the term *kilopond* will be used in this chapter. It is well known that $\dot{V}O_2$ increases at a linear rate with power output and that $\dot{V}O_2$ (ml·min^{-1}) can be estimated from cycle ergometer power output with the following linear equation (Jones & Campbell, 1982):

$$Y = 2X + 300 \tag{9.2}$$

where Y is $\dot{V}O_2$ expressed as ml·min^{-1}, 2 is the slope, X is ergometer power output expressed as kpm·min^{-1}, and 300 is the intercept. The relationship is shown graphically in Figure 9.1.

In a resting state, a human utilizes about 300 ml·min^{-1}; for each kpm·min^{-1} increase in power output, 2 additional ml·min^{-1} of oxygen are needed to meet the energy demands of exercise. For example, the steady-state $\dot{V}O_2$ energy cost of cycling at a

---

[2]A kilopond is equal to 2.2 pounds, or 1 kilogram.

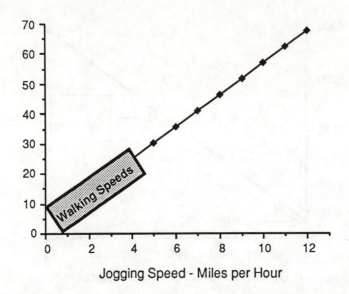

Figure 9.2   Conversion of jogging speed to $\dot{V}o_2$ by the ACSM equation. The jogging speed was transformed to miles per hour (mph) because meters per minute (m/min) is not a common unit of measurement. Jogging at 4 mph is a speed of 107.3 m/min while 12 mph is 321.9 m/min.

power output of 600 kpm·min^{-1} is 1500 ml·min^{-1}, 1200 ml·min^{-1} over the 300 ml·min^{-1} needed at rest:

$$Y = 2(600) + 300 = 1200 + 300$$
$$= 1500 \text{ ml·min}^{-1}$$

Example 2: Jogging

The American College of Sports Medicine (ACSM, 1987) has published a linear equation for predicting $\dot{V}o_2$ (ml·kg^{-1}·min^{-1}) from steady-state jogging pace. The linear equation is $Y = 0.2X + 3.5$, where X is jogging speed expressed in meters per minute (m·min^{-1}). The intercept of 3.5 represents the amount of oxygen utilized at rest,[3] expressed in ml·kg^{-1}·min^{-1}. For each m/min increase in jogging speed, the additional energy cost is a $\dot{V}o_2$ of 0.2 ml·kg^{-1}·min^{-1}; this is the slope of the linear equation, as shown in Figure 9.2.

---

[3]A $\dot{V}o_2$ of 3.5 ml·kg^{-1}·min^{-1} equals 300 ml·min^{-1} for a 189-lb person.

Defining the Slope and Intercept

For the examples shown in Figures 9.1 and 9.2, the slope of the line may be calculated by selecting any two values of X (i.e., X_1 and X_2) plus the corresponding values of Y (i.e., Y_1 and Y_2) and calculating the slope from:

$$b = (Y_2 - Y_1)/(X_2 - X_1). \tag{9.3}$$

For the cycle ergometer example, with power output values of 600 and 1200 $kpm \cdot min^{-1}$, the calculation of the slope is: $b = (2700 - 1500)/(1200 - 600) = 1200/600 = 2$. The intercept is defined as the point where the line crosses the Y axis, which is 300 (see Figure 9.1).

Statistical Definition of the Slope and Intercept

If two variables are perfectly correlated, a scattergram may be constructed and the slope defined by drawing a straight line through all points on the graph. This is illustrated in Figures 9.1 and 9.2. However, it is unlikely that one will encounter a perfect correlation using real data. A more typical example is illustrated with data shown in Table 9.1, which gives hydrostatically determined body density, percent body fat, and the sum of seven skinfold measurements.[4]

When the correlation is less than perfect, the slope and intercept can be calculated from the correlation coefficient, means, and standard deviations for the data sets. The slope and intercept are determined by:

$$b = r_{xy} (S_y/S_x) \tag{9.4}$$

$$c = \overline{Y} - b\overline{X} \tag{9.5}$$

where S_y is the standard deviation of the Y distribution, S_x is the standard deviation of the X distribution, and $\overline{Y}$ and $\overline{X}$ are the means of the distributions. The final form of the regression equation becomes:

$$Y' = bX + c \tag{9.6}$$

where Y' is the value estimated from X, termed the **independent variable** or the *predictor variable*. The term Y' is not the same as Y. The term Y symbolizes the **dependent variable** or the **criterion variable**. In contrast, Y' is an estimate of Y based on a person's score on X. The values of Y' can be used to define the **regression line**, which is often termed the *line of best fit*.

The calculation of the slope and intercepts are illustrated in Table 9.1. Both hydrostatically determined percent body fat and body density were used as the Y or

---

[4]These data were randomly selected from a large database (Jackson & Pollock, 1985).

Table 9.1. Determination of the Regression Equations for Predicting Percent Body Fat and Body Density from the Sum of Seven Skinfolds.

Subject	%Fat	BD	Σ7 Skinfolds	
1	13.27	1.0685	111	
2	11.50	1.0726	55	
3	13.61	1.0677	115	
4	8.59	1.0794	73	Percent Body Fat
5	6.22	1.0850	49	$b = r(S_Y/S_X)$
6	14.09	1.0666	115	$b = 0.879(8.55/54.64)$
7	16.45	1.0612	129	$= 0.138$
8	14.40	1.0659	79	
9	12.92	1.0693	49	$c = \overline{Y} - b\overline{X}$
10	11.71	1.0721	123	$= 16.395 - (0.138 \times 107.95) = 1.55$
11	19.28	1.0548	69	
12	12.75	1.0697	49	Body Density
13	21.34	1.0502	172	$b = -.879(0.0191/54.635)$
14	18.66	1.0562	122	$= -0.00031$
15	27.29	1.0371	193	$c = 1.06167 - (-.00031 \times 107.95)$
16	23.50	1.0454	135	$= 1.09513$
17	28.54	1.0344	174	
18	40.10	1.0100	237	
19	3.09	1.0925	44	
20	10.59	1.0747	66	
Mean	16.4	1.0617	107.9	
SD	8.6	0.0191	54.6	

criterion variable in order to illustrate the development of equations with a positive and negative correlation.[5] A graphic[6] representation of these data is shown in Figure 9.3.

Provided in Table 9.2 are the observed scores (Y), percent fat values predicted (Y') from X, the sum of skinfolds, and the differences between the predicted and actual scores ($e = Y - Y'$). These errors in prediction (e) are termed residual scores and are presented graphically in Figure 9.4.

Figure 9.4 is similar to the percent body fat graph presented in Figure 9.3, with the exception that Y', estimated percent body fat, and the residual score for one subject

---

[5]Percent body fat is calculated from %fat = (495/Body Density) − 450; thus, the correlation between the two is −1.00.

[6]All graphics were completed on Macintosh software developed by the Cricket Software Company, Malvern, PA. The graphics programs used were Cricket DRAW and GRAPH.

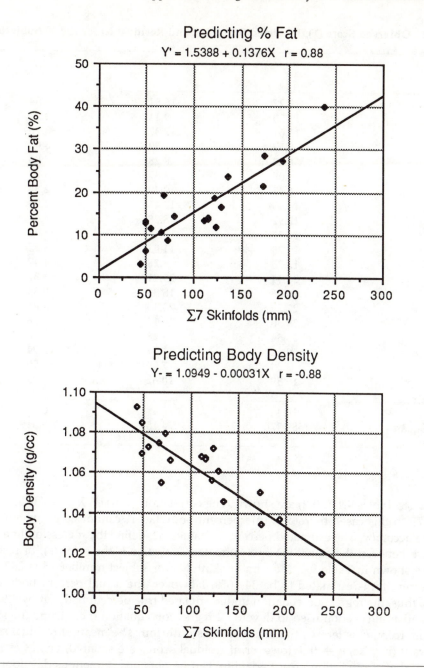

Figure 9.3 Scattergram and regression line for estimating hydrostatically determined percent body fat and body density from the sum of seven skinfolds. The data used to develop the graphs are provided in Table 9.1. (Graphs by MacASJ)

Table 9.2   Observed Score (Y), Predicted Score (Y'), and Residual (e) for the 20 Subjects

Subject	Y	Y'	(e = Y − Y')
1	13.27	16.81	−3.54
2	11.50	9.11	2.39
3	13.61	17.37	−3.76
4	8.59	11.59	−3.00
5	6.22	8.28	−2.06
6	14.09	17.37	−3.28
7	16.45	19.29	−2.84
8	14.40	12.41	1.99
9	12.92	8.28	4.64
10	11.71	18.47	−6.76
11	19.28	11.03	8.25
12	12.75	8.28	4.47
13	21.34	25.21	−3.87
14	18.66	18.33	0.33
15	27.29	28.10	−0.81
16	23.50	20.12	3.38
17	28.54	25.48	3.06
18	40.10	34.16	5.94
19	3.09	7.59	−4.50
20	10.59	10.62	−0.03
Mean	16.4	16.4	0
Sum of Squares	1389.776	1074.157	315.619

(number 18, Tables 9.1 & 9.2) are shown. The correlation between X and Y is less than 1.0 (0.879 in this case); therefore, true percent body fat, Y, cannot be estimated with complete accuracy. The estimated percent fat values, Y', define the regression line. The difference between the actual (Y) and estimated (Y') value is the error (e), or residual score. As shown in Table 9.1, the sum of skinfolds for subject number 18 is 237 mm; thus, percent fat is estimated to be 34.16%. However, the actual percent body fat is 40.10%; thus, the regression equation underestimated true percent body fat by 5.94%.[7]

The statistical criterion used to develop a regression equation (i.e., define the slope, b, and intercept, c) is termed the **least-squares criterion**. The mean of residual scores is always 0 (i.e., $\Sigma e/n = 0$). However, if residual scores are squared, i.e., $e^2 = (Y - Y')^2$, an index of prediction error variability can be obtained. Equations developed by

---

[7]The residual score for this person is 5.94% (e = 40.1 − 34.16 = 5.94).

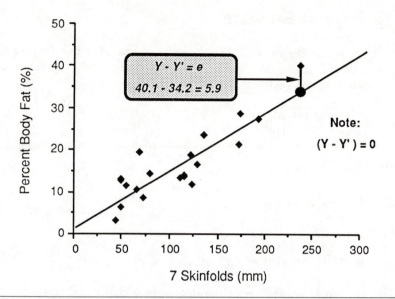

Figure 9.4   The scattergram and regression line formed by Y' and the definition of the residual score of one subject. (Graph by MacASJ)

the least-squares criterion result in the sum of the squared residuals, i.e., $\Sigma e^2 = \Sigma(Y - Y')^2$, being minimized.[8]

Provided at the bottom of Table 9.2 are the sum of squares (SS) for the three sources of variance in the regression model. The three sources of variance are:

Total observed score variance (SS_Y): $= \Sigma(Y - \overline{Y})^2$ (9.7)

Predicted score variance ($SS_{Y'}$) $= \Sigma(Y' - \overline{Y})^2$ (9.8)

Residual variance (SS_e) $= \Sigma(Y - Y')^2$ (9.9)

As shown in Table 9.2, the means of Y and Y' are equal, and the mean of e is zero. The sum of squares of each term is different, but: $SS_Y = SS_{Y'} + SS_e$ (1,389.78 = 1,074.16 + 315.62).

The proportion of the total variance in Y that is predictable from the regression equation is the coefficient of determination, r^2, and can be calculated from the sum of squares:

$r^2 = SS_{Y'}/SS_Y$
$r^2 = 1074.16/1389.78 = 0.760$, thus   (9.10)
$r_{xy} = \sqrt{0.760} = 0.879$

---

[8]The mathematical proof for the least squares criterion can be found in another source (Glass & Stanley, 1970, Appendix C).

Standard Error of Estimate

When the correlation is less than 1.0, Y cannot be estimated with complete accuracy. The standard error of estimate (SE_{est}) is the statistic used to quantify prediction accuracy. SE_{est} is calculated from the **residual scores**:

$$SE_{est} = \sqrt{[\Sigma(Y - Y')^2/(N-2)]} \tag{9.11}$$
$$SE_{est} = \sqrt{(315.62/18)} = \sqrt{17.53} = 4.19$$

An equivalent equation is:

$$SE_{est} = S_Y \sqrt{1 - r_{xy}^2} \tag{9.12}$$

where $S_Y = \sqrt{(SS_Y/N-2)}$
$$S_Y = \sqrt{(1389.78/18)} = 8.79 \tag{9.13}$$
$$SE_{est} = 8.79\sqrt{1 - 0.879^2} = 8.79\sqrt{0.23} = 4.19$$

The SE_{est} is a standard deviation of the degree to which the predicted scores vary from the actual scores. If the basic assumption of **homoscedasticity** is met, one can expect 68% of the actual scores (Y) to vary ± 1 SE_{est} from the regression line (Y') and 95% of the actual scores (Y) to be within ± 2 SE_{est} of the regression line. Homoscedasticity means *equal spread* and assumes that the variances of Y scores for each value of X are the same. This is difficult to see in small data sets and is therefore illustrated next with a large bivariate distribution.

Standard Error Example

In major health studies, body mass index (BMI), a weight-height ratio (Keys, Fidanza, Karvonen, Kimura, & Taylor, 1972), is used as an index of obesity.[9] Using a large database (Jackson & Pollock, 1985), hydrostatically determined percent body fat of men was estimated from BMI. The relationship between these variables is illustrated in Figures 9.5 and 9.6. The regression analysis produced the following: $Y' = 1.606(BMI) - 21.384$ and $SE_{est} = 6.0\%$ fat, where Y' is estimated percent body fat and X is BMI.

An inspection of Figures 9.5 and 9.6 shows that the plotted scores tend to be grouped in the middle of the bivariate distributions. This is expected when the variables are normally distributed. In addition to the regression line, the lines for ± 1 and ± 2 standard errors are plotted in Figure 9.6. As can be seen, very few scores fall beyond ± 2 standard errors. In theory, one would expect about 5% of the actual scores (Y) to deviate more than ± 2 standard errors from the predicted scores (Y'). The predicted scores, Y', mathematically define the regression line.

---

[9]Body mass index (BMI) equals weight in kilograms divided by height in meters squared (BMI = Wt/Ht^2).

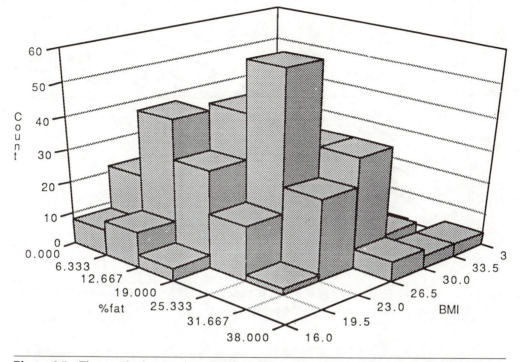

Figure 9.5 The graph shows a bivariate histogram of percent body fat and body mass index. Note how the cases cluster near the means of each variable (Percent Fat: Mean = 17.9, SD = 8.0; BMI: Mean = 24.5, SD = 3.4). (Graph by MacASJ)

Interpreting the Standard Error of Estimate

The accuracy of a regression equation is quantified with the SE_{est}. All other things being equal, the higher the correlation between X and Y, the lower the SE_{est}, and the more accurate the prediction. This can be illustrated with an example.

The field methods most often used to measure body composition include the use of skinfolds or some form of weight-height ratio like the BMI. It has been found (Jackson & Pollock, 1985) that the correlation between percent body fat and the sum of skinfolds is 0.90, compared to only 0.55 for BMI related to percent body fat. Thus, the SE_{est} for estimating hydrostatically determined percent body fat is 3.5% with the sum of skinfolds and increases to 6.0% for BMI.

The effect of the two equations' prediction accuracy for subjects with a hydrostatically measured percent body fat of 20% is illustrated in Figure 9.7. Shown are the 68% and 95% confidence bands for estimating an actual percent fat of 20%. Explained in another way, if the actual percent fat of 100 people was 20%, then 68% of the predicted

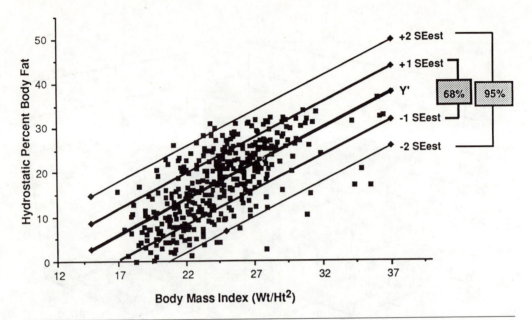

Figure 9.6   Bivariate plot of percent body fat and body mass index. The regression line and ±1 and ±2 standard errors are plotted on the scattergram. (Graph by MacASJ)

measurements (Y') would vary by the degree represented by the ± 1 SE_{est} confidence bands and 95% from the ± 2 SE_{est} confidence bands.

Figure 9.7 illustrates the error ranges for an actual percent body fat of 20%, but these confidence bands can be applied to any actual percent body fat value. For example, 68% of the skinfold percent fat estimates (i.e., ± 1 standard error) would be expected to vary from an actual percent body fat of, for example, 30% by the same magnitude, $\pm 3.5\%$ body fat. Thus, for all those with an actual percent body fat (Y) of 30%, 68% of the scores predicted from the sum of seven skinfolds (Y') would range from 26.5 to 33.5 percent and only 5% would vary beyond 23 to 37 percent fat.

The advantage of using the sum of skinfolds over body mass index can be seen in Figure 9.7. The skinfold prediction equations provide a more accurate estimate of true percent body fat. To illustrate, 5% of the BMI estimates (± 2 SE_{est}) would be in error by ± 12 percent fat. For those with an actual percent fat of 20%, 5% of the obtained percent fat estimates (Y') would be lower than 8% fat and higher than 32% fat.

Computer Regression Analysis Example

Although it is possible to calculate a simple linear regression equation by hand (see Table 9.1), it is somewhat laborious and subject to error. Numerous mainframe and

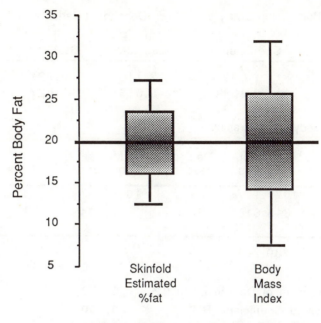

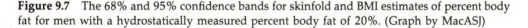

Figure 9.7   The 68% and 95% confidence bands for skinfold and BMI estimates of percent body fat for men with a hydrostatically measured percent body fat of 20%. (Graph by MacASJ)

microcomputer programs are available for these calculations. The sample regression computer output for a Macintosh regression program[10] is provided in Figure 9.8. Although the output of computer programs varies, the equation, ANOVA source table, and summary statistics tend to be common output of regression programs.

The terms for c (1.539) and b (0.138) are shown in Figure 9.8a.[11] The ANOVA and source data are furnished in Figure 9.8b. The F-ratio can be used to determine if the correlation (i.e., 0.879) is significantly larger than zero. The Coefficient of Determination (R^2) is the Coefficient of Correlation (R) squared, or can be calculated from the ANOVA sums of squares, i.e., $R^2 = 1074.157/1389.776 = 0.773$.

---

[10]*StatWorks: Statistics with Graphics for the Macintosh*, Cricket Software, Version 1.2. This program has an excellent regression program that is very easy to use.

[11]The computer example uses more precision than is used to illustrate the calculation of the slope and intercept in Table 9.2, which explains the slight difference in the obtained values.

a. Data File: Body Comp Example   Dependent Variable: % Fat

Variable Name	Coefficient	Std. Err. Estimate	t Statistic	Prob > t
Constant	1.539	2.116	0.727	0.477
$\Sigma7$ Skinfolds	0.138	0.018	7.827	0.000

b. Data File: Body Comp Example

Source	Sum of Squares	Deg. of Freedom	Mean Squares	F-Ratio	Prob>F
Model	1074.157	1	1074.157	61.260	0.000
Error	315.619	18	17.534		
Total	1389.776	19			

Coefficient of Determination (R^2)	0.773
Adjusted Coefficient (R^2)	0.760
Coefficient of Correlation (R)	0.879
Standard Error of Estimate	4.187
Durbin-Watson Statistic	2.374

Figure 9.8   Basic output of the Cricket StatWorks simple regression program.

All regression statistics are estimates of population parameters; thus, their stability is affected by the sample size used to develop the equation. The Adjusted Coefficient (R^2) provides an estimate to correct for sample size (N) and the number of independent variables (K) used in the development of the model. The equation is:

$$\text{Adjusted } R^2 = 1 - (1-R^2)\,[(N-1)/(N-K-1)] \qquad (9.14)$$

which is computed as:

$$\text{Adjusted } R^2 = 1 - (1-773)\,[(20-1)/(20-1-1)] = 0.760.$$

The SE_{est} (4.187) is provided at the bottom of Figure 9.8b. The SE_{est} can also be calculated by simply taking the square root of the error mean square: $SE_{est} = \sqrt{17.534} = 4.187$.

The Durbin-Watson Statistic is an advanced statistic that is used to determine if some of the basic assumptions are met. A discussion of the Durbin-Watson Statistic is beyond the scope of this chapter.

Table 9.3   Descriptive Statistics of Men and Women Used to Illustrate Body Composition Prediction Examples (Data from Jackson and Pollock, 1985).

Variables	Means (SDs in Parentheses)	
	Men ($N = 400$)	Women ($N = 283$)
Percent Body Fat (%)	17.9 (8.0)	24.4 (7.2)
$\Sigma 7$ Skinfolds (mm)	122.9 (52.0)	125.6 (42.0)
Body Mass Index (Wt/Ht^2)	24.4 (3.2)	20.2 (2.2)

Validity of Regression Equations

Regression equations are valid for use with subjects representative of the same population used to develop the equation. For example, body composition equations developed on a sample of men do not accurately estimate the percent body fat of women. Different equations are available for men (Jackson & Pollock, 1978) and women (Jackson, Pollock, & Ward, 1980). The problem is that the regression slope and intercept may differ, which produces systematic prediction errors. This can be examined by developing body composition prediction equations for men and women. Summarized in Table 9.3 are the body composition characteristics of men and women (Jackson & Pollock, 1985). The mean sum of seven skinfolds for the men and women were nearly identical, but the percent body fat of the women was nearly 7% higher than the men's. The BMIs of men and women are different.

Differences in Regression Slopes

Simple linear regression was applied to the male and female data predicting hydrostatically determined percent body fat from BMI. These results are shown in Figure 9.9. As can be seen, the slope of the men's and women's regression lines differs.[12] The correlation between percent body fat and BMI for women is higher ($r_{xy} = 0.70$) than for the men ($r_{xy} = 0.55$), because women have a higher percent body fat and a higher proportion of their body weight consists of fat. This results in the need for regression equations with different slopes and, usually, different intercepts. The gender specific equations are these:

Men: $Y' = 1.327(\text{BMI}) - 14.575$ 　　　　　　　　　　　　　　　　(9.15)

Women: $Y' = 2.172(\text{BMI}) - 21.411$ 　　　　　　　　　　　　　　(9.16)

Predicting the percent body fat of a man or woman with the equation developed on the other gender would produce systematic prediction errors. Using the gender specific

---

[12]The test for homogeneity of regression slopes is provided by Kerlinger and Pedhauzur (1973, pp. 267–271).

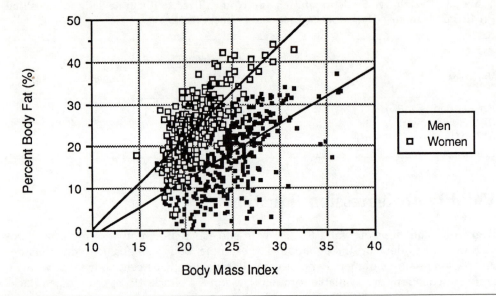

Figure 9.9 Scattergram and regression lines for estimating hydrostatically determined percent body fat of men and women from body mass index. (Data from Jackson & Pollock, 1985; graph by MacASJ)

equations, the estimated percent body fat for men and women for given BMI values are shown in Table 9.4.

The nature of the differences in slopes can be seen by examining the difference in percent body fat estimated for men and women, illustrated in Figure 9.9. As weight per squared meter of height increases, the difference in estimated percent body fat becomes larger. This numerically illustrates the difference in regression slopes.

Table 9.4 Percent Body Fat Estimated from Gender-Specific Body Mass Index Prediction Equations

| BMI | % Fat | | % Fat Difference |
	Women	Men	
20	22.0	12.0	10.0
25	32.9	18.6	14.3
30	43.7	25.2	18.5
35	54.6	31.9	22.7

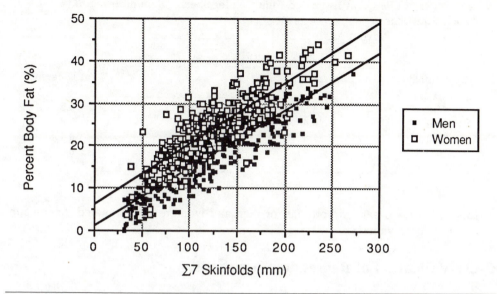

Figure 9.10   Scattergram and regression lines for estimating hydrostatically determined percent body fat of men and women from the sum of seven skinfolds. The equations are: Men: $Y' = 0.136(\Sigma 7) + 1.179$; Women: $Y' = 0.143(\Sigma 7) + 6.318$. (Graph by MacASJ)

Intercept Difference

A second condition that can produce systematic prediction errors is a similar regression slope but different intercepts. This also can be shown with the male and female body composition data. Provided in Figure 9.10 is a plot of the male and female data predicting the hydrostatically measured percent body fat from the sum of seven skinfolds. As can be seen, the slopes (*b*) of the men and women were nearly identical (0.136 and 0.1432, respectively), but the intercept[13] of the men (1.179) was about 5% lower than the intercept of the women (6.318).

The reason for the difference in intercepts can be traced to gender differences in the types of body fat. The fat compartment of the body consists of two types: essential fat and adipose tissue. Essential fat is internal and surrounds vital organs; adipose fat is next to the skin and is the component measured with the caliper. Women have more essential fat than men. The underwater weighing method measures essential fat; the skinfold caliper will not. Applying men's equations to women or women's equations to men would lead to a systematic prediction error of about 5.5 to 6.5 percent fat over ranges typically measured. This can be traced to intercept differences and is illustrated

---

[13]The test for homogeneity of regression intercepts is provided by Kerlinger and Pedhauzur (1973, pp. 237–238).

Table 9.5   Percent Body Fat Estimated from Gender Specific Sum of Seven Skinfold Prediction Equations

| Σ7 Skinfolds | (% Fat) | | % Fat Difference |
	Women	Men	
50	13.5	8.0	5.5
100	20.6	14.8	5.8
150	27.8	21.6	6.1
200	34.9	28.4	6.5

in Table 9.5, where percent body fat for men and women was estimated for the sum of seven skinfold values.

Cross-Validation of Regression Equations

Prediction equations are often developed to provide a valid and feasible method of measuring an important trait. For example, underwater weighing is expensive and time-consuming, whereas skinfold fat is easy to measure. The original research study used to develop the body composition regression equation involved measuring both skinfold and hydrostatic parameters, but in an applied study, only skinfolds are measured and percent body fat is then estimated. The original regression analysis provides evidence of an equation's validity, but the strongest evidence is obtained with cross-validation research.

A major limitation of the body composition regression equations published before 1978 was the lack of cross-validation research (see chapter 2 for a discussion of cross-validation). A step in the development of generalized skinfold prediction equations (Jackson & Pollock, 1978; Jackson, Pollock, & Ward, 1980) was cross-validation of the body composition equations. Cross-validation involves: (a) selecting a sample different from the one used to develop the original equation, (b) applying the developed equation to the data of the cross-validation sample, and (c) computing the correlation and standard error between the predicted and actual values.[14] The summary of the body composition cross-validation studies is published in another source (Baumgartner & Jackson, 1987, p. 252).

Advanced Regression Topics

The prediction of a dependent variable from an independent variable with a linear equation is useful for many prediction problems, but more complex regression models

---

[14]The cross-validation standard error is: $SE_{est} = \sqrt{[\Sigma(Y - Y')^2/(N)]}$

are often needed. The logic of simple linear regression analysis can be applied to multiple and polynomial regression models that have application to many exercise science problems. A third model, logistic regression analysis, has not been used but appears to be a valuable model for many exercise science questions. These models are discussed briefly next. The mathematics and computations of the models are complex and beyond the scope of this chapter. The approach is illustrative since advanced multivariate statistical courses are needed for individuals wishing to use these models.

Multiple Regression

Many exercise questions are complex, and several factors may be related to a dependent variable. That is, variation in the dependent variable (Y) is a function of concomitant variation in many independent variables (X_1, X_2, X_3 . . . X_k) acting simultaneously. The advantage of **multiple regression** is the use of several independent variables, resulting in a higher correlation and lower standard error and leading to improved prediction accuracy. A multiple regression equation will have one intercept and several bs, one for each independent variable. The general forms of two and three predictor multiple regression equations are:

$$Y' = b_1X_1 + b_2X_2 + c \tag{9.17}$$

$$Y' = b_1X_1 + b_2X_2 + b_3X_3 + c \tag{9.18}$$

The computer output for a multiple regression equation is similar to that obtained with a simple linear model, with the exception that several regression coefficients (i.e., bs) are obtained. To illustrate a multiple regression model, percent body fat was estimated from height (cm) and weight (kg) with a multiple regression equation. The StatWorks computer output is shown in Figure 9.11.

To illustrate the use of the equation, assume two men are the same height, 178 cm (70 in.), but the weight of one is 70 kg (154 lb) while the other is 90 kg (198 lb). Using the multiple regression equation, percent body fat would be estimated as follows:

$$
\begin{aligned}
Y' &= 0.538(\text{Wt kg}) - 0.402(\text{Ht cm}) + 47.961 \\
Y' &= 0.538(70) - 0.402(178) + 47.961 = 14.1\% \text{ fat} \qquad (9.19) \\
Y' &= 0.538(90) - 0.402(178) + 47.961 = 24.8\% \text{ fat}
\end{aligned}
$$

Polynomial Regression

The regression models discussed to this point assume a linear relationship. With some exercise science data, this is not the case. For example, when relating age and strength, the relation is linear for the ages of 10 through 17 but nonlinear for ages 10 through 65. Aging tends to be associated with a loss of lean body weight, which results in a loss of strength.

Data File: REG Cpt Major Data   Dependent Variable: %fat

Variable Name	Coefficient	Std. Err. Estimate	t Statistic	Prob > t
Constant	47.961	8.307	5.774	0.000
Ht - cm	-0.402	0.050	-7.985	0.000
Wt - kg	0.538	0.028	19.483	0.000

Data File: REG Cpt Major Data

Source	Sum of Squares	Deg. of Freedom	Mean Squares	F-Ratio	Prob>F
Model	12585.357	2	6292.679	189.981	0.000
Error	13149.733	397	33.123		
Total	25735.091	399			

Coefficient of Determination (R^2)	0.489
Adjusted Coefficient (R^2)	0.486
Coefficient of Correlation (R)	0.699
Standard Error of Estimate	5.755
Durbin-Watson Statistic	1.383

Figure 9.11   Basic output of the Cricket StatWorks multiple regression program.

The most commonly encountered type of **polynomial regression** calls for a quadratic regression equation, which yields a regression curve with a single bend. The general form of the equation for a quadratic regression is:

$$Y' = b_1X_1 + b_2X^2 + c \qquad (9.20)$$

where X_1 is the independent variable and X^2 is X_1 squared. If these two terms are expressed as X_1 and X_2, the quadratic regression equation takes the form of the two-predictor multiple linear regression equation:

$$Y' = b_1X_1 + b_2X_2 + c \qquad (9.21)$$

where $X_2 = X_1^2$.

It has been shown that with subjects varying greatly in age and body fatness, the relationship between the sum of seven skinfolds and hydrostatically determined percent body fat is quadratic rather than linear. This is shown is Figure 9.12. The polynomial regression line provides a more accurate fit of the data, especially when at the extremes

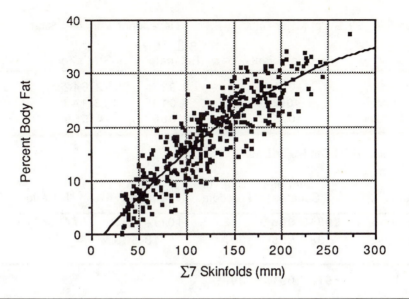

Figure 9.12   Scattergram and quadratic regression line for estimating the hydrostatically determined percent body fat of men from the sum of seven skinfolds. (Graph by MacASJ)

of the bivariate distribution. The computer output for Cricket StatWorks and the calculation of percent body fat with the polynomial equation is shown in Figure 9.13.

Logistic Regression Analysis

Logistic regression analysis has been used extensively by medical scientists to define cardiovascular disease risk factors (Kannel, McGee, & Gordon, 1976). This model is similar to the regression models discussed in this chapter, with the exception that the variable being predicted is categorical and not continuous like percent body fat.[15] In the cardiovascular disease example, the dependent variable is absence of disease or diagnosed disease.

The logistic model can be a simple, multiple, or polynomial regression model, and the solution yields a logistic value that can be used to estimate the probability that an event (e.g., presence of cardiovascular disease) would occur. The probability is determined by:

$$p = e^{-bx + c}/(1 + e^{-bx + c}), \tag{9.22}$$

where $bx + c$ is the regression equation derived by the logistic model and e is a constant of 2.718. The BMDP computer program PLR 14.5 (Engelman, 1985) can be used to

---

[15]Logistic regression and discriminant analysis are similar. Discriminant analysis is a statistical technique in which linear combinations of variables are used to distinguish two or more categories of cases; the logistic model is designed to estimate a probability of group membership.

Data File: REG Cpt Major Data   Dependent Variable: %fat

Variable Name	Coefficient	Std. Err. Estimate	t Statistic	Prob > t
Constant	-2.476	0.937	-2.642	0.009
$\Sigma 7$ Skinfolds	0.206	0.016	13.143	0.000
$\Sigma 7$ Skinfolds ^2	-0.000	0.000	-4.559	0.000

Data File: REG Cpt Major Data

Source	Sum of Squares	Deg. of Freedom	Mean Squares	F-Ratio	Prob>F
Model	20348.006	2	10174.003	749.771	0.000
Error	5387.085	397	13.569		
Total	25735.091	399			

Coefficient of Determination (R^2)	0.791
Adjusted Coefficient (R^2)	0.790
Coefficient of Correlation (R)	0.889
Standard Error of Estimate	3.684
Durbin-Watson Statistic	1.567

Figure 9.13   Basic output of the Cricket StatWorks polynomial regression program.

develop logistic equations. Logistic regression analysis was used in a preemployment study (Laughery & Jackson, 1987) designed to determine if isometric strength could be used to estimate the probability that a person was physically capable of transporting boxes up and down stairs at a defined pace. The isometric strength tests are summarized in another source (Baumgartner & Jackson, 1987, pp. 190–193).

The criterion for a productive, physically fit applicant was developed by defining a minimal work rate and determining physiological response of the subject to the work rate. Heart rate and work rate were measured during a 5-min bout. Based on various forms of data, a pass-fail criterion was developed to represent a reasonable work rate where a subject was working largely aerobically. The test consisted of two loads: a 35-lb box and a 50-lb box. The logistic equations to estimate the criterion of work from isometric strength are

35-lb transport $Y' = 0.016(X) - 2.78$ (9.23)

50-lb transport $Y' = 0.017(X) - 5.21$ (9.24)

where X is the sum of isometric strength. The logistic curves for these two transports are provided in Figure 9.14. The equation provides a probability, based on isometric

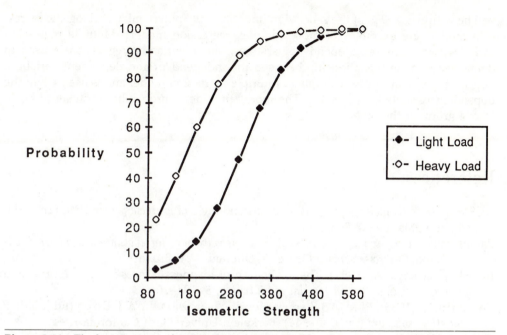

Figure 9.14   The logistic curves for estimating from isometric strength the probability of reaching the 35- and 50-pound box carry criteria. (Graph by MacASJ)

strength, that a person would be a productive, physically capable worker. The curves for both the 35-lb, and 50-lb loads are provided. To illustrate, for a person who scored 300 on the sum of isometric strength, approximately 88.7% of the subjects ($Y' = 0.016 \times 300 - 2.78 = 2.02$, $p = 88.7\%$) could be expected to achieve the 35-lb criterion, but only 44.5% would be expected to achieve the more difficult 50-lb criterion ($Y' = 0.017 \times 300 - 5.21 = -0.11, p = 44.5\%$). Said differently, the probability of someone with 300 pounds of isometric strength meeting the criteria is 88.7% and 44.5% for the 35-lb and 50-lb weight loads respectively.

Conclusion

Regression analysis is a statistical model that can be used to predict performance on a dependent variable from one or more independent variables. A simple linear regression model includes a regression slope and intercept. The slope is the rate at which the dependent variable changes with the independent variable, and the intercept represents the value of the dependent variable for a value of *0* on the independent variable. The prediction accuracy of a regression equation is quantified by the standard error of estimate (SE_{est}). About 67% of the predicted values will be ± 1 SE_{est} and about 95%

will be within $\pm 2 \, SE_{est}$ of the regression line. Multiple, polynomial, and logistic regression models are examples of more complex regression models. Multiple regression includes two or more independent variables, and polynomial regression is used to define the nonlinear relationship between the independent and dependent variables. Logistic regression can be a simple or multiple regression model and is used when the dependent variable is categorical. The model provides a probability estimate of being in one group or the other.

References

ACSM. (1987). *Guidelines for graded exercise testing and exercise prescription* (2nd ed.). Philadelphia: Lea & Febiger.

Baumgartner, T.A., & Jackson, A.S. (1987). *Measurement for evaluation in physical education and exercise science* (3rd ed.). Dubuque, IA: Brown.

Brozek, J., & Keys, A. (1951). The evaluation of leanness-fatness in man: Norms and intercorrelations. *British Journal of Nutrition, 5*, 194–206.

Engelman, L. (1985). PLR 14.5 Stepwise logistic regression. In W.J. Dixon (Ed.), *BMDP statistical software* (pp. 330–344). Berkeley: University of California Press.

Glass, G.V., & Hopkins, K.D. (1984). *Statistical methods in education and psychology* (2nd ed.). Englewood Cliffs, NJ: Prentice-Hall.

Glass, G.V., & Stanley J.C. (1970). *Statistical methods in education and psychology.* Englewood Cliffs, NJ: Prentice-Hall.

Jackson, A.S. (1984). Research design and analysis of data procedures for predicting body density. *Medicine and Science in Sports and Exercise, 16*, 616–620.

Jackson, A.S., & Pollock, M.L.. (1978). Generalized equations for predicting body density of men. *British Journal of Nutrition, 40*, 497–504.

Jackson, A.S., & Pollock, M.L. (1985). Practical assessment of body composition. *The Physician and Sportsmedicine, 13*, 76–90.

Jackson, A.S., Pollock, M.L., & Ward, A. (1980). Generalized equations for predicting body density of women. *Medicine and Science in Sports, 12*, 175–182.

Jones, N.L., & Campbell, E.J.M. (1982). *Clinical exercise testing.* Philadelphia: W.B. Saunders.

Kerlinger, F.N., &. Pedhauzur, E.J. (1973). *Multiple regression in behavioral research.* New York: Holt, Rinehart and Winston.

Keys, A., Fidanza, F., Karvonen, M.J., Kimura, N., & Taylor, H.L. (1972). Indices of relative weight and obesity. *Journal of Chronic Disease, 25*, 329–343.

Kannel, W.B., McGee, D., & Gordon, T. (1976). A general cardiovascular risk profile: The Framingham study. *American Journal of Cardiology, 38*, 46–51.

Laughery, K.R., & Jackson, A.S. (1987). *Preemployment physical test development for Stewart, Utilities and Warehouse jobs.* Houston: Rice University, Center of Applied Psychological Sciences.

Lohman, T.G. (1981). Skinfolds and body density and their relation to body fatness: A review. *Human Biology, 53*, 181–225.

Statview 512+ [Statistical package for Macintosh]. (1986). Calabasas, CA: Brain Power, Inc.

StatWork: Statistics with graphics for the Macintosh [Statistical package for Macintosh]. (1985). Philadelphia: Cricket Software.

Tabachnick, B.G. , & Fidell, L.S., (1976). *Using multivariate statistics*. New York: Harper and Row.

Supplementary Readings

Bulbulian, R., Johnson, R.E., Grubes, J.J., & Darabos, B. (1987). Body composition in paraplegic athletes. *Medicine and Science in Sports and Exercise, 19,* 195–220.

Cooper, K.H. (1968). A means of assessing maximal oxygen intake. *Journal of the American Medical Association, 203,* 201–204.

Draper, N., & Smith, H. (1984). *Applied regression analysis*. New York: Wiley.

Jackson, A.S., & Pollock, M.L. (1982). Steps toward the development of generalized equations for predicting body composition of adults. *Canadian Journal of Applied Sport Science, 7,* 187–196.

Jackson, A.S., Pollock, M.L., Graves, J.E., & Mahar, M.T. (1988). Reliability and validity of bioelectrical impedance in determining body composition. *Journal of Applied Physiology, 64,* 529–534.

Kline, G.M., Porcall, J.P., Hintgermeister, R., Freedson, P.S., Ward, A., McCarron, R.E., Ross, J., & Rippe, J.M. (1987). Estimation of $\dot{V}O_2$max from one mile track walk, gender, age and body weight. *Medicine and Science in Sports and Exercise, 19,* 253–259.

Roscoe, J.T. (1969). *Fundamental research statistics for the behavioral sciences*. New York: Holt, Rinehart and Winston.

Analyzing Change

Robert W. Schutz
University of British Columbia

The Problem

A very large part of exercise and sport science research and evaluation activities is directed at change. That is, we study growth, fatigue, learning and forgetting, training, velocity and acceleration, behavior modification, weight loss, and the effects of interventions on numerous physical, physiological, social, and behavioral variables. The measurement and analysis of this change, however, has been a nagging and persistent problem for statisticians, researchers, and educators for at least 60 years. Although there are many ways to measure change, and even more ways to statistically analyze these measures, the most common technique is to calculate a **gain** or **change score** by subtracting an **initial score** from a **final score**. It is the analysis and interpretation of this deceivingly simple measure that causes many of the problems in the analysis of change. Very briefly, these problems are: gain scores are generally unreliable, they are often negatively correlated with initial values, and the **value** or **worth** of X units of change is often perceived to be dependent on the initial value (it being more difficult to change near the top of the scale). Cronbach and Furby, in their classic 1970 treatise on change, concluded ". . . that gain scores are rarely useful, no matter how they may be adjusted or refined," and, "It appears that investigators who ask questions regarding gain scores would ordinarily be better advised to frame their questions in other ways" (p. 80). Eighteen years and approximately 200 methodological papers later, despite a number of statistical and computational advances, the situation remains basically unchanged, as indicated by Bryk and Raudenbush's (1987) assertion that we still are unable to accurately measure the true relationship between change and initial status. Although some recent advances have been made in identifying the causes of the erratic and biased nature of change scores, and a number of new and promising statistical techniques have been proposed, these new procedures have not been readily adopted by the empiricist. This chapter contains a brief overview of the major issues in the analysis of change and a nontechnical presentation of strategies for dealing with the statistical analysis of change data.

Scope and Restrictions

A comprehensive treatment of the topic of change could include such concerns as: measurement issues in obtaining change indicators, the classical problem of the statistical analyses of pre-post designs, the analysis of repeated measures designs involving measures at more than two time periods, design and analyses of longitudinal research, evaluation of change (e.g., grading), curve fitting, time series analyses, probabilistic approaches (e.g., stochastic modeling), and repeated measures structural equation modeling. The primary focus of this chapter will be on pre-post designs because they are the most commonly employed experimental designs and also the ones that cause the most problems. Some attention is given to repeated measures designs and to the issue of evaluating change scores for the purpose of grading. The topic of longitudinal design and analysis, although one of primary importance in some of our areas of study, is not addressed. It deserves much more attention than can be given here, and there are many excellent texts devoted to the topic (e.g., Nesselroade & Baltes, 1979; Plewis, 1985). The measurement problems associated with change can also be important, especially the **physicalism-subjectivism dilemma** (Bereiter, 1963), which deals with the issue of whether equal change scores at various points on the scale account for equal changes in the phenomenon being measured. Unfortunately, space limitations require that this too be omitted—Bereiter (1963) and Cronbach and Furby (1970) provide a full explanation of this issue. The remaining topics require a mathematical sophistication that could go beyond what is assumed of the readers of this text.

Analysis Issues: Overview and Chronological Review

There is such a vast amount of published literature on the analysis of change, most of it too technical for the researcher and practitioner and with little consensus among the authors, that it would be virtually impossible to fully document the status of the topic in this chapter. Presented below is a brief summary of the more influential work on the statistical analysis of change. Because the behavioral psychometricians and the life science methodologists have worked somewhat independently of each other, separate sections are devoted to each area. A brief synthesis of the published work in physical education is also given. This historical overview is followed by specific recommendations for analyzing change for each of the five types of studies where change analysis is required.

Behavioral Sciences

The early publications were primarily concerned with the correlation between initial score and **gain score**, where gain equals posttest minus pretest (hereafter referred to as $G = Y - X$). Thorndike (1924) and Zieve (1940) showed that a negative correlation between G and X existed in most empirical data, and that caution must be observed in interpreting these G scores. In the 1950s and 1960s extensive work was done by Lord and DuBois to develop procedures for adjusting G scores so they would be independent of initial scores. Lord (1956) proposed a **true change** score, which was the difference between the estimated true Y and X score, i.e., both X and Y were corrected for errors of measurement. DuBois (1957) and Manning and DuBois (1962) developed a **residual gain** score in which that portion of Y that could be linearly predicted from X was removed from Y. This resulted in a G score that was uncorrelated with X. Tucker, Damarin, and Messick (1966) then presented a **base-free** or **true residualized gain** score that was uncorrelated with the true X score (Lord's and DuBois's derived gain scores were independent of raw X scores). A number of statisticians (e.g., O'Connor, 1972) have taken issue with this base-free measure, and it is rarely used today. In the 1970s there were three influential publications that examined the broader issue of the statistical analyses of change, the most notable being the frequently cited paper by Cronbach and Furby (1970). Although Cronbach and Furby presented a thorough analysis of previously published gain score adjustments, proposed a modification of Lord's true gain score, and related the type of gain score to the purpose of the research question, their work is most often cited for their rather strong conclusion that (a) calculating gain scores and attempting to transform them into some psychometrically sound adjusted gain scores is almost always unsatisfactory, and (b) researchers should attempt to rephrase their research questions so that gain score analyses are not required. Linn and Slinde (1977) provide a clear distinction between change scores for the purpose of testing for significance between groups and for the purpose of identifying individual differences (correlational studies). They are not much more encouraging than Cronbach and Furby, in that they conclude that "problems in measuring change abound and the virtues in doing so are hard to find" (p. 147). For most situations they recommend using regression analysis rather than computing some type of adjusted gain score.

The 1980s have seen a tempering of the rather extreme positions taken in the earlier publications. Zimmerman and Williams (1982) and Williams, Zimmerman, and Mazzagatti (1987) have shown that the mathematical conditions under which the previous work was performed are overly restrictive and do not reflect the actual distributions found in most empirical data sets. The earlier papers often assumed the conditions of equal variances at X and Y, uncorrelated errors, and virtually no variance in the true change. Relaxing some of these overly restrictive mathematical assumptions led to the conclusion that raw gain scores can be appropriate in a number of situations. Rogosa and colleagues, in three very substantial pieces of work, take issue with some of the extremely unlikely situations proposed by Zimmerman and Williams, but support their general conclusions (Rogosa, Brandt, & Zimowski, 1982; Rogosa & Willett, 1983, 1985). They indicate that because most previous studies used examples in which true change exhibited little variation across individuals it was to be expected that this lack of interindividual variability in change would result in a difference score that was unable to adequately distinguish the true change among individuals. With respect to correlational issues, they make a clear distinction between the analysis of individual differences in the amount of change and the analysis of individual differences in the parameters of a particular model for individual change. An important conclusion of their work is that "the importance of obtaining observations on each individual at more than two time points cannot be overstated" (Rogasa & Willet, 1985, p. 225).

In summary, there has been extensive theoretical work done on the problems inherent in the analysis of change. It is apparent that there is no one best method, and that each particular research question requires its unique approach. Although there is no consensus as to what these most appropriate approaches are, the suggested procedures given later in this chapter appear to have considerable support.

Life Sciences

Historically the life, physical, and medical sciences have not been as concerned with statistical issues as the behavioral sciences, perhaps because of the assumed greater reliability of the dependent measures used. However, the problem of negative correlations between initial values and amount of change is one that has plagued physiologists and psychophysiologists for many years. Wilder appears to have had a lifelong obsession with this issue, as indicated in his detailed documentation of more than 400 reported studies in which his "Law of Initial Value" is shown to hold (Wilder, 1967). This book and most of his periodical publications (e.g., Wilder, 1957; and his earlier works in German) identify studies in which those subjects who score high at the start of an intervention (on blood pressure, galvanic skin response, heart rate, etc.) generally record the smallest change in response to the imposed stressor, drug, or treatment. This **ceiling effect** leads to the negative correlation between initial status and gain. Wilder offered little in the way of remedies for this situation other than careful examination of the data and cautious interpretations, but Lacey (1956) extended Wilder's work and proposed a solution in the form of the "Autonomic Lability Score" (ALS). The ALS used the initial score to adjust the final score, the adjustment being a function of the correlation between the two, and then standardized the resultant adjusted final score so that it had a mean of 50 and a standard deviation of 10. If we use psychometric terminology, Lacey's ALS is the T-score form of the residual gain score. It is interesting that the behavioral and life science researchers worked quite independently of each other on this common problem. Although some papers refer to work in the other field (e.g., Rogosa and Willett [1985] acknowledge Lacey and Wilder), there is a discouragingly small amount of cross-disciplinary communication. Recent publications on the Law of Initial Value (Myrtek & Foerster, 1986; Scher, Furedy, & Heslegrave, 1985) fail to reference any of the psychometric work on the analysis of change.

Physical Education and Exercise Science

Although publications in our research journals reflect considerable statistical and methodological sophistication, we, like other behavioral and life scientists, have generally ignored the issue of measurement of change. Examination of 20 measurement and research methods texts in physical education indicated an almost complete disregard for the issue of change. Exceptions are measurement texts by Baumgartner and Jackson (1987), Mood (1980), and Safrit (1986), in which the unreliability of change scores is noted within discussions on grading and evaluation. Thomas and Nelson's (1985) research methods text includes a comment on the unreliability of difference scores emanating from a pre-post research design. No one offers any solutions.

In our periodical literature, methodologists (Dotson, 1973; Schutz, 1978) have reviewed specific aspects of the analysis of change, identified the problems, and suggested the solutions advocated in the psychometric literature. Morrow and Frankiewicz (1979), Schutz and Gessaroli (1987), and Stamm and Safrit (1975) have published methodological papers on the statistical analysis of repeated measures designs. In some of our subdisciplines, researchers have grappled with problems specific to the measures used in their field. For example, in motor learning Carron and Marteniuk (1970) and Schmidt (1972) addressed the problem of measuring the amount of learning that occurs when many trials are performed. Using only the first trial as a pretest score usually gives a very unreliable score, but using the mean of the first 5 or 10 trials results in a pretest score that, although more reliable, includes part of the actual learning. Kroll (1966) applied classical test theory to gains in strength and concluded that the data were sufficiently reliable to permit valid use of change scores. Finally, in the context of grading in physical education, Hale and Hale (1972) proposed a method for equating change scores that were derived from different initial levels of skill.

Analysis Issues: Suggested Procedures

The following sections present recommended statistical procedures for dealing with data involving measures of change. Because the method of analysis should always be determined by the research questions being asked, two main categories of analyses are developed. The first deals with data in which the primary purpose of the research is to test for differences among groups. Within this category an important distinction is whether the groups have been formed by random assignment of subjects (as in most experimental studies) or already exist (e.g., males and females, high-, medium-, and low-stressed individuals, obese and nonobese subjects). The second major category deals with studies in which individual differences constitute the focus of the research questions. In this situation the researcher may wish to identify those individuals who exhibited the most or least change, or to determine which other variables correlate most strongly with change in the dependent variable. The recommendations given are based on the works of dozens of methodologists over the past 30 years, but most notably on the following publications: Cronbach and Furby (1970), Linn and Slinde (1977), Maxwell and Howard (1981), and Rogosa and Willett (1983, 1985).

Two sample data sets were simulated to provide the bases for empirical examples throughout this chapter.[1] The data sets are purposely small ($n = 8$) so that readers can readily perform their own calculations. The consequence of such small sample sizes are spuriously high multiple correlations in the regression analyses and low power in the ANOVAs. The data are assumed to be pretest (X) and posttest (Y) scores on a test in which the maximum possible score is 50. In Group 1 the pretest scores are relatively low ($M = 30$), thus allowing for considerable improvement by all subjects. In Group 2 the pretest mean is approaching the maximum ($M = 40$), and thus it is impossible for some subjects to show improvement. As a consequence, the pre-post correlation is higher in Group 1 than in Group 2 ($r_{xy} = .72$ and $.46$, respectively). As will be shown, this is an important consideration in the analysis and interpretation of change.

The appropriate statistics have been calculated for many, but not all, of the proposed methods for examining change. In most cases the results are presented in tabular form and discussed briefly in the text. For topics such as repeated measures MANOVA and applying a correction for attenuation no examples are provided, because they would consume far too much space or be unnecessarily repetitive. No examples are provided for the methods presented under Case 4 (each method would require a complete chapter).

The raw data are presented in Table 10.1, along with a number of the derived change scores and the three concomitant variables used in the Correlational Studies section.

Case I: Group Differences in Pre-Post Designs

One-group design Given the situation where a single group of subjects have been tested pre and post, and the question of interest is "Has there been a change in performance?", then the recommended analysis is the common one-sample *t*-test. Two possible problems exist: (a) lack of variance in the calculated difference score brought about by unreliability of the measure, and (b) regression to the mean if the group was identified for treatment because of extreme (low or high) performance. With respect to the former,

---

[1]I would like to acknowledge and thank Hanjoo Eom for his assistance in the preparation of the numerical examples used throughout this chapter.

Table 10.1 Raw Data and Derived Change Scores

Group, Subject	Age	Height	Weight	X	Y	G	G_x	HH_{100}	HH_{1000}
G1:									
S1	30	156	62	31	40	9	4.3	22.6	17.9
S2	28	159	64	13	18	5	−4.7	2.0	0.6
S3	24	183	71	39	41	2	−0.5	7.4	7.0
S4	34	163	70	37	42	5	1.9	17.8	16.6
S5	29	177	70	40	45	5	2.8	23.5	25.1
S6	29	179	73	33	38	5	0.8	12.3	9.5
S7	40	175	77	17	35	18	9.4	20.5	11.6
S8	26	167	74	30	21	−9	−14.0	− 9.0	− 4.5
Mean:	30	170	70	30	35	5.0	0.0	12.2	10.5
SD:	5	10	5	10	10	7.5	6.9	11.4	9.6
G2:									
S1	30	156	62	41	45	4	1.5	19.7	21.3
S2	28	159	64	23	38	15	−0.1	25.0	16.7
S3	24	183	71	49	50	1	4.0	8.9	12.9
S4	34	163	70	47	48	1	2.6	7.4	9.8
S5	29	177	70	50	49	−1	2.7	−8.9	−12.9
S6	29	179	73	43	40	−3	−4.2	−12.8	−12.9
S7	40	175	77	27	45	18	5.7	51.6	46.1
S8	26	167	74	40	31	−9	−12.3	−22.6	−17.9
Mean:	30	170	70	40	43.3	3.3	0.0	8.5	7.9
SD:	5	10	5	10	6.5	9.1	5.8	23.8	21.6

Note. X: Pretest score, Y: Posttest score, G: Simple gain score $(Y - X)$, G_x: Raw residualized gain $(Y - Y')$, and HH: Hale & Hale index $(S_{max} = 100$ or $1000)$.

the classical unreliability of difference-score problem comes into play. The reliability of a difference score can be expressed as

$$r_{dd} = (r_{xx'} - r_{xy})/(1 - r_{xy}), \tag{10.1}$$

where r_{dd} is the reliability of the difference score (post-pre, Y-X), $r_{xx'}$ is the reliability of the pretest (and assumed to be equal to the reliability of the posttest in this formulation), and r_{xy} is the correlation between X and Y. As is apparently obvious, the lower the value of $r_{xx'}$ the lower the value of r_{dd} (for any fixed r_{xy}), and the higher the value of r_{xy} the lower the value of r_{dd} (for any fixed $r_{xx'}$). For example, if $r_{xx'} = .80$ and $r_{xy} = .75$, then $r_{dd} = .20$. Although such $r_{xx'}$ and r_{xy} combined values would be unlikely in any empirical study (usually r_{xy} is quite a bit smaller than $r_{xx'}$), difference scores are generally quite unreliable. Researchers have known this for many years, and consequently some of them have been reluctant to use these simple difference scores in statistical analysis. However, while this unreliability will definitely cause biased interpretations with individual difference studies, it is not a major problem in analyzing differences between means. Overall and Woodward (1975) and others have shown that a rather strange paradox exists in that the lower the reliability of the difference score the greater the statistical power of the t-test (or F-test). This results from the fact that the denominator in the equation for a repeated measures statistical test (t, F) is a direct function of the reliability of the pre to post change score. The denominator of the one-sample t-test is a function of S_d^2, where

$$S_d^2 = S_x^2 + S_y^2 - 2r_{xy}S_xS_y \qquad (10.2)$$

Thus it can be seen that the larger the r_{xy} the smaller the value of S_d^2, and therefore the larger the calculated t statistic. Consequently, because r_{dd} is negatively related to r_{xy}, the more unreliable the difference score the greater the power of the statistical test. It must be noted, however, that although the one-sample t-test is a suitable analytical procedure to assess the statistical significance of a pretest-posttest design, such a design does *not* permit inferences regarding causality—history, maturation, differential attrition, and so forth, could have caused the significant change in behavior. One must also recognize that with pretest-posttest studies in which the value of r_{xy} approaches that of $r_{xx'}$ and $r_{yy'}$, the value of r_{dd} approaches zero, thus yielding extremely high statistical power. In such cases one can still be confident of the reliability of the statistical significance, but substantive significance should certainly be examined as well (e.g., calculate effect sizes).

As mentioned above, a potential problem exists if subjects have been chosen because they scored at the extreme of the population distribution. Such is often the case when selecting subjects for weight-loss programs, stress reduction, fitness enhancement, and so forth. In this case the **regression to the mean** effect is going to bias the results. Subjects who score in the top or bottom 10%, as determined by a single administration of some test, are likely to exhibit some regression to the mean on a second testing. Thus low-fit individuals almost always show some improvement on retesting when improvement is judged by a change in the group mean. The inclusion of a control group with the same initial status is desirable, but if that is not possible then the recommended solution is to give the pretest a second time. The scores on the first pretest are used to select the extreme subjects, and these subjects are tested a second time, with the second set of scores serving as the pretest score in the eventual pre-post analysis. If it is not possible to include a control group or to administer a second pretest, then it is questionable if a study to assess change in an extreme group should be conducted. The recommendation here is that it should not be conducted.

As can be seen in Table 10.2, the ceiling effect in Group 2 results in a lower S_y and a lower r_{xy} (and consequently a larger S_d) than exists in Group 1. This results in a larger mean square error for Group 2 and less power in the F-test (but because of small n, the Group 1 effect was nonsignificant also). Due to the lower r_{xy}, however, the reliability of the difference score is higher in Group 2 (.63 vs. .28), as is the magnitude of r_{xG}.

Table 10.2   Relevant Statistics for Pre-Post Comparisons

Statistic	Group 1	Group 2
Pretest (X): Mean	30.0	40.0
SD	10.0	10.0
Posttest (Y): Mean	35.0	43.25
SD	10.0	6.5
r_{xy}	0.72	0.46
S_d	7.5	9.1
r_{xG}	−0.37	−0.77
$r_{dd}{}^a$	0.28	0.63
F (pre vs. post)	3.59	1.03
MS_{error}	27.90	41.00
p	.10	.34
Effect size [$(M_Y - M_X)/S_X$]	0.50	0.325

[a]Assuming that $r_{xx'} = r_{yy'} = .80$.

Thus the ceiling effect has caused: (a) a loss in power of the F-test, (b) a decreased r_{xy} and therefore an increase in the calculated r_{dd} (but this is of little benefit), and (c) an increase in the dependence of improvement on the initial score.

Two or more groups: Random assignment With two or more experimental groups, subjects having been randomly assigned to these groups, and pretest and posttest measures available, the research question is usually something like, "Is there a difference among the groups in the amount of change from pretest to posttest?" Given proper experimental controls, any differences can be attributed to the treatments administered. As with the single-group design, any unreliability in the change scores (if they are calculated) brought about by a high r_{xy} serves only to maximize the power of the statistical test. Traditional ANOVA procedures are a suitable method of analysis in this situation.

Two or more groups: Nonrandom assignment In many instances it is not feasible to randomly assign subjects to treatment groups—the groupings are determined by some a priori condition such as location, gender, age, or etiology. Under such conditions it is quite likely that the groups are not equal on the pretest. This is where regression toward the mean and the Law of Initial Values cause problems; the group with the highest initial mean will probably show the least change. An individual with a high resting heart rate will not show the same treatment-induced heart rate elevation as someone with an initial low resting rate. A subject who makes many errors on the first trial is likely to show a greater reduction in errors than a subject who made very few errors initially. Thus with preformed groups there exists a high probability that the groups will not be equal to start with, and the problem is one of making the proper adjustments for these preexisting group differences. Early investigators of this problem (Cronbach

Table 10.3   ANOVA and ANCOVA for a 2-Group Pre-Post Design

Source	df	MS	F	p
ANOVA				
Group (G)	1	666.1	4.87	.045
SwG	14	136.7		
Time (T)	1	136.1	3.96	.067
G×T	1	6.1	0.18	.680
SwG×T	14	34.4		
ANCOVA				
Group (G)	1	30.3	0.63	.444
Zero Slope	1	367.2	7.55	.017
SwG	13	48.6		
Equality of slopes	1	62.8	1.32	.270
Error	12	47.5		

& Furby, 1970; Lord, 1969) concluded that although it was possible to use adjustments such as residual gain scores or true gain scores, there is really no adequate solution. Unfortunately, we still do not have any clearly accepted technique to do this. ANCOVA appears to be a commonly used analysis in many fields, but it generally is not a suitable analysis, because one of the assumptions of ANCOVA is that the subjects are randomly assigned to groups. With preformed groups the distribution of X may differ among groups, and an adjustment for a pretest score of 20 in one group cannot be equated to a similar adjustment in another group ($X = 20$ could be the lowest score in one group, the highest in another). As is pointed out later in this chapter, the analysis of change becomes much more valid with an increase in the number of testing sessions. Richards (1975) has shown that ANCOVA can provide valid tests of differential change among preformed groups only if there are multiple testing periods. In conclusion, if one is forced to use a pretest-posttest design with preformed groups and if these groups exhibit considerable differences on pretest, then there is no theoretically acceptable method of analysis. A two-way mixed model ANOVA may be the best solution, because it will provide statistical tests of the significance of differential change—but interpretations are open to criticism.

Given the large pretest differences, Group 1 and Group 2 could reflect two groups that were nonrandomly assigned to treatments. The ANOVA results in Table 10.3 indicate that the significant difference between the groups is due primarily to pretest differences. There is no differential change over time, as indicated by the nonsignificant Groups × Time interaction. This analysis is probably inappropriate, given the very large pretest differences and the ceiling effect present in Group 2. The ANCOVA results show that there is no significant difference in the posttest scores once the linear component of the pretest differences is taken out ($p = .44$). Given that the *zero slope effect* is significant ($p = .017$), indicating a reliable XY linear relationship, and the assumption of equal r_{xy} within each group is met ($p = .27$), this analysis is appropriate in this case.

Case 2: Individual Differences

Identifying individuals In research and in practice it is occasionally desirable to identify individuals who have exhibited exceptional change, either very large or very small. We may wish to isolate those subjects who failed to show any learning, to identify subjects who recorded large blood pressure increases, or, as is often the case in school settings, to determine a change (learning, improvement) score for each member of a sample. It should be noted that this is a different process from the situation in which an investigator attempts to identify the *type* of individuals who exhibit the most or the least change—that sort of problem is dealt with in the following section on correlates of change. In some situations it may be appropriate to use the simple raw gain score ($G = Y - X$). If the reliability of the measure is high, there are true individual differences in change (as reflected by large variance in the G scores), and the intent is to determine which individuals gained the most or least, then the simple G score is certainly appropriate. However, it is frequently the case that the measure is quite unreliable, thus yielding G scores that are very unreliable. Identifying, rewarding, or penalizing individuals on the basis of such scores would certainly be unjust. Additionally, in cases where **ceiling** and **floor effects** are present, resulting in the Law of Initial Values phenomena, it is often desirable to take into account the magnitude of the pretest score. How to do this has been the focus of controversy since the beginning of time (or so it seems). There are a number of possible approaches.

Raw gain. Early investigators of the measurement of change were generally unanimous in their conclusion that one should never use the raw gain score. More recently (Rogosa & Willett, 1983; Zimmerman & Williams, 1982) it has been pointed out that these early investigators used situations that are not common to most empirical data. It is now known that when X is quite reliable ($r_{xx'} > .7$) and r_{xy} is not unduly large relative to $r_{xx'}$, thus reflecting true interindividual differences in change, the raw gain score is an acceptably reliable indicator of true change. However, if initial scores are not equal, then *evaluation* of these change scores may be difficult, even though they are reliable measures. As was seen in our examples (Table 10.2), the r_{dd} for Group 1 is a rather low .28 but increases to .63 for Group 2 due to the much lower r_{xy}.

Raw residualized gain. When it is desirable to remove the advantage or disadvantage due to initial status, then a transformed score referred to as a **residualized difference score** or **raw residualized gain score** is preferred over a simple gain score. This residualized gain (G_x) score is obtained by subtracting the predicted Y score (Y_p) from the observed Y score, where the Y_p is computed from the ordinary simple linear regression equation predicting Y from X. That is, Y_p is the posttest score with X partialled out. The difference, $Y - Y_p$, is a measure of the degree to which an individual gained more or less than would be expected given his or her initial status. This G_x score is uncorrelated with X and has been shown to be considerably more reliable than the simple G score (Williams, Zimmerman, & Mazzagatti, 1987). Table 10.1 contains the calculated G_x scores for all subjects.

Hale and Hale Index. In 1972, Hale and Hale published a paper in which they proposed an "exponential modification" of improvement that would "convert into comparable terms the large increase of the novice and the smaller increase of the student who started with a high level of skill" (p. 113). They imply that such a score, which they refer to as the "weighted improvement percentage score," is necessary for valid grading in activity classes. There is no evidence that this procedure is being used in practice, but because its use is recommended in a number of our measurement texts (Baumgartner & Jackson, 1987; Eckert, 1974; Safrit, 1986) it deserves comment.

First, one must question the implication that it is necessary or desirable to grade improvement. *Measurement* of improvement is required for feedback to both instructor and student, as it is a necessary component of the learning process. *Evaluation* of improvement, however, is quite a different matter, and perhaps this aspect of the total assessment program should be an individual responsibility. In most other fields within the educational system we do not attempt to grade on improvement, but rather on status. It is recommended here that raw gain improvement scores be reported, along with normative data (if appropriate), but that status rather than improvement be the measure on which grading is based. Second, Hale and Hale state that their derived score converts improvement into "comparable terms." But comparable on what basis— potential, initial level, previous improvement? They have chosen initial level, with the implicit assumption that initial level is perfectly correlated (nonlinearly) with attainable status. This appears to be a tenuous assumption. Finally, the derivation of the equations presented by Hale and Hale are based on arbitrary assumptions, they make no reference to or acknowledgment of any previous psychometric work on change analysis, and their results have not been subjected to any type of empirical validation. For example, we do not know if an exponential curve is the most appropriate nonlinear function for skilled performance; perhaps a logistic, power, or double exponential function would provide a better fit for performance variability. The theory is based on an assumed *interindividual* distribution whereas the application is to *intraindividual* change. Application of the equations requires an estimate of some "limiting" score, a maximum or minimum best possible performance. Hale and Hale suggest using a world record, if available; if not, they suggest a T-score of 100. This arbitrary selection of a parameter can cause very different final improvement scores. Table 10.1 includes the Hale and Hale scores for all subjects using the suggested S_{max} values of both 100 and 1000.

Hale and Hale are to be commended for attempting to solve a difficult problem and for the sophisticated approach they adopted. However, it is questionable if we should be grading on the basis of improvement. If in fact one does have valid reasons for doing so, then further theoretical and empirical work needs to be done. Given the present state of the art, the residualized gain score presented above appears to be the most valid measure of change that is uncorrelated with initial status.

Examples. Table 10.1 contains the individual values and means for the four measures

Table 10.4 Correlations Among Raw Scores and Derived Change Measures (Group 1 above diagonal, Group 2 below diagonal)

Group 2	X	Y	G	Group 1 G_x	HH_{100}	HH_{1000}
X		.72	−.37	.00	.23	.47
Y	.46		.38	.68	.81	.86
G	−.77	.21		.93	.77	.53
G_x	.00	.89	.64		.92	.75
HH_{100}	−.64	.33	.95	.71		.94
HH_{1000}	−.56	.36	.87	.69	.98	
Age	−.39	.23	.60	.47	.67	.64
Height	.39	.32	−.20	.15	−.20	−.20
Weight	.06	−.10	−.14	−.14	−.09	−.07

of change (G, G_x, HH_{100}, HH_{1000}), and Table 10.4 gives the correlations between these measures and with the pretest and posttest values. The values in Table 10.1 are presented so that readers can practice and check calculations of these indices. Additionally, some interesting comparisons are possible with individual data (e.g., compare S_5 and S_6 in Group 1; see S_5 in Group 2).

With respect to G and G_x, the correlations in Table 10.4 reveal what one would expect. The amount of gain is inversely related to the pretest level, and this is most pronounced in Group 2, where some subjects were already near the maximum possible score at pretest. Thus any *evaluation* of G must take pretest levels into account. The residualized gain (G_x) removes the pretest influence and thus is uncorrelated with pretest values. If the pretest-posttest relationship were actually linear, this would be the appropriate measure; however, it is obviously nonlinear at the upper end of the scale. The Hale and Hale indices take this nonlinearity into account but assume a specific type of exponential relationship. The finding that the Hale and Hale indices correlate positively with X for Group 1 but strongly negatively with X for Group 2 leaves interpretation of their index open.

Correlational studies Frequently a researcher is interested in determining the characteristics of individuals with a given pretest score who benefit the most from a treatment. In this type of correlational study, testing whether the treatment has an overall effect is generally not an issue, as it is already established that, for example, the fitness program causes fitness changes, the enhanced feedback accelerates learning, or the progressive relaxation procedures reduce perceived stress. What we want to know is what *type* of individuals show the greatest (or least) change as a result of the intervention, thus permitting the prediction of change. This is a completely different question from that addressed previously, in which we were attempting to identify which specific individuals showed the greatest change. Conceptually, what we want to do is examine the correlations between the amount of change and a number of concomitant variables (hereafter referred to as the set V), but at the same time control for any relationship between pretest levels and the magnitude of change.

Simple gain score correlations. The most obvious procedure is to calculate a simple G score and correlate it with V; however, two problems suggest that this is often an unsatisfactory method. As noted earlier, gain scores are often negatively correlated with initial status, and as the concomitant variables are usually measured at the same time as the pretest, the errors of measurement in the pretest are correlated with the errors of measurement in V. This usually results in a spurious negative correlation between G scores and V. The second problem arises in the presence of unreliability of measurement in one or more of the pretest, posttest, or concomitant variables. This, too, will negatively bias the correlations. If the reliabilities are known the correlation between the hypothetical true scores (T_x, T_y) can be calculated with the standard **correction for attenuation** formula (Allen & Yen, 1979, p. 98):

$$r_{T_x T_y} = \frac{(r_{xy})}{(r_{xx'} r_{yy'})^{1/2}} \tag{10.3}$$

for all correlation coefficients. Although correction for attenuation is recommended in a number of situations (e.g., see following sections), it is of dubious value in this case, because the former problem of correlated errors remains. Consequently, in agreement with Cronbach and Furby (1970), Linn and Slinde (1977), and many others, it is recommended that the calculation of simple gain scores *not* be performed in correlational studies of change.

Part and partial correlations. One possible solution is to use the residual gain score, G_x, rather than the simple G score, and correlate it with the other variables of interest. This results in a *part* correlation in which the pretest score is partialled out of the posttest score, yielding a residual that is then correlated with V. Alternately, one could compute the more commonly used *partial* correlation in which the linear relationship associated with the pretest is partialled out of both the posttest and the other variables. Theoretically, this gives a correlation between the posttest and V for any fixed value of the pretest. Unfortunately, the negative bias introduced by unreliablility is as much of a problem with partial correlations as with simple difference scores. Thus, when dealing with measures known to have low reliabilities, one should correct all correlations for attenuation before calculating the partial correlations. In general, the research questions posed by most investigators are probably better answered with partial correlations than with part correlations.

Regression approach. Hummel-Rossi and Weinberg (1975), following Cronbach and Furby's general recommendations, suggest using a stepwise multiple-regression approach to identify the correlates of change. Such a procedure avoids the need to calculate any sort of difference score. The posttest is used as the dependent variable, with the pretest and V being the independent variables. The pretest is forced into the regression equation as the first independent variable, with the concomitant variables entering freely in a stepwise fashion based on the usual criteria for entry. The variables that enter the equation are those that are significantly related to the posttest score, having controlled for pretest. The first variable to enter freely is obviously the most important

Table 10.5   Regression Equations to Identify Correlates of Change

Method	Dependent Variable	X	Age	Height	Weight	R^2
(a) Simple gain	G		.84	.33	−.63	.52
(b) Part correl.	G_x		.99	1.11	−1.23	.81
(c) Partial correlation	G_x		.92	1.10	−1.22	.81
(d) Hierarchical regression	Y	.49	.89	.97	−1.09	.84

Note. Entries are standardized regression coefficients.

correlate of change; but care must be taken in making relative comparisons of the importance of the remaining variables, because multicollinearity (intercorrelation among the independent variables) could hide some strong zero-order relationships. Hummel-Rossi and Weinberg recommend correcting for attenuation in the presence of unreliable measures. This regression approach is the recommended method for determining the correlates of change.

Examples. Table 10.1 contains raw data and descriptive statistics for the set V of concomitant variables. The raw scores and the correlations with the pretest are identical for the two groups. The correlations among the three variables and with all other variables (for Group 2 only), are presented in Table 10.4. In general, older people scored lower on X but had the greatest gain, and height and weight tended to be negatively related to improvement. The problem is to identify the characteristics that predispose individuals to show improvement, controlling for initial level influences. Table 10.5 presents the results of the four procedures described above. The simple gain approach is included only for comparative purposes, because it is not a recommended procedure. For methods (b) and (c) identified in Table 10.5, the pretest effect was partialled out of the gain score, yielding G_x as the dependent variable. Additionally, for (c) the pretest was partialled out of each one of the three concomitant variables (using $V - V_p$, where V_p is predicted from X using simple linear regression). In all four procedures all variables were forced into the equation regardless of the F-to-enter value. As an aside, it is interesting to note that all beta coefficients are significant in the final equations, but some would not have entered if a stepwise procedure had been utilized (i.e., it is an interesting regression example as well).

The results are consistent across all four methods in this particular case, i.e, all three variables are related to the amount of change that occurred. In general, regardless of any pretest-posttest linear relationship, older and taller subjects show greater positive change, but heavier people are less inclined to exhibit improvement.

Case 3: Designs with Multiple Repeated Measures

The problems inherent in the measurement of change are greatly reduced when we have measures at more than two time periods. Although multiple observations are common in motor learning studies, longitudinal studies, and in some types of experimental and evaluation studies, most studies are based on the classical pre-post design. Because of this and because the problems of regression to the mean, unreliability of difference scores, and Law of Initial Values are most pronounced in the pre-post design, the emphasis in this chapter is on that situation. Recent literature on the analysis of change indicates that valid assessments of change require multiple observations—for testing group differences and for individual difference studies. Consequently, a few brief comments on the multiple repeated observations designs are given.

Testing for group differences The statistical analysis of repeated measures designs involving many trials or testing sessions has both disadvantages and advantages over the pre-post analysis. The main advantage is that multiple observations provide an indication of the shape of the learning curve, whereas a pre-post design automatically assumes a linear change. A situation could exist where all treatment groups started and ended at identical levels; but one group had strong initial learning and then plateaued, another group exhibited a constant linear change, and the third group showed little change over the early stages but then an exponential increase in the later stages. Multiple observations over the duration of learning would be necessary to detect these important differences. Another advantage is that the effect of unreliability diminishes with repeated testing (it will be reflected in the error term of an ANOVA, but should not bias the main effects or interaction). A disadvantage of multiple repeated measures is that the additional assumption of *sphericity* is required for valid F-tests on the repeated measures factor(s). In particular, it is assumed that variances and covariances (correlations) are similar for all groups (technically, it is the transformed orthonormalized variance-covariance matrices that are assumed to exhibit this pattern). Violation of the sphericity assumption usually leads to an inflation in the calculated F-ratios. Researchers may protect against this bias by using a MANOVA procedure to analyze their repeated measures designs or by using the Huynh-Feldt adjusted p values within the usual ANOVA. Methodologists have recently been extolling the virtues of these techniques and encouraging their use in a variety of scientific disciplines, e.g., psychology (O'Brien & Kaiser, 1985), physiology (Vasey & Thayer, 1987), growth and development (Hertzog & Rovine, 1985), and exercise science (Schutz & Gessaroli, 1987). Refer to these publications for numerical examples of a variety of repeated measures analyses.

Individual differences With respect to determining the correlates of change, Rogosa and Willet (1985) state that "the common longitudinal design which obtains just two observations on each individual (and which, at best, allows estimation of only the amount of change) is rarely adequate for the study of systematic individual differences in growth. The importance of obtaining observations on each individual at more than two points cannot be overstated" (p. 225). Rogosa and Willett recommend modeling individual change with linear and nonlinear functions and using parameter estimations as the indicators of the nature and degree of change. It is interesting to note that this was the approach adopted over 30 years ago by Henry and DeMoor (1956) in their classic paper on lactic-alactic debt, but it has been used rather infrequently since. Rogosa and Willett also present some rather surprising data that show how the time at which the measures are taken can have major effects on the correlation of change with other variables. Thus it is especially important that we not rely on only two time periods.

Case 4: Some Nontraditional Approaches

The assessment of change through the use of classical experimental and quasi-experimental designs followed by statistical tests on group means is certainly the most common procedure in the behavioral and life sciences. Additionally, correlational procedures are frequently employed to examine correlates of change. However, there exist a number of alternative procedures for examining change that are not so common. Many of these techniques require data sets beyond what is often available and require statistical methodologies that are not readily accessible (or understandable). What follows is a partial listing of these alternative approaches and a brief description of their purpose. Interested readers are encouraged to pursue the suggested references for a more complete description.

Hierarchical linear models Bryk and Raudenbush (1987) advocate the application of **hierarchical linear models** (HLM) for analyzing change. These procedures, which are somewhat similar to ANOVA methods, are claimed to permit a more detailed examination of both the correlates of change and the identification of change (as well as its prediction). A distinct advantage of the HLM approach is that, unlike ANOVA, it does not require the same number of repeated measures for each individual (the time periods between the repeated measures can also vary). This would be of special value in studies that require individual assessments in field settings.

Failure rates In some studies the dependent variable of interest is measured on a nominal scale, i.e., the subject did or did not quit smoking, achieve a criterion, or maintain an exercise program. In such instances it is common to use the concept of *failure rate* and define it as the percentage of individuals who fail to meet the standard at a certain point in time. Maltz and McCleary (1977) propose an alternative measure of failure rate that is based on the distribution of failures over time rather than at a single point in time. These concepts would be appropriate in research involving behavioral modification and perhaps even with criterion-referenced skill assessment.

Stochastic models The availability of stochastic models for the analysis of change has been with us for a long time (e.g., Goodman, 1962), but researchers have yet to include it in their repertory of statistical tools. Stochastic models permit statements about the probability of an individual achieving any one of a number of possible scores at some time in the future, given his or her current score. It is assumed that an individual possesses a characteristic in the form of a distribution of possible observed scores. This is in contrast to the more common deterministic models that are based on the concept of a true score with observed deviations from the true score representing error scores. Schutz (1970a, 1970b) presented the theory of stochastic processes to physical educators, provided suggestions for the application to sport and exercise science, and analyzed and revised a sport scoring system using Markov chain procedures, a type of stochastic model. Little if any further application of stochastic processes appears to have taken place in our field. The large number of observations required make it somewhat impractical for empirical work, and the lack of standardized computer software undoubtedly discourages its general use. Mathematical psychologists use it extensively in developing and testing mathematical models of learning (e.g., Townsend & Ashby, 1982).

Rate of change   Kissane (1982) suggests that we may be able to avoid some of the classical problems in the meaurement of change by studying the rate of change rather than just the amount of change. While this concept is in accord with that of others who have recommended using mathematical functions such as learning curves, Kissane's approach is unique in that he utilizes latent trait theory to overcome the inequality-of-scale dilemma brought about by floor and ceiling effects. This methodology, like most of the more elaborate models of change analysis, requires multiple observations throughout the learning or change period. As measures of change are taken before and after a treatment, this technique would seem to be especially useful for measuring change in attributes that already are undergoing a natural change, as is the case in many studies involving children.

Time series analysis   Time series analysis is an especially useful tool in studies incorporating few subjects but many observations per subject. Although it could be construed as falling within the field of stochastic modeling, the application is quite different from the Markov model type of application presented above. Time series analysis generally requires at least 50 trials per subject and can be applied to the data of a single subject or a group of subjects. It is a type of curve-fitting procedure that takes into account the serial (trial-to-trial) dependency of the trials. Econometricians have used time series extensively to chart, compare, and predict stock prices and other economic indices. Spray and Newell (1986) provide an example of how time series analysis can lead to conclusions different from a traditional ANOVA approach when examining the effect of knowledge of results on motor learning.

Structural equation models   The common statistical tools of the last 50 years (*t*-tests, ANOVA, MANOVA, and correlation/regression) are gradually being replaced by more sophisticated techniques such as those mentioned above. However, the primary statistical tools of the next 20 or more years will undoubtedly be those falling within the general area of structural equation modeling. Causal modeling, path analysis, specification searches, covariance structure analysis, cross-lagged panel correlations, and confirmatory factor analysis all have some identification with this methodology. The highly sophisticated and popular system developed and marketed under the title of LISREL (Linear Structural Relations) by Jöreskog and his colleagues (e.g., Jöreskog & Sörbom, 1984) should now be familiar to most readers of social science and behavioral science research. No attempt is made here to describe the theory or application of structural equation modeling, but readers should be alert to its potential usefulness for analyzing change. Recent developments have enabled us to apply LISREL to longitudinal designs in order to test models of the interrelationships among change and a number of correlates. For example, a study of changes in participation in physical activity brought about by an educational program, while accounting for the correlates of knowledge about health and physical activity, exercise opportunity, fitness level, and peer-group activity, could be analyzed appropriately with causal modeling techniques. LISREL and other similar techniques, such as Bentler's EQS (Bentler, 1985), permit reasonably strong conclusions regarding causal relationships when applied to data that have been collected at two or three time periods. Structural equation modeling is certainly the most promising technique available for identifying the relative importance of pretest, concomitant variables, and interventions as contributors to the process of change, and it is the recommended tool for the sophisticated researcher. An excellent series of articles in a special issue of *Child Development* (February, 1987) provides a good starting point for the interested reader.

Conclusion

The measurement and analysis of change, a necessary component of many research studies, has been shown to be a process fraught with difficulties. In experimental studies, different levels of initial status cause problems in comparing the amounts of change exhibited by different experimental and control groups. In correlational studies the unreliability of change scores results in a negative bias in correlations between measures of change and other explanatory variables. There is no generally agreed-upon best method of analysis to overcome these problems, and different research questions require different measurement and analysis strategies. In this chapter procedures are suggested for the analysis of change for five situations inherent in two distinct types of research studies: (a) testing differences among means (for the single-group design, two or more groups with random assignment of subjects to groups, and two or more preformed groups), and (b) examining individual differences (identifying extreme individuals and determining correlates of change). Each of these five situations requires a different form of statistical analysis, but two overriding principles emerge that are recommended when measuring change: (a) use reliable measures and (b) obtain measures at more than two points in time. A number of less commonly used procedures are identified that permit the analysis and interpretation of change from different perspectives. Structural equation modeling is viewed as the methodology of the future and is highly recommended for multiple-variable studies of change.

References

Allen, M.J., & Yen, W.M. (1979). *Introduction to measurement theory*. Monterey, CA: Wadsworth.

Baumgartner, T.A., & Jackson, A.S. (1987). *Measurement for evaluation in physical education and exercise science*. Dubuque, IA: Brown.

Bentler, P.M. (1985). *Theory and implementation of EQS: A structural equation program.* Los Angeles: BMDP SoftStatistical Software Inc.

Bereiter, C. (1963). Some persisting dilemmas in the measurement of change. In C.W. Harris (Ed.), *Problems in Measuring Change* (pp. 3–20). Madison: University of Wisconsin Press.

Bryk, A.S., & Raudenbush, S.W. (1987). Application of hierarchical linear models to assessing change. *Psychological Bulletin, 101*, 147–158.

Carron, A.V., & Marteniuk, R.G. (1970). An examination of the selection of criteria scores for the study of motor learning and retention. *Journal of Motor Behavior, 2*, 239–244.

Cronbach, L.J., & Furby, L. (1970). How should we measure "change"—or should we? *Psychological Bulletin, 74*, 68–80.

Dotson, C.O. (1973). Analysis of change. In J. Wilmore (Ed.), *Exercise and sport sciences reviews*, (Vol. 1, pp. 393–419). New York: Academic Press.

DuBois, P.H. (1957). *Multivariate correlational analysis.* New York: Harper.

Eckert, H.M. (1974). *Practical measurement of physical performance.* Philadelphia: Lea & Febiger.

Goodman, L.A. (1962). Statistical methods for analyzing processes of change. *American Journal of Sociology, 68*, 57–78.

Hale, P.W., & Hale, R.M. (1972). Comparison of student improvement by exponential modification of test-retest scores. *Research Quarterly, 43*, 113–120.

Henry, F.M., & DeMoor, J. (1956). Lactic and alactic oxygen consumption in moderate exercise of graded intensity. *Journal of Applied Physiology, 8*, 608–614.

Hertzog, C., & Rovine, M. (1985). Repeated-measures analysis of variance in developmental research: Selected issues. *Child Development, 56*, 787–809.

Hummel-Rossi, B., & Weinberg, S. (1975). Practical guidelines in applying current theories to the measurement of change. Part 1, Part 2. *JSAS Catalog of Selected Documents in Psychology, 5*, 226 (ms#916).

Jöreskog, K.G., & Sörbom, D. (1984). *LISREL VI: Analysis of linear structural relationships by the method of maximum likelihood.* Mooresville, IN: Scientific Software.

Kissane, B.V. (1982). The measurement of change as the study of the rate of change. *Educational Research and Perspectives, 9*, 55–72.

Kroll, W. (1966). Application of an elementary model for assessing change to an isometric measurement schedule. *Research Quarterly, 37*, 61–65.

Lacey, J.I. (1956). The evaluation of autonomic responses: Toward a general solution. *Annals of the New York Academy of Sciences, 67*, 123–164.

Linn, R.L., & Slinde, J.A. (1977). The determination of the significance of change between pre-and posttesting periods. *Review of Educational Research, 47*, 121–150.

Lord, F.M. (1956). The measurement of growth. *Eductional and Psychological Measurement, 16*, 421–437.

Lord, F.M. (1969). Statistical adjustments when comparing pre-existing groups. *Psychological Bulletin, 72*, 336–337.

Maltz, M.D., & McCleary, R. (1977). The mathematics of behavioral change. *Evaluation Quarterly, 1*, 421–438.

Manning, W.H., and Dubois, P.H. (1962). Correlational methods in research on human learning. *Perceptual and Motor Skills, 15,* 287–321.

Maxwell, S.E., & Howard, G.S. (1981). Change scores—Necessarily anathema? *Educational and Psychological Measurement, 41,* 747–756.

Mood, D.P. (1980). *Numbers in motion: A balanced approach to measurement and evaluation in physical education.* Palo Alto, CA: Mayfield.

Morrow, J.R., & Frankiewicz, R.G. (1979). Strategies for the analysis of repeated and multiple measures designs. *Research Quarterly, 50,* 297–304.

Myrtek, M., & Foerster, F. (1986). The law of initial value: A rare exception. *Biological Psychology, 22,* 227–237.

Nesselroade, J.R., & Baltes, P.B. (1979). *Longitudinal research in the study of behavior and development.* New York: Academic Press.

O'Brien, R., & Kaiser, M. (1985). MANOVA method for analyzing repeated measures designs: An extensive primer. *Psychological Bulletin, 97,* 316–333.

O'Connor, E.F. (1972). Extending classical test theory to the measurement of change. *Review of Educational Research, 42,* 73–97.

Overall, J.E., & Woodward, J.A. (1975). Unreliability of difference scores: A paradox for measurement of change. *Psychological Bulletin, 82,* 85–86.

Plewis, I. (1985). *Analysing change: Measurement and explanation using longitudinal data.* Chichester, England: Wiley.

Richards, J.M. (1975). A simulation study of the use of change measures to compare educational programs. *American Educational Research Journal, 12,* 299–311.

Rogosa, D.R., Brandt, D., & Zimowski, M. (1982). A growth curve approach to the measurement of change. *Psychological Bulletin, 90,* 726–748.

Rogosa, D.R., & Willet, J.B. (1983). Demonstrating the reliability of the difference score in the measurement of change. *Journal of Educational Measurement, 20,* 335–343.

Rogosa, D.R., & Willet, J.B. (1985). Understanding correlates of change by modelling individual differences in growth. *Psychometrika, 50,* 203–228.

Safrit, M.J. (1986). *Introduction to measurement in physical education and exercise science.* St. Louis: Mosby.

Scher, H., Furedy, J., & Heslegrave, R. (1985). Individual differences in phasic cardiac reactivity to psychological stress and the law of initial value. *Psychophysiology, 22,* 345–348.

Schmidt, R.A. (1972). The case against learning and forgetting scores. *Journal of Motor Behavior, 4,* 79–88.

Schutz, R.W. (1970a). Stochastic processes: Their nature and use in the study of sport and physical activity. *Research Quarterly, 41,* 205–212.

Schutz, R.W. (1970b). A mathematical model for evaluating scoring systems with specific reference to tennis. *Research Quarterly, 41,* 552–561.

Schutz, R.W. (1978). Specific problems in the measurement of change: Longitudinal studies, difference scores, and multivariate analyses. In D. Landers and R. Christina (Eds.), *Psychology of motor behavior and sport—1977* (pp. 151–175). Champaign, IL: Human Kinetics.

Schutz, R.W., & Gessaroli, M.E. (1987). The analysis of repeated measures designs involving multiple dependent variables. *Research Quarterly for Exercise and Sport, 58,* 132–149.

Spray, J.A., & Newell, K.M. (1986). Time series analysis of motor learning: KR versus no-KR. *Human Movement Science, 5,* 59–74.

Stamm, C.L., & Safrit, M.J. (1975). Comparison of significance tests for repeated measures ANOVA designs. *Research Quarterly, 46,* 403–409.

Thomas, J.R., & Nelson, J.K. (1985). *Introduction to research in health, physical education, recreation and dance.* Champaign, IL: Human Kinetics.

Thorndike, E.I. (1924). The influence of chance imperfections of measures upon the relationship of initial score to gain or loss. *Journal of Experimental Psychology, 7,* 225–232.

Townsend, J.T., & Ashby, F.G. (1982). Experimental test of contemporary mathematical models of visual letter recognition. *Journal of Experimental Psychology: Human Perception and Performance, 8,* 834–864.

Tucker, L.R., Damarin, F., & Messick, S. (1966). A base-free measure of change. *Psychometrika, 31,* 457–473.

Vasey, M.W., & Thayer, J. (1987). The continuing problem of false positives in repeated measures ANOVA in psychophysiology: A multivariate solution. *Psychophysiology, 24,* 479–486.

Wilder, J. (1957). The law of initial value in neurology and psychiatry. *Journal of Nervous and Mental Disease, 125,* 73–86.

Wilder, J. (1967). *Stimulus and response. The law of initial value.* Bristol, England: Wright.

Williams, R.H., Zimmerman, D.W., & Mazzagatti, R.D. (1987). Large sample estimates of the reliability of simple, residualized, and base-free gain scores. *Journal of Experimental Education, 55,* 116–118.

Zieve, L. (1940). Note on the correlation of initial scores with gain. *Journal of Educational Psychology, 31,* 391–394.

Zimmerman, D.W., & Williams, H. (1982). A note on the correlation of gains and initial status. *Journal of General Psychology, 107,* 203–207.

CHAPTER 11

New Approaches to Solving Measurement Problems

Judith A. Spray
The American College Testing Program

Psychometrics, the study of the measurement of human psychological behaviors from the cognitive and affective domains, has served as a primary source for the theory and techniques that have been used by physical educators to measure human behavior in the motor (or, more appropriately, psychomotor) domain. Past and present reliance on such concepts as validity and reliability (through the formulation and use of the Spearman-Brown prophecy formula, coefficient alpha, Kuder-Richardson equations 20 and 21 [see chapter 12], the correction for attenuation, and the upper bound for test validity) come from the assumptions and results of classical test theory. However, the psychometrics field has undergone radical change within the past ten years, influenced by an increasingly expanding knowledge base developed over the previous 20 years. For the most part, physical education has ignored these new developments, even for the measurement of the shared psychological behaviors in the affective and cognitive domains.

Physical educators, especially those who study measurement as an area of specialization, need to become familiar with these advances and techniques in psychometric theory for consideration of their implementation in shared behavior domains. It is even possible that such advances might be useful in the measurement of psychomotor skills (Spray, 1987).

This chapter presents some of the introductory, theoretical developments of the primary psychometric advancement—item response theory—and some of its applications in terms of item banking, computerized adaptive testing, and mastery testing. Similarities between some of these applications of item response theory and sequential testing of psychomotor skills, a testing plan that has already appeared in the physical education literature, are presented, and implications for directions of future research toward the application of sequential testing to adaptive or tailored testing of psychomotor skills are given.

Item Response Theory Versus Classical Test Theory

Item response theory (IRT) is an attempt to go beyond the more traditional or classical test theory framework in order to get more out of the answers on test questions or **item responses** given by examinees. Item response theory does this, as the name implies, by treating each separate test item and each individual's response to that item as a source of information about the testing situation (i.e., about the true but unknown ability of the examinee and about the characteristics of the test item itself). In contrast classical *test* theory attempts to make these same general types of inferences about items and abilities by inferring from total test score information obtained from a group of examinees. This is also implied in the name, *test* theory. One of the basic differences, then, between item response theory and test theory is the level at which these inferences are made. In some respects this is similar to a physicist's attempt to understand matter by studying the behavior of matter either at the molecular level or at the atomic or subatomic level. Items are the basic building blocks of tests, and item responses are the basic building blocks of observed test scores. In order to understand the interaction of tests and examinees, it makes some sense to observe this interaction at its most basic level.

Unfortunately, there is a price for this degree or level of understanding. Sometimes the price is easily met; at other times the price is too steep, and consequently the information at this level is unobtainable. However, many professionals who are involved at some level in test-construction or test-usage activities are willing to pay this price, because the quality of the information, about either the examinees or the test, more than makes up for the cost.

The price is in terms of the assumptions required about the examinee $\times$ item response interaction. Occasionally these assumptions can be tested to determine if they are reasonable. Often they cannot, and the validity of the information gained by the employment of IRT may be in doubt in these instances. Alternatively, the use of classical theory in its weakest form requires very few assumptions concerning either the examinees or the test scores. Therefore, one can either use classical test theory with very few assumptions and learn something about a group of examinees and a total test, or use IRT with the possible requirement of many more assumptions and learn even more about individual examinees and individual test items.

To get a better understanding of the differences between IRT and classical test theory, consider how the latter uses testing information to quantify or measure examinees' ability. First, it usually is assumed that an examinee's ability is not measurable directly but can be measured indirectly, through the **observed score**. It is also assumed that, unless the testing situation is perfectly reliable, some error in the observed test score prevents us from knowing an examinee's actual or **true score**. We could get perfect test reliability by giving an n-item test, with no error in any of the n items, or we could give a test consisting of an infinite number of imperfect test items. Because we are usually faced with some middle ground, we can give n-item tests that contain error and estimate the amount of the error, thereby estimating the examinee's true n-item test score. This estimate of error in the observed test score is usually assumed to be the same for all examinees. Perhaps more important, the estimate of true score is based on these particular n test items. It is a total score on a zero-to-n scale. Generalizations made from this true score can only be made to other k-item tests, which are in some sense equivalent to the one administered, where k is greater than, equal to, or less than n.

IRT makes the assumption that a single trait, ability, or skill underlies each examinee's performance on each item on a test. This single ability is also unknown and is not directly measurable. In fact it has been referred to as a **latent trait** for this very reason. Unlike the true score scale, however, the latent trait scale (usually designated by the Greek symbol θ) is assumed to be infinite in length and therefore not bound by a finite test length. In addition, the amount of error in the observed test score is assumed to be a function of the latent ability, θ. In other words, error in the observed test score varies according to ability. Classical test theory allows for this variability but requires very strong distributional assumptions concerning test scores.

The real advantage of IRT in terms of measuring an examinee's ability from responses to test items is that the ability construct is not limited or bound to a particular test, but can be measured by any collection of test items, considered as separate units, and assumed to be measuring the same unidimensional trait or ability. This is an important distinction between IRT and classical test theory, because it creates the possibility of measuring θ by administering different collections of test items to different examinees—perhaps even creating tests that are optimal in some sense for each individual. The critical assumption required by the use of IRT in this context is the unidimensionality of θ. The items on a given test must measure the same, single latent trait (unless a more complicated multidimensional item response theory application is used).

Classical test theory and IRT also differ in the way item characteristics are defined. The two traditional item characteristics commonly used in item analyses are (a) item difficulty, as measured by the proportion of examinees in a given group who correctly answered the item, and (b) item discriminating power, or the tendency of examinees in the higher ability range to answer the item correctly more frequently than other examinees with lower ability. The latter characteristic is usually measured by a point-biserial or biserial correlation coefficient. Like the true score measure of ability, these item characteristics are functions of the total test score and the group of examinees as a whole. Change the test items or change the group of examinees on which these scores are dependent, and the item characteristics, as measured by these indices, could change radically.

The traditional definition of item difficulty is also hard to justify, because, like an error score, the item difficulty supposedly describes the difficulty for all examinees, regardless of ability level. And yet we intuitively think that a test item can be more difficult for lower-ability examinees than for those with higher ability.

In an IRT framework, item difficulty is usually measured on the same scale as ability. Item difficulty can then be assessed in terms of the examinee's θ value relative to the fixed value of difficulty for that item. The item difficulty value or parameter is usually symbolized by b; more specifically, the jth item's difficulty is b_j. We can assess the relative difficulty of an item with difficulty, b_j for an examinee with ability, θ_i, as follows. If θ_i is greater than b_j, then this item is relatively *easy* for this examinee. If θ_i is smaller than b_j, then the item is relatively *difficult* for this examinee. When $\theta_i = b_j$, the item has *moderate* difficulty for this examinee. In this way an item with fixed difficulty, b_j, can have different relative difficulty levels for different examinees.

IRT Models

IRT uses concepts, such as examinee ability and item difficulty, to describe mathematically the way in which an examinee with ability θ_i will respond to an item with difficulty b_j. This examinee $\times$ item interaction is usually described by an IRT *model*. The model describes the probability of an examinee with ability θ_i answering item j in a particular manner or with a particular response. For **dichotomously scored** items, this probability is usually given as the probability of a *correct* response. A plot of these probabilities as a function of ability is called an *item characteristic curve* or ICC.

The form of an actual ICC function is probably not terribly important, but some overall characteristics of the curve should be noted. First, the probability scale is bounded by 0 and 1, while the θ scale is infinite. This means that the shape of the curve necessarily must be nonlinear. Second, it makes some sense to think of the curve as being a monotonic function of ability. As θ increases, the probability of a (correct) response for item j or $P_j(\theta)$ should also increase, approaching 1 as θ approaches $+\infty$. If a correct response can be obtained by all examinees with some nonzero probability value c (for example, by guessing at the choices offered in a multiple-choice format), then $P_j(\theta)$ approaches this value of c as θ approaches $-\infty$. This value of c is sometimes referred to as a lower asymptote or *guessing parameter*.

Table 11.1   Values of $P_j(\theta)$ for Three Different Items, Where $P_j(\theta)$ Is the 1-PLM

| | Values of $P_j(\theta)$ | | |
| | b_j | | |
θ	.5	.0	-1.0
-2.0	.08	.12	.27
-1.0	.18	.27	.50
.0	.38	.50	.73
1.0	.62	.73	.88
2.0	.82	.88	.95

One reasonable form of an ICC is a logistic curve of the following general form:

$$P_j(\theta) = c + \frac{(1 - c)}{1 + e^{-(\theta - b_j)}} \qquad (11.1)$$

For situations where $c = 0$ (i.e., where guessing is not possible), this reduces to a simpler form involving only the b parameter and examinee ability, θ. This model is referred to as the one-parameter logistic model, or 1-PLM, and is given by the following:

$$P_j(\theta) = \frac{1}{1 + e^{-(\theta - b_j)}} \qquad (11.2)$$

The plot of the ICC for a 1-PLM with a given value for b (say $b = .5$) shows how the curve defines item difficulty differently for different examinees with varying abilities. The trait or θ scale and the b parameter scale (recall that they are the same scale) are usually defined as a standard scale with 0 mean and standard deviation equal to 1. This scale has nothing to do with the normal probability distribution and does *not* imply that any given group of examinees must have a normal distribution for θ. On the contrary, with IRT the distribution of θ is immaterial. The item difficulty, as defined by the b parameter, remains constant regardless of which group of examinees responds to the test item. This is sometimes referred to as item **parameter invariance.**

For this particular 1-PLM with $b = .5$, the probabilities for a correct response or $P_j(\theta)$ increase as θ increases, as seen in Table 11.1, column 2. Again this shows the monotonicity of the 1-PLM. In columns 3 and 4 of Table 11.1, the values of $P_j(\theta)$ are given for items $b = .0$ and $b = -1.0$, respectively. For a given θ value, say $\theta = -2.0$, $P_j(\theta)$ increases as b becomes smaller relative to θ. This is true for any value of θ given in Table 11.1 and for any value of θ in general.

For any 1-PLM, the point on the ICC at which there is a 50-50 chance of answering the item correctly is called the *point of inflection.* A perpendicular line dropped from this point to the θ scale will intersect the horizontal axis at $\theta = b$.

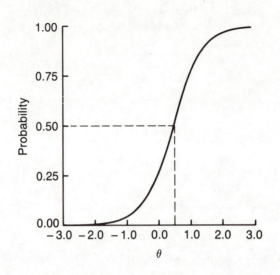

Figure 11.1   Item characteristic curve of a two-parameter logistic model with $a = 2.125$ and $b = .5$.

For an n-item test one would have n separate ICCs, one for each test item. An IRT definition of an examinee's true score would be the sum of the n $P_j(\theta)$ values across the n items:

$$T(\theta_i) = \sum_{j=1}^{n} P_j(\theta_i) \tag{11.3}$$

Thus, within an IRT framework it is possible to define examinee ability at either the true score level *or* at the latent trait level. This is not the case with classical test theory.

In IRT a test item's discriminating power is defined by the steepness of the ICC. Most IRT models can change the steepness of this curve by incorporating a second parameter into the equation for $P_j(\theta)$. Usually this is done only when it is hypothesized that some of the n items have steeper slopes (and therefore, *more* discriminating power) than other items on the test. If all n items are thought to have the same discriminating power, then the 1-PLM should model the examinee-by-item response interaction well. If item discrimination does vary within a test, then a two-parameter model such as the 2-PLM can be used. (See Figure 11.1). An example of such a model is

$$P_j(\theta) = \frac{1}{1 + e^{-a_j(\theta - b_j)}} \tag{11.4}$$

where the discrimination parameter, a_j is usually defined to be a positive value with larger a parameters indicating more discrimination (i.e., a sharper distinction between

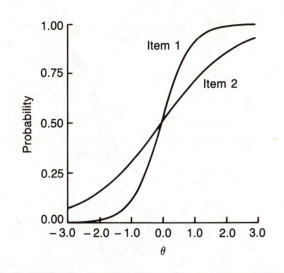

Figure 11.2   Two items with identical b parameters but different a parameters.

high and low values of θ). Figure 11.2 shows the ICCs of two items with the same b values ($b = .0$) but with different a values, where $a_1 > a_2$. Therefore, there is a sharper distinction between high and low θ values on item 1 than on item 2.

A three-parameter version of the IRT logistic model, the 3-PLM, incorporates all three item parameters (a, b, and c) and is hypothesized to fit item response data in which the items on a test have different levels of item discriminating power and a nonzero lower probability asymptote, at least for some items. The 3-PLM is given by

$$P_j(\theta) = c_j + \frac{1 - c_j}{1 + e^{-a_j(\theta - b_j)}} \qquad (11.5)$$

Figure 11.3 contrasts the ICCs of a 2-PLM with a 3-PLM, with $b = .5$ and $a = 1.25$ for both models but with $c = .20$ rather than zero, as in the 2-PLM version.

Estimation

In actual applications of IRT to real item response data, the item parameters and the examinees' abilities are estimated. Most estimation procedures require the use of computer programs that solve rather complicated systems of nonlinear equations. Many of these programs require further assumptions regarding the use of the IRT models. For example, almost all programs assume that, for each examinee, responses to each of the n items are independent of all other responses for that examinee. This is called the *assumption of local independence*.

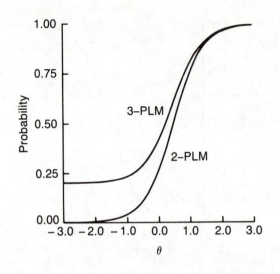

Figure 11.3   Two-parameter logistic ICC versus three-parameter logistic ICC with nonzero c.

Although the methodology and theory required to obtain estimates of item and ability parameters are beyond the scope of this chapter, a simplified and somewhat heuristic approach to the estimation problem is presented in this section. The estimation problem is made more or less complicated by the choice of IRT model used for the actual estimation procedure. A general rule is that estimation becomes more difficult as the number of item parameters in the model increases. This implies that a one-parameter model is less complicated to estimate than a two-parameter model, for example. Estimation is also made much simpler if the item parameters are known and only the ability parameters must be estimated. For the purposes of simplification and illustration, the case of known item parameters will be assumed for the following example.

Maximum Likelihood Estimation

Most parameter estimation procedures are based on the concept of *likelihood*. The likelihood concept provides a quantitative answer to the question, "How likely is it that an examinee with ability θ_i produced the n responses on a test?". For example, suppose two items had item characteristic curves defined by the one-parameter logistic model (1-PLM) with $b_1 = -1.0$ and $b_2 = 0.5$. If local independence held so that for a given ability value θ_i, the response to item 2 did not depend on the response to item 1 or vice versa, then the probability of any two responses occurring together would be equal to the product of each response occurring separately.

Table 11.2 gives some selected values of θ_i, along with the corresponding probabilities for items 1 and 2 of success (P_1 and P_2) and failure (Q_1 and Q_2), where $Q_j(\theta) = 1 - P_j(\theta)$. These values come directly from the equation of the 1-PLM.

Table 11.2   Success and Failure Probabilities for Two Items at Different Abilities

θ	P_1	P_2	Q_1	Q_2
-1.00	.50	.07	.50	.93
$-$ .50	.70	.15	.30	.85
$-$ .25	.78	.22	.22	.78
.00	.85	.30	.15	.70
.25	.89	.40	.11	.60
.50	.93	.50	.07	.50
1.00	.97	.70	.03	.30

Now, suppose that one observes responses (1, 0) indicating a correct answer for item 1 and an incorrect answer for item 2. Under the 1-PLM with these known item parameters, what is the most likely value of θ_i associated with an examinee with this observed response string? The likelihood of this response string is P_1Q_2; this product is called a *likelihood function* of the unknown ability trait, θ_i. Likelihood values $L(\theta_i) = P_1Q_2$ are given in column 2 of Table 11.3. The likelihood function appears to reach a maximum value at $\theta = -.25$.

For another response string (0, 1) (i.e., an incorrect response on item 1, a correct response on item 2), values of $L(\theta_i) = Q_1P_2$ appear in column 3 of Table 11.3. Notice how small these values are relative to the likelihood values in column 2. This makes sense in terms of the items, when one considers that item 1 is easier than item 2. Therefore, the response string (1, 0) is more likely to occur than (0, 1).

Table 11.3   Likelihood Functions $L(\theta)$ of Response at Different Ability Levels

θ	$L(\theta)$ (1, 0)	(0, 1)	(0, 0)	(1, 1)
-1.00	.465	.035	.465	.035
$-.50$	.595	.045	.255	.105
$-.25$	.608	.048	.172	.172
.00	.595	.045	.105	.255
.25	.534	.044	.066	.356
.50	.465	.035	.035	.465
1.00	.291	.021	.009	.679

Estimates of θ_i for which $L(\theta_i)$ reaches a maximum are called **maximum likelihood estimates** (MLEs) of θ and are symbolized by $\hat{\theta}$. For one-parameter IRT models, examinees with the same number-correct score, X_i, will have the same estimates of ability from the maximum likelihood estimation procedure. In this example, the response strings (1, 0) and (0, 1) yield the same estimate of ability, $\hat{\theta} = -.25$.

When the item parameters are not known, they must be estimated from the response data as well. This is called **item calibration**. Although the invariance principle suggests that the value of item parameters should not change according to the group tested, it is important to realize that during an initial calibration the items should fit the ability of the examinees. This means that the items should not be too difficult or too easy for those examinees who provide the item response data for the calibrations. Otherwise, the item characteristic curves, which are determined from the item **parameter estimates**, may be distorted and may represent an unrealistic version or model of the item-by-examinee interaction.

Although some leading authorities suggest that the sample size, in terms of both examinees *and* items, should be fairly large for calibration purposes, others think that the minimal sample sizes could be as small as 200 examinees and as few as 10 items (Lord, 1983). Certainly these minimum numbers depend on many factors, including the IRT model to be fit and the estimation procedure to be used. The most popular computer programs used to calibrate items and estimate trait scores (e.g., Logist, Bilog) usually require group sizes in excess of 1,000; 2,000 appears to be a popular minimum for many 3-PLM calibrations that use MLE (Mislevy & Bock, 1984; Wingersky, Barton, & Lord, 1982).

Item Parameter Estimation Errors

One method of evaluating the usefulness of IRT item-parameter calibrations is to observe the minimum standard errors associated with the estimates. These standard errors are usually printed as part of the item calibration output in most programs used for this purpose (e.g., Logist, Bilog).

These standard errors give some indication of the precision of the item parameter estimates. In general, the estimates have a larger error associated with them when any of the following conditions hold: (a) the sample size, N, is small; (b) the number of parameters in the IRT model, m, is large; (c) c, the pseudo-guessing parameter value increases; (d) a, the discriminating power of the item decreases; and (e) b, the item difficulty decreases, or the item becomes easier.

Goodness-of-Fit Evaluation

Another method of evaluating the results of IRT item calibrations is to assess a measure or measures of the *goodness-of-fit* of the data to the item characteristic curve, as defined by the item parameter estimates and the ability or trait estimates. There are many statistics or indices available that purport to measure the degree to which the $P_j(\theta)$

values, as hypothesized by the IRT model, actually fit the *proportion-correct* values at various levels of $\hat{\theta}_i$. Many of these indices are based on chi-square procedures; most of the acceptable statistics are defined and compared, via a computer simulation study, in an article by McKinley and Mills (1985).

Steps to Take in Conducting an IRT Calibration

Although the actual process of obtaining item parameter and ability parameter estimates depends on the specific situation, it is possible to list in general terms the basic steps one would follow in using IRT.

1. Initially hypothesize an IRT model for the data to be collected. This is a tentative model and may have to be changed if the data do not fit the model.
2. Collect the item response data.
3. Use one of the available IRT computer programs to estimate item parameters and ability parameters from these item responses.
4. Evaluate the model's fit to the data by observing (a) the standard errors of the estimates and (b) some overall index of fit, such as a chi-square statistic. If the fit is good, the estimates can be regarded as true parameters. If the fit is not good, hypothesize a new model and return to step 3.

It should be noted that some psychometricians (Wright & Masters, 1982) advocate that when there is a model-data mismatch or lack of fit, the data should be discarded *until* the model fits the data. Although there are usually some extreme outliers in almost any data set, most leading authorities suggest that if the data do not fit the hypothesized model, a more appropriate model should be used.

IRT Applications

The psychometric literature describes many applications of IRT to current assessment problems in the cognitive and affective behavior domains. Among these applications are those that may be useful to physical educators; these include item banking, computerized adaptive testing, mastery testing, attitude assessment, and the measurement of change.

Item Banking

The phrase *item banking* refers to the calibration and creation of large pools of test items for use in the construction of tests according to some predetermined specifications. The creation of **item banks** is actually a prerequisite for the implementation of IRT-based computerized adaptive tests and mastery tests.

Usually, good item banks contain many more items than the number required for any single test. It is important to note that item calibrations should periodically be performed again on the items within the pool to prevent item parameter *drift*—the tendency for item parameters to change over time (Rentz, 1978). The causes of these parameter changes can include compromising the item (i.e., deliberately or inadvertently releasing the items to future examinees), modifying the items, or changing the test administration procedures (e.g., penalizing for guessing).

In addition to the construction and administration of computerized adaptive and mastery tests, item banking makes it possible to construct tests that are more parallel in terms of the difficulty and discrimination distributions of the items. It is also useful in constructing tests that must meet certain minimum information requirements. IRT yields a measurement of how well the observed test score, X_i, provides information about the latent variable, θ_i. If X_i provides a lot of information so that θ_i is estimated very precisely, then the standard error of estimate of θ_i will be small. Conversely, if X_i provides very little information about θ_i, the standard error of estimate of θ_i will be large. It is possible to construct tests using this information approach. For example, one might specify that a test have better measurement (i.e., smaller standard errors) at the center of the ability range than at the extremes.

Computerized Adaptive Testing

Tests that consist of those test items that provide the most information for *each* examinee's ability can be constructed from calibrated item pools. Such tests are usually referred to as **tailored tests**, meaning that the items have been chosen specifically for the individual with $\theta = \theta_i$. The tests are tailored to each ability in that the items selected are those that provide the most precision at $\theta = \theta_i$. Of course θ_i is never known, and the problem becomes one of selecting items that yield the most precision at $\theta = \hat{\theta}_i$.

To begin a tailored test, examinees usually are administered items at random from those that maximize information around $\theta = .00$. Obviously no estimate of θ exists before the administration of the first item, so this first item is usually selected to be of medium difficulty at or near an average ability value. Because θ_i must be estimated from the item responses and because subsequent items are to be selected for administration on the basis of having an estimate of θ_i at hand, an impossible, circular problem in the application of tailored testing seems to exist. The problem can be handled if (a) the kth item is administered on the basis of the latest estimate of θ, say $\hat{\theta}_{k-1}$; (b) the estimate of θ is then updated to include the latest item response; and (c) based on this estimate of ability, $\hat{\theta}_k$, the next item is selected from the item pool as the one that provides the most information at $\theta = \hat{\theta}_k$. This process continues until some level of precision in the measurement of θ has been reached, or perhaps some maximum number of test items to be administered has been exceeded.

The many computations required between item administrations and the necessity of a search algorithm to locate the best test items in the pool make these tailored tests possible only with the aid of a computer. Hence, such tests are known as computerized adaptive tests (CAT). CAT administrations are **sequential tests**, meaning that the number of test items administered to examinees taking the test may vary.

The primary feature of a CAT is that the items tend to be neither too difficult nor too easy for each examinee. If the items have been calibrated using an IRT model for which $c = 0$, then those items in the pool that offer the examinee a 50-50 chance of selecting the correct response will maximize information for these examinees. For non-zero c values, this optimal difficulty level of the items is $\frac{1}{2}(1 + c)$ (Lord, 1980). Estimates of θ can be obtained using the usual MLE methods or by using a Bayes procedure developed especially for CAT situations by Owen (1975).

Mastery Testing

Traditional criterion-referenced or **mastery tests** require that a domain of educational objectives be measured by a domain of test items. Tests are constructed that theoretically represent the objectives domain with a sample of test items. A cutoff score, usually given as a proportion of test items to be answered correctly from the entire domain of test items, is set before testing. For example, in the typical 2-state mastery testing situation, a single cutoff score, π_c, is established. A k-item mastery test is administered to an examinee, and if the proportion of correct responses on the test from the examinee exceeds or equals π_c, then the examinee is classified as a master. Otherwise the examinee is classified as a nonmaster.

IRT methods offer a valuable tool in selecting items from the item domain in mastery testing. Assume that the n items in the pool, or the item domain, have been calibrated and reasonable item parameter estimates exist for each of these n items. A mastery test of k items is to be administered to a group of examinees. A single cutoff score, π_c, has been established, where π_c is the proportion of items in the domain that an examinee is expected to answer correctly in order to be classified as a master.

IRT methods can be used to select the optimal k items for this mastery test. The items are optimal in that they will be the k items from the n-item pool that yield the most information (i.e., the most precision) at the θ value that corresponds to π_c.

The advantage gained in using this IRT-based item selection process is that misclassification errors can be minimized around the cutting score. Testing plans that incorporate the setting of misclassification errors before testing using this IRT item selection plan are documented in Hambleton and DeGruijter (1983), Lord (1980), and Reckase (1983). The latter two are sequential testing plans based on sequential probability ratio tests (SPRT). All of these IRT-based approaches to item selection and test administration offer improvements over the random selection, construction, and observed-score evaluation of traditional mastery testing.

Attitude Assessment and the Measurement of Change

Two interesting uses of IRT pertain to (a) the assessment of attitude using a rating or Likert-type scale and (b) the measurement of latent-trait change over time. The models used in these examples and the discussion of these uses of IRT models are fairly simple. Readers interested in more complex models and applications should consult Andrich (1978b), Wright and Matthews (1982), or Fischer (1983).

Both of the examples presented here are based on a general form of the one-parameter model:

$$P_j(\theta_i) = \frac{e^{(\theta_i - \beta_j)}}{1 + e^{(\theta_i - \beta_j)}} \tag{11.6}$$

As in previous notation, the ith examinee's latent trait is represented by θ_i and the item parameter is denoted by β_j.

For the purposes of this discussion, each item offers an s-choice or s-category selection of scaled attitude intensity levels. An example of a 4-category scale would be: (1) strongly disagree, (2) disagree, (3) agree, and (4) strongly agree. At best such a scale is only ordinal, and although *points* or scores may be assigned to each of the s categories (e.g., 0, 1, 2, 3), the interpretation of any function of these item scores (e.g., total scale score) may be questionable if the interpretation is made on an interval scale. The typical practice of analyzing total-scale scores with statistical tests that assume an interval scale is also controversial.

Andrich (1978a, 1978b, 1979) has proposed an IRT model for rating scales based on the general one-parameter model given above. The application of such a model to attitude-scale data offers several advantages over traditional procedures. First, the data determine the step sizes between categories. This implies that if the scale reflects an interval measurement situation, the data will reflect this property. A second feature is that the attitude (trait) parameter for each respondent is estimated and interpreted on an interval scale, independent of the ordinal property of the observed total-scale score. Finally, a score for each θ_i is available for *each* category on *each* item. Other models that can be used in attitude assessment via rating scales have been proposed by Samejima (1969), Jansen (1986), and Masters (1982).

Similar models can be used to assess change. Fischer (1983) proposed what he terms a "family of linear logistic models" to measure the change of θ_i over time. In other words, one could estimate an individual ability before some treatment or intervention at time t_1 and after treatment at time t_2, and observe any systematic change in θ_i. The change in θ_i is assumed to be linear, but the effect of such a change on $P_j(\theta_i)$ from t_1 to t_2 is nonlinear. This feature of the models discussed in this chapter makes IRT the perfect vehicle for studying improvement in some sports skills, as discussed by Hale and Hale (1972).

Psychomotor Assessment

The preceding examples of applications of IRT to measurement problems have involved only the cognitive and affective behavior domains. It is reasonable to ask if IRT is useful in assessing psychomotor behaviors, such as sports skills, gross or fine motor tasks used in motor behavior laboratory settings, or fitness test items. This remains an unanswered question, although some preliminary research has been attempted (Costa, Safrit, & Cohen, 1987; Safrit, Costa, & Cohen, in press).

There are several differences, for example, between a written or cognitive test that consists of n separate items and a psychomotor skills test that consists of only a single test item repeated for n trials. The assumptions of most IRT models also include requirements about local independence, an assumption that may be violated within an n-attempts model of a single task. Finally, once a written test item has been calibrated, the usual assumption is that the test item does not change between administrations, making the item parameter estimates somewhat stable across different tests for different populations of examinees. Alternatively, a skill test item may vary considerably between testing administrations because of changes in the environment or in the equipment used to execute the skill. But this may not be important if the only purpose is to administer a test in order to estimate skill ability *at that moment* under those conditions.

The applicability and usefulness of IRT to these testing situations remains an open issue. Future researchers in measurement in physical education must answer these questions. However, models are already available for multiple-attempt, single-item tests (**MASI tests**, as opposed to the single-attempt, multiple-item, or **SAMI tests** discussed previously).

These IRT models for MASI tests have two things in common. First, the multiple attempts at a single task can be thought of as independent, dichotomously scored Bernoulli trials with a success probability, $P(\theta)$, constant across all trials. Second, this success probability, $P(\theta)$, approaches zero as θ approaches $-\infty$ (i.e., there is no lower, nonzero asymptote, because there is no random guessing).

Given these conditions, three models could be used in the MASI testing of psychomotor skills. The first is the binomial trials model discussed by Andrich (1978c) and Wright and Masters (1982). This model would be useful for fixed-length tests that consist of n attempts, each scored dichotomously as successful or unsuccessful (i.e., 1 or 0).

The second model, the Poisson model, discussed by Jansen (1986), Lord and Novick (1968), and again by Wright and Masters (1982), would be used in situations in which one is counting the number of successful attempts observed within a fixed time period. Here the number of successes is not bounded by a fixed number of attempts. The number of successfully performed sit-ups or push-ups observed in 60 seconds would fall into this MASI testing model.

The third model is the trials-to-criterion (TTC) or inverse binomial model discussed by Feldt and Spray (1983), Shifflett (1985), and Wetherill (1975). This is a sequential testing plan that requires the number of successful attempts, the *criterion* or c, to be established in advance. Examinees take this test by performing X attempts until c successes are observed. The models are all similar statistically, and in certain cases each can be shown to be a special case of the others.

Sequential Testing of Psychomotor Skills

Testing plans that allow an examinee to take only a certain number of trials of a psychomotor skill or a certain number of items on a written test, where the number of trials or items is a function of the examinee's ability, are referred to as *sequential testing plans*. Sequential tests are terminated by a *stopping rule*, which is determined by the precision required in the test.

Two sequential plans have already been discussed in this chapter. CAT administrations are IRT-based sequential plans in which the examinees receive only enough items to adequately estimate their latent trait or ability. The stopping rule for most CAT administrations is the observation of a minimal value of the standard error of $\hat{\theta}$.

The trials-to-criterion or TTC testing plan discussed previously is also sequential. It should be noted that the TTC plan is not adaptive because *all* examinees receive the same test item with the same difficulty. However, it is sequential in that those examinees with higher skills (i.e., larger values of θ) will reach c successes sooner than examinees with lower abilities.

The TTC plan has been studied rather extensively in conjunction with its use in psychomotor skills testing. Feldt and Spray (1983) compared the TTC testing plan to the more traditional binomial or fixed-length plan and showed that the latter produced higher values of traditional, overall test reliability for most true score distributions. TTC plans were preferred for certain negatively skewed true score distributions.

Spray, Sorenson, and Hooper (1985) illustrated an empirical procedure for determining an optimal value of c for a TTC MASI test and also presented an example of the TTC approach in the validation of the sensitivity of a psychomotor test to the discrimination of the skill levels of children in elementary school. Shifflett (1985) compared several methods of estimating the internal consistency of a test administered via the TTC plan and reported that an unbiased estimator similar to the binomial model's KR-21 equation performed better than Cronbach's alpha or parallel forms estimators.

It should be pointed out that in all of these studies, TTC was used *only* in a classical, strong true score theory setting. Estimation of latent abilities, θ, and item difficulty was not considered. In retrospect, the usefulness of the TTC plan may be with its use in MASI IRT testing. Future research using TTC plans probably should incorporate the estimation of θ and item difficulty for the reasons outlined in the beginning of this chapter.

Another sequential testing plan, the sequential probability ratio test (SPRT), has also been used for testing psychomotor skills. Shifflett, Hooper, Jackson, and Spray (1982) showed how the SPRT procedure could be used to administer a badminton short-serve test. And Safrit, Wood, Ehlert, Hooper, and Patterson (1985) applied the SPRT to a golf skills test.

Unlike the TTC plan, which is primarily an estimation procedure (Wetherill, 1975), the SPRT, first presented by Abraham Wald (1947), was designed to test a simple statistical hypothesis. For example, a simple hypothesis involving a coin toss might be that the true probability of observing a single toss as *heads* is .5 versus the alternate choice, .1. Stated another way, if π is the probability of observing *heads* then

$H_0: \pi_0 = .5$

versus

$H_1: \pi_1 = .1.$

If ten tosses have been made and ten *tails* have been recorded, how likely is the observation of ten *tails* under H_0 versus H_1? Because likelihood is simply the product of the individual probabilities, under H_0 the probability of *tails* is $1 - \pi_0$, or .5. The likelihood of ten *tails* would be $(.5)^{10}$, or approximately .001. The likelihood of ten *tails* under H_1 is $(1 - \pi_1)^{10}$ or $(.9)^{10}$, which is approximately .349. In other words, after ten tosses, the evidence of observing ten straight *tails* favors H_1 over H_0. The quantitative evidence of H_1 over H_0 can be written as the ratio of the two likelihoods, $L(\pi_1)$ and $L(\pi_0)$, or $L(\pi_1)/L(\pi_0)$. This is referred to as a *likelihood ratio*.

One might ask if there could be some number of coin tosses less than ten that would still provide overwhelming evidence of π_1 over π_0. For example, even after only three tosses, $L(\pi_0)$ is .125 and $L(\pi_1)$ is .729. The likelihood ratio .729/.125 is greater than 5.8, so that H_1 is almost six times more likely to be true than H_0. Is another toss necessary, or is the evidence sufficient to choose H_1 after only three tosses?

The SPRT procedure developed by Wald offers a test of $L(\pi_1)/L(\pi_0)$ following each trial. If the usual error rates in hypothesis testing are set before starting the testing, so that

Prob (choosing $\pi_1|\pi_0$ is true) $= \alpha$

and

Prob (choosing $\pi_0|\pi_1$ is true) $= \beta$,

then SPRT establishes two values, B and A, where

$B = \beta/(1 - \alpha)$

and

$A = (1 - \beta)/\alpha.$

If after each trial the likelihood ratio is greater than B but less than A, then another trial must be taken. However, testing may terminate if the likelihood ratio is (a) smaller than B or (b) greater than A. The decision will be in favor of H_0 for (a) and H_1 for (b). In actual testing situations, H_0 and H_1 usually represent upper and lower bounds for cutoff proportions in mastery testing situations. As soon as π_0, π_1, α, and β are established, the stopping rule for the SPRT is determined.

The SPRT procedure has been used in a classical test theory sense, in that only observed, total test scores are recorded. It is possible to use SPRT in an IRT setting with adaptive testing. Reckase (1983) showed how the SPRT procedure could be used adaptively to make pass-fail decisions and to estimate θ with test items that have been calibrated using the 3-PLM.

The use of these two sequential testing plans, TTC and SPRT, represented early attempts by physical education measurement specialists to incorporate *one* feature of adaptive testing (i.e., variable length as a function of ability) into the testing of psychomotor skills. The other features of adaptive testing, such as those that involve item selection based on (a) the match between examinee ability and item information and (b) ability-difficulty estimation, need to be incorporated into these sequential plans in the future. Only then will the *full* benefits of adaptive, sequential testing be available for the measurement of psychomotor skills.

Conclusion

Item response theory offers several advantages over the traditional or classical test theory approach to measurement. Examinees' abilities are measured on an interval scale that is *test-free* and not dictated by the items on the test, and item characteristics are defined as *population-free*, completely apart from the examinees who take that item. These so-called invariance principles make it possible to describe the interaction of a single examinee with a single test item by way of an IRT model. The most common IRT models are the logistic one-, two-, and three-parameter models. The models are completely described by their item parameters (for example, the a, b, and c parameters in the three-parameter logistic model).

Item parameters and examinees' abilities are estimated from the actual item response data. Parameter estimates, usually obtained by the method of maximum likelihood estimation, are used to construct item banks and to administer computerized adaptive tests and mastery tests. The estimates can also be used to measure change in an examinee's ability over time, to measure attitude, and to estimate examinees' psychomotor abilities in multiple-attempt, single-item skills tests (MASI tests).

The IRT-based procedures can be compared with two sequential testing plans used to test psychomotor skills: the trials-to-criterion (TTC) test and the sequential probability ratio test (SPRT). The sequential plans, while somewhat adaptive to the individual needs of each examinee in terms of test length, have yet to incorporate the features of a truly adaptive, IRT approach to measurement.

References

Andrich, D. (1978a). A rating formulation for ordered response categories. *Psychometrika*, 43, 561–573.

Andrich, D. (1978b). Application of a psychometric rating model to ordered categories which are scored with successive integers. *Applied Psychological Measurement*, 2, 581–594.

Andrich, D. (1978c). A binomial latent trait model for the study of Likert-style attitude questionnaires. *British Journal of Mathematical and Statistical Psychology*, 31, 84–98.

Andrich, D. (1979). A model for contingency tables having an ordered response classification. *Biometrics*, 35, 403–415.

Costa, M.G., Safrit, M.J., & Cohen, A.S. (1987). *The appropriateness of two item response theory models for measurement of motor behavior.* Manuscript submitted for publication.

Feldt, L.S., & Spray, J.A. (1983). A theory-based comparison of the reliabilities of fixed-length and trials-to-criterion scoring of physical education skills tests. *Research Quarterly for Exercise and Sport, 54*, 324–329.

Fischer, G.H. (1983). Some latent trait models for measuring change in qualitative observations. In D.J. Weiss (Ed.), *New horizons in testing: Latent trait test theory and computerized adaptive testing* (pp. 309–329). New York: Academic Press.

Hale, P.W., & Hale, R.M. (1972). Comparison of student improvement by exponential modification of test-retest scores. *Research Quarterly, 43*, 113–120.

Hambleton, R.K., & DeGruijter, D.N.M. (1983). Application of item response models to criterion-referenced test item selection. *Journal of Educational Measurement, 20*, 355–367.

Jansen, M.G.H. (1986). A Bayesian version of Rasch's multiplicative Poisson model for the number of errors of an achievement test. *Journal of Educational Statistics, 11*, 147–160.

Lord, F.M. (1980). *Applications of item response theory to practical testing problems.* Hillsdale, NJ: Lawrence Erlbaum Associates.

Lord, F.M. (1983). Small N justifies Rasch model. In D.J. Weiss (Ed.), *New horizons in testing: Latent trait test theory and computerized adaptive testing* (pp. 51–61). New York: Academic Press.

Lord, F.M., & Novick, M.R. (1968). *Statistical theories of mental test scores.* Reading, MA: Addison-Wesley.

Masters, G.N. (1982). A Rasch model for partial credit scoring. *Psychometrika, 47*, 149–174.

McKinley, R.L., & Mills, C.N. (1985). A comparison of several goodness-of-fit statistics. *Applied Psychological Measurement, 9*, 49–57.

Mislevy, R.J., & Bock, R.D. (1984). *BILOG, maximum likelihood item analysis and test scoring: Logistic model.* Mooresville, IN: Scientific Software, Inc.

Owen, R.J. (1975). A Bayesian sequential procedure for quantal response in the context of adaptive mental testing. *Journal of the American Statistical Association, 70*, 351–356.

Reckase, M.D. (1983). A procedure for decision making using tailored testing. In D.J. Weiss (Ed.), *New horizons in testing: Latent trait test theory and computerized adaptive testing* (pp. 237–255). New York: Academic Press.

Rentz, R.R. (1978, March). *Monitoring the quality of an item pool calibrated by the Rasch model.* Paper presented at the meeting of the National Council on Measurement in Education, Toronto, Ontario, Canada.

Safrit, M.J., Costa, M.G., & Cohen, A.S. (in press). Item response theory and the measurement of motor behavior. *Research Quarterly for Exercise and Sport.*

Safrit, M.J., Wood, T.M., Ehlert, S.A., Hooper, L.M., & Patterson, P. (1985). The application of sequential probability ratio testing to a test of motor skill. *Research Quarterly for Exercise and Sport, 56*, 58–65.

Samejima, F. (1969). Estimation of latent ability using a response pattern of graded scores. *Psychometrika Monograph, 34*(17).

Shifflett, B. (1985). Reliability estimation for trials-to-criterion testing. *Research Quarterly for Exercise and Sport, 56*, 266–274.

Shifflett, B., Hooper, L., Jackson, S., & Spray, J. (1982, April). *A sequential criterion-referenced badminton short-serve test*. Paper presented at a meeting of the AAH-PERD National Convention, Houston.

Spray, J.A. (1987). Recent developments in measurement and possible applications to the measurement of psychomotor behavior. *Research Quarterly for Exercise and Sport, 58*, 203–209.

Spray, J.A., Sorenson, C., & Hooper, L.M. (1985). Inverse sampling procedures for criterion-referenced testing of motor or sport skills in the elementary school. *Motor Skills: Theory Into Practice, 8*, 103–112.

Wald, A. (1947). *Sequential analysis*. New York: Wiley.

Wetherill, G.B. (1975). *Sequential methods in statistics* (2nd ed.). London: Chapman and Hall.

Wingersky, M.S., Barton, M.A., & Lord, F.M. (1982). *LOGIST user's guide*. Princeton, NJ: Educational Testing Service.

Wright, B.D., & Masters, G.N. (1982). *Rating scale analysis*. Chicago: Mesa Press.

Supplementary Readings

Allen, M.J., & Yen, W.M. (1979). *Introduction to measurement theory*. Belmont, CA: Wadsworth.

Andrich, D. (1988). *Rasch models for measurement*. Newbury Park, CA: Sage.

Hambleton, R.K., & Swaminathan, H. (1985). *Item response theory: Principles and applications*. Boston: Kluwer-Nijhoff.

Kane, M.T. (1987). On the use of IRT models with judgmental standard setting procedures. *Journal of Educational Measurement, 24*, 333–345.

SECTION

V

Applied Measurement and Evaluation

In the current era of *accountability*, a question of great import in school and nonschool settings concerns the extent to which program objectives are being met. Traditionally physical educators have outlined program objectives in three domains: cognitive, affective, and psychomotor. This section addresses testing and measurement in each domain. In addition, attention is given to methods of program evaluation and to the use of computer technology in measurement and testing.

Chapters 12, 13 and 14 focus on the application of measurement in the cognitive, affective, and pychomotor domains. In chapter 12, Dale Mood presents a persuasive discussion linking the purposes and underlying meaning of knowledge tests to the use of appropriate test construction procedures. Similarly Jack Nelson, in chapter 13, targets the importance of constructing affective tests with proven validity and reliability, pointing out the pitfalls in constructing affective tests and presenting measures of affect in physical education and exercise science that were constructed using sound measurement procedures. Larry Hensley and Whitfield East present in chapter 14 an overview of psychomotor testing in the instructional process, with emphasis on significant trends in measuring sports skills, physical fitness, and motor abilities. These authors also, through a discussion of grading practices in physical education, bring home the significance of the material presented in chapters 12 and 13 in evaluating student achievement.

Accountability has little meaning unless the quality of programs can be assessed. In chapter 15, Rosemary McGee brings a wealth of knowledge and experience to an excellent discussion of program evaluation, ranging from descriptions of various evaluation models to steps in the evaluation process and measurement considerations in program evaluation.

Two of the greatest barriers to the widespread use of appropriate testing, measurement, and evaluation practices in field settings are the time-consuming nature and quantitative complexity of these taks. In chapter 16, Harry King examines the application of computer technology to these and other problems in testing and measurement, discussing topics that range from computerized data collection and data reduction to the decision making process.

CHAPTER 12

Measurement Methodology for Knowledge Tests

Dale P. Mood
University of Colorado

The measurement of **knowledge** is an *indirect* process. Knowledge is not tangible. It cannot be weighed or assessed through the use of some mechanical instrument. The use of a written test to measure knowledge is based on the assumption that responses made to a written item reflect to some degree the amount of knowledge achieved. Thus it is important to understand the relationship between the tasks presented on a test and the mental process that the test is intended to measure. The indirect nature of this measurement process also has implications for the methods of assessing its efficacy.

The collection of items comprising a written test must be considered a sample of an infinite number of possibilities that could be assembled. Thus, knowledge testing is an *incomplete* process. The worth of any sample is directly proportional to its representativeness of the population from which it is drawn. The written-test constructor must select an appropriate set of questions depending on the knowledge to be assessed. Procedures have been developed, such as the use of a **table of specifications**, to facilitate this important process.

Typically scores on a knowledge test reflect an interval scale. That is, although the scoring procedure provides equally spaced units along a scale, there is no true zero point. Because any particular written test is but one of an infinite number of possible samples, a score of zero does not necessarily indicate the examinee has no knowledge of the content measured by the test. Thus ratios cannot be constructed from written test results (i.e., it is not correct to state that an examinee who scored 40 has twice as much knowledge as another who scored 20). Knowledge tests thus provide *relative* measurements that are situation specific and must be interpreted in relation to some reference group. A particular written-test score has no inherent meaning of its own. It takes on meaning only when compared with other scores and when the nature of the examinees is known (Marshall & Hales, 1971).

The purpose for constructing and administering a knowledge test has important ramifications for its interpretation. Ebel and Frisbie (1986) identified three broad categories encompassing the reasons knowledge test scores are obtained: (a) to compare an individual's performance to a particular content area, (b) to compare performance with other individuals in a group, or (c) to compare performance with a cutoff score. The first category is characterized by the desire to compare an individual's performance to a precisely defined group of abilities or area of knowledge. The second category, commonly labeled **norm-referenced**, is applicable when maximizing the amount of discrimination among examinees with respect to the knowledge being assessed. **Criterion-referenced tests**, the third category, are most often used to classify individuals as masters and nonmasters or as having passed or failed on the basis of the score achieved. This type of test is also referred to as a **mastery test**. These introductory measurement concepts are not discussed in detail here; however, it is important to understand that the interpretation of a knowledge test score is influenced by several measurement concerns in addition to the purpose of the test. The two most important knowledge test qualities are **reliability** and **validity**. These are usually, though not exclusively, assessed through statistical procedures.

Reliability of a test is examined by assessing its consistency. A perfectly reliable test would yield identical results at every administration, assuming no changes took place among the examinees tested. Unfortunately perfectly reliable tests of any kind, and in particular knowledge tests, exist only in theory because of the inevitable presence of measurement error. The sources and consequences of measurement error are a major focus of the remainder of this chapter.

Reliability of Knowledge Tests

Importance

The correlation between a set of knowledge test scores for a group of examinees and a second set of knowledge test scores on an equivalent test obtained independently from the same group of examinees is called a *reliability coefficient* (see chapter 3). This coefficient is an important statistical index of the quality of a written test, because a measuring device that is not reliable, whatever other attributes it may have, is worth very little. As necessary as reliability is to the quality of a knowledge test, it is not a sufficient condition. A highly reliable test may measure precisely some trivial or inconsequential attribute. For this reason test validity (discussed later) must also be considered. Students, teachers, and researchers should examine reliability evidence when making important decisions on the basis of scores from knowledge tests—especially as the seriousness of the decision increases.

An examination of the procedure to estimate reliability reveals several important implications. First, reliability changes when it is assessed under varying conditions, i.e., a test does not have only one reliability but rather this quality is situation specific. Second, the statistic used to express test reliability can be obtained through the use of various procedures (e.g., correlation, ANOVA). Thus interpretation of a reliability coefficient is dependent on knowledge of the properties of the correlation coefficient. For example, because it reflects relative rather than absolute agreement between pairs of scores, the size of the differences between one individual's two scores as compared with the differences among various individuals' scores affects the magnitude of the coefficient. If small changes occur between scores for one individual when compared with larger differences among examinees, the coefficient will be relatively high; the opposite relationship will produce a low coefficient. Thus if the range of talent in a group of examinees is small, the reliability coefficient would be expected to be smaller than if the range of talent is large. Finally, the definition of reliability indicates that to calculate a reliability coefficient it is necessary to obtain an equivalent and independent measure of the same characteristic for each examinee. The approaches to accomplishing this task produce various methods of estimating reliability.

Methods of Estimating Reliability

The usual result of a knowledge test is the assignment of a score to each examinee based on the number of correct responses. This is called the *observed score* (X) and can be thought of theoretically of consisting of two parts: a *true score* (T) and an *error score* (E). This relationship is expressed as:

$$X = T + E \tag{12.1}$$

It represents the essence of a conceptional domain known as classical test theory. The implications of classical test theory for the estimation of reliability are discussed in chapter 3 and chapter 11. If classical test theory assumptions are accepted, it is possible to partition the variance of the obtained scores into two parts. It will be equal to the sum of the true score variance and the error score variance:

$$\sigma_X^2 = \sigma_T^2 + \sigma_E^2 \tag{12.2}$$

where σ_X^2 is the variance of the observed scores, σ_T^2 is the variance of the true scores, and σ_E^2 is the variance of the error scores.

Reliability can be defined as the ratio of the true score variance to the obtained score variance:

$$r = \frac{\sigma_T^2}{\sigma_X^2}$$
(12.3)

There are several sources of measurement error in knowledge tests, and many attempts have been made to categorize them. This is complex because factors contributing to error variance in some situations may contribute to true score variance in others. Also, all potential sources of error are not present in every test situation. Because various methods used for calculating a reliability coefficient take different error sources into account, it is important to identify which reliability coefficient has been employed. In this section three potential error sources—the examinee, the test, and the scorer—are discussed, and the methods for calculating the appropriate reliability coefficient are presented.

Examinee reliability. The most obvious way to assess test consistency is to administer the same test twice and calculate the correlation coefficient for the resulting two sets of scores. This is called **test-retest** reliability. Although use of this technique is logical and appropriate for traits that remain stable over time, it is not recommended for examining the reliability of knowledge tests for several reasons. There is the problem of how much time should elapse between test administrations. If too much time is permitted, score changes may be a result of learning, and thus true differences might be interpreted as error. In addition, it is unlikely that examinees' answers on the second administration of the same test would be independent of their first answers. Remembering their first answers would undoubtedly influence their second response, especially if the interval between test administrations was short. Administering the same test again does not provide evidence about possible consistency had a different sample of questions been selected. To provide this type of evidence, two separate but similar forms of a test must be constructed. If the two forms are built around the same table of specifications and if each examinee completes both forms of the test, the correlation coefficient between the resulting two sets of scores is called the **equivalent forms** reliability coefficient. With this procedure almost all possible sources of measurement error can influence the resulting scores, and thus a high equivalent-forms reliability coefficient is very meaningful. The makers of commercial standardized tests usually employ this technique for estimating reliability. Unfortunately there is rarely time either to administer the same test twice (test-retest) or to construct a second, similar test (equivalent forms) solely for the purpose of estimating reliability. Therefore, other techniques have been devised involving a single administration of the test and the use of scores from various divisions of the test to estimate reliability.

Test reliability (internal consistency). If it is possible to divide a test into two comparable halves, the **split-halves** technique can be used to estimate reliability. For each examinee two scores are obtained, one for each half of the test, and a correlation coefficient is calculated from the two sets of scores for the group. If pairs of items can be located on the test that are comparable in content, difficulty, and discriminating ability, two roughly equivalent halves of the test can be formed by putting one of each pair of items on each half of the test. Another common procedure is to simply split the test by placing odd numbered items on one half and even numbered items on the other. Once the correlation between the two halves is obtained, a further correction is required. Because reliability is a function of test length and because the correlation obtained using the split-halves procedure is based on half as many items as the whole test, this reliability estimate should be corrected using the Spearman-Brown prophecy formula. This equation can be used to estimate the reliability of a lengthened or shortened test given the reliability of the original test. In the case of the split-halves procedure, this equation takes the following form:

$$r_{(est)} = \frac{2\ r_{(obt)}}{1 + r_{(obt)}} \qquad\qquad (12.4)$$

where $r_{(est)}$ is the estimate of the lengthened test and $r_{(obt)}$ is the reliability of the half test.

For example, if the correlation between the two halves of a test is .60, the estimate of the reliability for the entire test is:

$$r_{(est)} = \frac{2\ (.60)}{1 + .60} = \frac{1.2}{1.6} = .75$$

If a reliability estimate is desired for a dichotomously scored test, that is, each answer is scored 1 if correct and 0 if not correct, another procedure can be used called the *KR20*. It is so named because it was the 20th equation in an article by Kuder and Richardson (1937). Any test can be split in half using many combinations of items, with the number of combinations increasing dramatically as the test length increases. Mathematically KR20 yields a reliability estimate that is the average of all possible split-half correlations that could be calculated for a test. Because the average of a set of numbers is always smaller than those values above the mean, KR20 is a conservative reliability estimate. The equation for the KR20 is as follows:

$$r = \frac{k}{k-1}\left[1 - \frac{\Sigma pq}{S^2}\right] \qquad\qquad (12.5)$$

where k is the number of items on the test, p is the proportion of correct responses to a test item, q is the proportion of incorrect responses to a test item ($p + q$ always equals 1), and S^2 is the variance of the test scores.

A disadvantage of KR20 is the requirement of calculating the values of p and q for each test item. An alternate equation, KR21, can be used if it can be assumed that the test items do not differ greatly in difficulty. The KR21 equation is as follows:

$$r = \frac{k}{k-1}\left[1 - \frac{\overline{X}\ (k-\overline{X})}{k\ S^2}\right] \qquad\qquad (12.6)$$

where k is the number of items on the test, $\overline{X}$ is the mean score on the test, and S^2 is the variance of the test scores.

For example, the reliability estimate for a 60-item test having a mean of 40 and a standard deviation of 5 is

$$r = \frac{60}{59}\left[1 - \frac{40(60-40)}{60(5)^2}\right] = 1.02\left[1 - \frac{800}{1500}\right] = .48$$

The KR21 is an underestimate of the reliability coefficient when the test items vary widely in difficulty, but its computational ease makes it a valuable statistical tool.

If a test is not scored dichotomously, it is possible to estimate a reliability coefficient using Cronbach's alpha (1951). This statistic is often used to examine the reliability of questionnaires that usually provide ordinal data. The KR20 is a special case of this coefficient. The equation is

$$\alpha = \frac{k}{k-1}\left[\frac{S_X^2 - \Sigma S_j^2}{S_X^2}\right] \qquad (12.7)$$

where k is the number of items on the test, S_j^2 is the variance of a test item, and S_X^2 is the variance of the total scores on the test.

Analysis of variance may also be used to obtain Cronbach's alpha coefficient to estimate the reliability of a test (or questionnaire) if the data are considered to be interval in nature. This is accomplished by obtaining the summary table for a two-way analysis of variance, where each examinee is considered to be a level of one independent variable and each test item is a level of the other factor. The dependent variable is the score each examinee received on each item. Coefficient alpha is calculated from

$$\alpha = \frac{MS_s - MS_i}{MS_s} \qquad (12.8)$$

where α is coefficient alpha, MS_s is the mean square for examinees, and MS_i is the mean square for interaction.

The hypothetical data in Table 12.1 illustrate the use of the above two equations to obtain α and to confirm their equivalence. For convenience of illustration, these data are abbreviated in number of examinees and test items.

Using equation 12.7:

$$\alpha = \frac{4}{3}\left[\frac{23.14 - 7.69}{23.14}\right] = (1.33)(.668) = .89$$

Using equation 12.8:

$$\alpha = \frac{6.94 - .76}{6.94} = \frac{6.18}{6.94} = .89$$

Scorer reliability. If a test is scored independently by two different examiners, the correlation between the resulting two sets of scores provides evidence of the objectivity

Table 12.1   Hypothetical Data to Illustrate the Calculation of Coefficient Alpha

Examinees	Scores for 4 Items				
	1	2	3	4	Total
A	5	4	5	6	20
B	2	4	3	2	11
C	5	6	5	6	22
D	7	6	5	7	25
E	3	4	4	3	14
F	6	6	5	4	21
Total	28	30	27	28	113

Values required for equation 12.7
$k = 4$, $S_X^2 = 23.14$, $\Sigma S_j^2 = 7.69$

Values required for Equation 12.8

Source of Variation	df	SS	MS
Among Examinees	5	34.71	6.94
Among Items	3	0.79	.26
Interaction	15	11.46	.76
Total	23		

(i.e., scorer reliability) of the scoring procedure. This correlation is typically more important for essay tests than for objective tests, because the scoring procedure for the former type is more open to variability.

Summary of methods of estimating reliability. Methods of estimating test reliability are not equivalent, because they account for different types of error. The test-retest method does not include possible errors from a poor sampling of potential test items but does reflect errors stemming from variations in test administrations and day-to-day changes in examinees. The internal-consistency methods (split-halves, KR20, KR21, alpha) do not reflect item sampling errors nor day-to-day changes in examinees or test administration. They are, however, practical measures of how similarly examinees perform on different but similar test items. The equivalent forms reliability coefficient reflects errors of sampling, day-to-day variation, and variations in the testing environment, and thus is probably the most complete and valuable method. It is not, however, a very practical approach in most situations. Scorer reliability is an assessment of the objectivity of the scoring procedure and does not reflect test or examinee reliability.

Standard Error of Measurement

When a knowledge test is administered and scored, the only data available are the obtained scores, which almost surely contain some measurement error for some or all examinees. A reliability coefficient can provide an indication of how much (or how little) error is present overall but not for each individual examinee. The error associated with an individual's obtained score can be explained using a statistic called the *standard error of measurement*, which is actually the standard deviation of the error scores. Calculation and interpretation of this statistic are described in chapter 3.

Factors Affecting Written Test Reliability

Test reliability is situation specific, because several factors influence its value. Some factors are related to the test items, some to test administration, and some to characteristics of the examinees. If the test items are homogeneous in content, highly discriminating, and of middle difficulty, the test will be more reliable than if the items are heterogeneous in content, only moderately discriminating, and of quite varied difficulty. If a test is long and administered in such a way that few examinees finish it (a **speed test**), it will be more reliable than if it is short and nearly all examinees complete it. Finally, if the examinees have a wide range of talent in the area being measured, the test will be more reliable than if the group is homogeneous in ability.

Test items. A 50-item test constructed to measure basketball rules will almost always be more reliable than a 50-item test covering sports rules. Examinees who know basketball rules well would score high consistently; on a more general test, different examinees could do well on some parts and poorly on others, resulting in little overall discrimination among examinees and leading to inconsistent (unreliable) evaluation.

This chapter discusses item discrimination and difficulty later in detail, but from logic it is obvious that if a test is made up of highly discriminating items (those that are effective in identifying who does or does not understand a particular concept) then the test will discriminate among examinees. Such a test would be likely to place the examinees in the same order if retested, thus increasing its reliability. If every examinee answers an item correctly (or incorrectly) the item has contributed nothing to the reliability of the test. If approximately equal numbers of good and poor students answer a question correctly, the question will not contribute much to the discrimination among students. However, this is not common. It is more often the case that a larger proportion of the correctly responding examinees are the better examinees and a larger proportion of the incorrectly responding examinees are the poorer examinees. The difficulty of the item is related to its potential discrimination power and thus to the test reliability.

Test administration. A special case of the Spearman-Brown prophecy formula was presented earlier to estimate test reliability when test length is doubled. The general form of this formula is

$$r_{(est)} = \frac{N \cdot r_{(obt)}}{(N-1)(r_{(obt)}) + 1} \tag{12.9}$$

where $r_{(est)}$ is the estimate of reliability of the lengthened test, N is the number of times a test is lengthened, and $r_{(obt)}$ is the reliability of the original test.

For example, if an original test containing 10 items has a reliability of .40, adding 20 more items (thus tripling the length of the test) having statistical characteristics similar to the initial 10 items would yield a new estimated reliability of

$$r_{(est)} = \frac{3(.40)}{2(.40) + 1} = \frac{1.20}{1.80} = .67$$

Of course, this equation is based on the assumption that the increased test length would not alter the examinees' approach to the test in some important way (e.g., boredom, fatigue).

Speed tests—those containing more items than possibly can be completed in the time allotted—generally have higher reliabilities than nonspeed tests, which are completed by almost all the examinees. For the most part this increase in reliability is spurious, because speed-test scores are a function not only of the examinees' ability to complete items correctly but also how fast they can work. To demonstrate why this reliability is spurious, consider the result of using one of the split-halves methods to estimate reliability. The two estimates of speed (one-half the number of items answered) necessarily turn out to be identical if an even number of questions were completed and different by one if an uneven number of questions were answered. When this speed factor is intermingled with the number of correct responses on each half of the test in the reliability calculations, the results are spuriously high. Because of the problem with reliability estimates and the necessity of applying a correction-for-guessing formula to speed tests (to prevent a test-wise student from marking answers to the otherwise uncompleted portion of the test and thus increasing his or her score by some factor close to chance on those final items), speed tests usually are not recommended except in specific situations.

Range of talent. A hypothetical test constructed for 3rd-grade students would be expected to have a higher reliability if administered to a group of K–6 students than if administered to a group of 3rd-grade students. This is because the 6th-grade students on the average should consistently score higher than the 5th-grade students and so on down to the kindergartners. If administered again, the test would be expected to place students fairly consistently in the same relative order. It is more difficult for this pattern to occur if the range of talent is smaller and the scores are thus closer together. With a narrow range of talent, a small score difference from one administration of the test to another could alter an examinee's relative position to a greater extent than when a wide range of talent is present. Mathematically this effect can be demonstrated by defining reliability as the ratio of true score variance to obtained score variance. If the range of talent is increased, true score variance should increase but measurement errors should not be affected. Table 12.2 shows reliability estimate increases for a hypothetical situation.

Reliability of Criterion-Referenced Tests

Although variations exist, the typical criterion-referenced test has a cutoff score; examinees scoring at or above this point are termed masters and those below it, nonmasters. The reliability of such a test is a function of the consistency with which

Table 12.2   An Example to Demonstrate How Range of Talent Affects Reliability Estimate

Smaller Range of Talent	Wider Range of Talent
$S_T^2 = 20$	$S_T^2 = 30$
$S_E^2 = 5$	$S_E^2 = 5$
$S_X^2 = 25$	$S_X^2 = 35$
$r = \dfrac{20}{25} = .800$	$r = \dfrac{30}{35} = .857$

examinees are classified rather than with their actual scores. Chapter 7 discusses the reliability of criterion-referenced tests.

Validity of Knowledge Tests

Validity is defined as the degree to which a test measures what it is intended to measure. Knowledge tests usually try to measure some cognitive ability. The precision with which the cognitive ability is measured is the concept of reliability previously discussed. Thus reliability is a necessary, though not sufficient, condition to achieve validity. However, if the test does not measure what it is intended to measure (no matter how reliably it may measure something), it is useless. The concept of written-test validity appears to be quite straightforward, but it is a rather complex topic and has been the center of discussion for many years.

Like reliability, validity must be thought of as being situation specific. In other words, a test may be more or less valid in one situation than another, and it is necessary to examine validity from the perspective of the interpretation of the test scores. For example, a test that is determined to be a valid measure of an examinee's current mathematical ability may or may not be a valid predictor of future achievement in this area. Several types of evidence can be collected to examine the validity of a test. Typically this evidence is categorized as **content-related validity**, **criterion-related validity**, or **construct-related validity**. Refer to chapter 2 for a discussion of the type of evidence used to examine criterion- and construct-related validity.

Content Validity

The concept of validity, like reliability, applies to all types of measurement. When the measurements are derived from a knowledge test, the most important evidence of validity is that of content validity. There is some controversy regarding the definition and even the existence of the concept of content validity. The traditional view holds that if it were absolutely certain that the content of the test accurately represented the domain in question, other types of validity evidence would be superfluous. Unfortunately, content-related evidence is subjective in nature and somewhat difficult to obtain, except through a careful inspection of the test items and a clearly defined goal for the purpose of the test. In fact, difficulty in determining acceptable definitions of content validity produces various conclusions about this concept.

Fitzpatrick (1983), in a review of various definitions of content validity, concluded that no appropriate rationale for defining this term exists, and therefore it should be deleted from the vocabulary of test specialists. She described content validity according to elements dealing with (a) the sampling adequacy of test content; (b) the sampling adequacy of test responses, i.e., whether the responses required of an examinee reflect the behaviors that the test has been designed to assess; (c) the relevance of test content to a content universe, i.e., whether the *important* elements of the universe are measured; (d) the relevance of test responses to a behavioral universe, i.e., whether the test responses are *important* to whatever is being measured; (e) the clarity of content domain definitions; and (f) the technical quality of test items. Fitzpatrick argued that each of these notions should be seen as definitions of concepts other than content validity. She suggested that sampling adequacy of test content should be associated with the term *content representativeness*. Relevance of test content should be called just that; *content relevance* and the clarity of domain definition, while important, should be discussed under the term *domain clarity* and not *content validity*. The sampling adequacy of test responses and the relevance of these responses were viewed as dimensions of construct validity and not content validity. Finally, although the technical quality of test items was essential, it affected all aspects of a test and should not be considered to reflect any form of validity.

Most traditional test specialists would probably agree with Fitzpatrick's conclusions regarding sampling adequacy of test response, relevance of test responses, and technical quality issues. However, while it may be more an issue of semantics than substance, the notions of sampling adequacy of test response, relevance of test content, and clarity of domain definition are still held by many to be the fundamental aspects of content validity. This was clearly expressed by Ebel (1983), when he argued that content validity should be thought of as *intrinsic rational validity*. Evidence for its existence should consist of a detailed and specific rationale for the test consisting of a definition of the ability to be measured, a clear description of the tasks to be assessed, and an explanation of the reasons for using these tasks to measure such an ability. If these are available, he contended, experts in the subject matter of the test will be able to judge its worth; ultimately expert judgment determines the validity of a test.

Validity of Criterion-Referenced Tests

Validity of a criterion-referenced test is reflected by the degree to which scores on the test can be used to infer an examinee's placement on the criterion measure. As with norm-referenced tests, various types of validity evidence exist for criterion-referenced tests; they can be evaluated both logically and empirically. Techniques for and information about assessing the validity of criterion-referenced tests are contained in chapter 6.

Selection of a cutoff score to separate masters from nonmasters is embedded in the validity issue. Various procedures, none of which are entirely satisfactory because of the many variables to be considered, have been suggested to establish a cutoff score. Some of these include selecting: (a) the score at the overlap point of the two frequency polygons, representing the performances of two groups previously selected by some experts as being masters and nonmasters; (b) a measure of central tendency for a group that experts have judged to be borderline between master and nonmaster; and (c) the score that represents the 25th percentile of all those who have passed the course. Another approach is to have a group of experts examine the test and make judgments about the score to be expected from a minimally competent examinee.

Nedelsky (1954) and Angoff (1971) suggested similar procedures, involving experts judging which incorrect responses for each multiple-choice item minimally competent examinees could eliminate. The cutoff score is then determined by computing the expected-chance score for the test, assuming the minimally competent examinees will guess blindly at the remaining responses. Another somewhat similar technique was proposed by Ebel (1972), where judges are first required to categorize questions in terms of difficulty and importance, then decide the percentage that minimally competent examinees should pass in the various categories; finally the cutoff score is determined from these percentages, calculating the total number of items that these students should complete correctly on the whole test. Ebel's procedure may be used with other than multiple-choice tests.

The accuracy of the cutoff score for a particular purpose is refered to as *validity*. Thus validity is dependent on a test's purpose, and a test does not have a general validity but rather a specific validity for each particular situation for which it is used.

Test and Item Analysis

Many important decisions are often made on the basis of scores resulting from knowledge tests. Therefore, it is important to have confidence in these measuring devices and to know they are as accurate as possible. For this reason, the overall test and the items that comprise it should be analyzed for maximum efficiency. This section gives procedures for examining the items of a test designed to maximally discriminate among examinees. The procedures presented here by no means cover the entire range of options, but they represent a reasonably simple yet complete approach to the task.

Item Analysis Procedures

The steps and directions listed below to analyze a test item belong to a conceptual domain generally referred to as *classical test theory*. There are analogous techniques in a relatively recent development called *item response theory,* also known as *latent trait theory* (see chapter 11). This approach, by adding some assumptions to those inherent in classical test theory, permits the measurement process to focus on examinees and test items, and the resulting statistics are not derived from a single population and a particular test. Unfortunately, the use of item response theory procedures usually requires large (500 or more) sample sizes, large numbers of items, and computer programs for solving systems of nonlinear equations iteratively. Because these conditions are not common, the classical test theory procedures are presented here.

Step 1: Administer and score the tests.

Step 2: Order the answer sheets according to score from highest to lowest.

Step 3: Separate the answer sheets into three subgroups:

a. The *upper group* consists of the upper (approximately) 27 percent of the answer sheets.

b. The *middle group* consists of the middle (approximately) 46 percent of the answer sheets.

c. The *lower group* consists of the same number of answer sheets as placed in the upper group.

Only the answer sheets of the two extreme groups are used in the item analysis. As a compromise between having as many responses as possible and maximizing the differences between the types of responses, test authorities suggest the two groups consist of the 27 percent of the answer sheets located at the two extremes of the score scale. Generally, as long as an equal number occurs in each of the two groups, the use of the most convenient number of answer sheets between 25 and 33 percent for each group is satisfactory. For example, if 60 answer sheets were available for analysis, the highest and lowest 15-20 could be used.

Step 4: Count and record for each test item the frequency of selection of each possible response by the upper group.

Step 5: Count and record for each test item the frequency of selection of each possible response by the lower group.

Steps 4 and 5 require the most time-consuming portion of the item analysis. Several procedures can help reduce the tedium of this task. Possibilities include using previously prepared scorecards for each item, using a typewriter to speed the process of recording responses (five adjacent keys can be used to represent each of five possible responses, for example, so that responses can be tabulated without lifting the eyes from the answer sheet); having one person read and another record; or, if possible, using an optical scanner to have a computer accomplish these steps.

At the completion of step 5 the necessary data are available to calculate indexes of difficulty and discrimination for each item. An example of a possible organization of these data is shown in Table 12.3.

These data are used in the following paragraphs to illustrate the calculation of the **difficulty index** and the **discrimination index** and the use of the response pattern to improve an item. These data were obtained from an item included on a nationally standardized test of knowledge of physical fitness, administered to college senior physical education majors (Mood, 1971). The left side of the table displays the initial draft

Table 12.3   Data Organization for Item Analysis

First Draft: In the opinion of most authorities, three of the following factors have contributed to a lowering of the national level of physical fitness. Which has *NOT* had this effect?

  A. An increase in life-span.

  B. A decrease in the physical effort required for daily living.
  C. An increase in the number of occupations involving sedentary activity.
*D. An increase in school consolidation.

Revision: In the opinion of most authorities, three of the following have contributed to a lowering of the national level of physical fitness. Which has *NOT* had this effect?

  A. An increase in the number of senior citizens.
  B. A decrease in the physical effort required for daily living.
  C. An increase in the number of occupations involving sedentary activity.
*D. An increase in school consolidation.

Item 5 Test: Form D Trial, Date: 9/70, N: 185

Item 25 Test: Final Form A, Date: 9/70, N: 1,112

Responses:	A B C D E Omit	Disc.	Diff.	Responses:	A B C D E Omit	Disc.	Diff.
Upper 27% = 50	28 2 1 19 0		36%	Upper 27% = 300	69 10 5 216 0		53%
Lower 27% = 50	24 8 1 17 0	.04		Lower 27% = 300	89 52 54 104 1	.37	

of the question and the response pattern of 185 examinees. On the right side, the revised question and the resulting response pattern from a national sample of 1,112 examinees are displayed.

Step 6: Calculate and record the index of difficulty for each item. Substitution into Equation 12.10 results in the calculation of this index:

$$DI = \frac{U_c + L_c}{U_n + L_n} \times 100 \tag{12.10}$$

where *DI* is the index of difficulty, U_c is the number of examinees in the upper group answering the question correctly, L_c is the number of examinees in the lower group answering the question correctly, U_n is the number of examinees in the upper group, and L_n is the number of examinees in the lower group (recall that $U_n = L_n$). Inspection of this equation reveals that the index of difficulty is actually the percentage of students answering the question correctly. Thus, the higher the difficulty index the easier the question. The following examples using the data displayed in Table 12.3 illustrate the use of the index of difficulty, Equation 12.10. First draft results in $N = 185$; therefore 50 examinees are represented in each extreme group ($185 \times 27\% = 50$):

$$DI = \frac{19 + 17}{50 + 50} \times 100 = \frac{36}{100} \times 100 = 36\%$$

Revised results show $N = 1,112$; therefore 300 examinees are represented in each extreme group ($1,112 \times 27\% = 300$):

$$DI = \frac{216 + 104}{300 + 300} \times 100 = \frac{320}{600} \times 100 = 53\%$$

The maximum amount of discrimination can occur only when an item has an index of difficulty of 50%. If this criterion could be met by every question on a test, the group mean score of such a test would necessarily be equal to one-half the number of items on the test. For example, the mean score of such a test containing 80 items would be 40. However, this interpretation does not take chance into account. On an 80-item multiple-choice test where each item has four possible responses, random marking of the answer sheet should produce approximately 20 correct responses. Thus, considering chance, the mean score of the test described here should be 50. This is calculated by determining the score falling halfway between the chance score and the highest possible score. If the difficulty index of each of the 80 items was 62.5%, the mean score for the test would be 50 ($80 \times 62.5\% = 50$).

Obviously it is not possible, especially on the first draft, to produce an item with a predetermined difficulty index. To maximize discrimination power, an item should be written in such a way that half or slightly more than half of the examinees will answer it correctly. One further point should be noted. Maximum discrimination can *only* occur for an item of middle difficulty, but meeting this condition does not necessarily guarantee that it will occur.

Step 7: Calculate and record the index of discrimination for each item. Equation 12.11 is used to determine this index:

$$ID = \frac{U_c - L_c}{U_n \text{ or } L_n} \tag{12.11}$$

where ID is the index of discrimination, U_c is the number of students in the upper group answering the item correctly, L_c is the number of students in the lower group answering the item correctly, U_n is the number of students in the upper group, and L_n is the number of students in the lower group ($U_n = L_n$). The denominator for this equation is not the sum of the number of students in both groups, but is the number in one group (either, since $U_n = L_n$). The following examples, again using the data presented in Table 12.3, illustrate the use of the index of discrimination equation.

First draft results: $N = 185$; therefore for each extreme group, $N = 50$:

$$ID = \frac{19 - 17}{50} = \frac{2}{50} = .04$$

Revision results: $N = 1,112$; therefore for each extreme group, $N = 300$:

$$ID = \frac{216 - 104}{300} = \frac{112}{300} = .37$$

The criterion used to examine the discriminating power of an item is usually the test on which the item appears. In general, if the examinees who did well on the entire test did well on the item and the examinees who did poorly on the entire test did poorly on the item, the item is considered a good discriminator. If approximately the same number of upper-group and lower-group examinees answer an item correctly, it is considered to possess little or no discriminatory power. Finally, if the item is answered correctly by more of the lower-group than the upper-group examinees, it is considered to be a negative discriminator.

The index of discrimination presented here is known as the *Net D* and is only one of several discrimination indexes that have been devised. The Net D is relatively simple to calculate, uses the same data as the difficulty index, and is fairly simple to interpret.

The higher the value of the Net D the higher the discriminating power of the item, and the Net D equation can produce a negative value indicating an item that discriminates negatively. In fact, the value obtained is actually the *net percentage* of positive discriminations achieved by an item. That is, the value of ID is actually the percentage obtained when the difference resulting from subtracting all negative discriminations from all positive discriminations is divided by the total number of possible discriminations. The following example illustrates the meaning of the Net D obtained for any item:

	Upper group $N = 3$	Lower group $N = 3$
Answered Correctly	2 Students (Cell A)	1 Student (Cell B)
Answered Incorrectly	1 Student (Cell C)	2 Students (Cell D)

No discriminations occurred between the students in Cells A and B because all these examinees answered the item correctly $(2 \times 1) = 2$. Similarly, no discriminations occurred between the students in Cells C and D, because all these students answered the item incorrectly $(1 \times 2) = 2$. Total neutral discriminations is $2 + 2$, or 4. The discriminations that occurred between the students in Cells A and D are considered positive because of the groups in which these students have been placed based on their total test scores. Altogether a total of 4 (2×2) positive discriminations occurred. Conversely the discrimination that occurred between the students in Cells B and C is considered negative. The total number of discriminations that could occur with three students in each group is 9 (3×3). Of these 9, 4 were positive, 1 was negative, and 4 were neutral. Subtracting the 1 negative discrimination from the 4 positive discriminations results in a *net* of 3 positive discriminations. The ratio of net positive discriminations to the total possible (3/9) is .33. Using the Net D equation 12.11 results in this same value.

$$ID = \frac{4 - 1}{9} = \frac{3}{9} = .33$$

Although it is desirable to keep the index of difficulty of an item slightly above 50% for an achievement test, the index of discrimination should be as high as possible. Generally most test-construction authorities agree that an item having a discrimination index of .40 or higher is a very good one. Items having an index of discrimination below .20, and especially those with negative discrimination indexes, are poor and probably should be discarded. Discrimination indexes between .20 and .40 are considered acceptable but generally indicate possible revision as the value approaches .20. Items that are negative discriminators are usually ambiguous (especially to the better students) or tricky.

Step 8: Examine the pattern of responses to determine how an item might be improved.

Although it is often difficult to understand why certain responses are selected or ignored and even more difficult to determine possible alterations of the responses or stem that will improve an item, examination of the response patterns often suggests possibilities. For example, the first response for the initial draft of the item displayed in Table 12.3 was chosen by over 50% of the students, although it was the incorrect response. Rewording this incorrect response in the revision resulted in the correct response becoming more attractive than the first response, especially to the students in the upper group. The changes in the difficulty and discrimination indexes indicate that the alteration of this one response improved the item considerably.

Item Analysis of Criterion-Referenced Tests

The item-analysis indexes described above can be used for assessing the quality of items on a criterion-referenced written test, but these indexes are interpreted differently from norm-referenced tests. For example, difficulty indexes for criterion-referenced tests are expected to be very high, especially if the examinees are well prepared. Although the difficulty index may not be useful for identifying items that are too easy, items that are too difficult for this type of a test can be identified. Items with high difficulty indexes should not automatically be considered good unless a high proportion of the examinees answered correctly because they mastered the concept being measured. The test developer must show that the results were not the result of unrealistic incorrect responses or internal clues.

The Net D is not very useful for criterion-referenced tests. However, if it reveals any negatively discriminating items, they should be omitted or revised. A good item on this type of test could easily result in a Net D value of zero or near zero because typical score distributions from criterion-referenced tests are negatively skewed and low in variability. Another approach suggested by Ebel and Frisbie (1986) is to use the phi coefficient to determine the amount of association between two dichotomous measures. In this case the two dichotomies would be correct or incorrect on the item and master or nonmaster on the test. The data in Table 12.4 illustrate the use of this statistic in this situation. The letters identify the cells of the table.

Table 12.4   Example of Phi Coefficient to Examine Discrimination Power of an Item from a Criterion-referenced Test

		Test		
		Master		Non-master
Test Item	Correct	A	64	B 23
	Incorrect	C	17	D 46

$$\Phi = \frac{AD - BC}{\sqrt{(A+B)(C+D)(A+C)(B+D)}}$$

$$\Phi = \frac{(64)(46) - (17)(23)}{\sqrt{(64+23)(17+46)(64+17)(23+46)}}$$

$$\Phi = \frac{2944 - 391}{\sqrt{(87)(63)(81)(69)}}$$

$$\Phi = \frac{2553}{\sqrt{5534.7}} = .46$$

The phi coefficient can be interpreted somewhat like a correlation coefficient, with high positive values belonging to the most desirable items.

Conclusion

The overall judgement of the quality of a knowledge test involves many factors and the use of both logical and empirical data. A well-constructed test displays balance and relevance, so that the test items represent adequately the domain being measured and the tasks required of the examinee are representative of the behavior to be assessed. The use of a table of specifications (see chapter 2) helps ensure that these qualities are achieved.

A knowledge test that is appropriate for a group of examinees will consist primarily of middle-difficulty items, and the items will be *fair*. Only middle-difficulty items can discriminate well among examinees. The inclusion of an item that every examinee answers correctly cannot be defended from the standpoint of reliability or discrimination, although its use could be argued for validity purposes. Fair items are ones for which examinees have been prepared, and all possible care has been taken to eliminate ambiguity and trickery. If an examinee knows the correct answer to a test item but misses it due to unfairness, it actually lowers the reliability of the test.

If the purpose of the test is to *discriminate* among examinees regarding their ability on whatever is being measured, then each item must possess the discriminatory characteristics. If test items are written in such a general way that a test-wise novice can score considerably better than chance on the test, the test is low in *specificity*. When this occurs it is impossible to distinguish high scores due to high ability in whatever is being measured and high scores due to general intelligence. To avoid this, test items should be made as specific to the topic being measured as possible.

An *efficient* test is one constructed to provide a large number of independent assessments of each examinee per unit of testing time. A test that is very efficient will almost always have high reliability, but it is not wise to sacrifice relevance and balance for the sake of efficiency. Issues such as cost and time are relevant to test *practicability*. This is an important area for consideration when examining a particular knowledge test for possible use, but it is not necessarily related to the quality of the test.

Finally, the most important characteristics of a knowledge test are *reliability* and *validity*. These, of course, are related to the factors discussed above. If it cannot be shown that a knowledge test actually measures what it is intended to measure and does so consistently, then it is of no use as a measuring device.

References

Angoff, W.H. (1971). Scales, norms, and equivalent scores. In R.L. Thorndike (Ed.), *Educational measurement* (2nd ed.) (pp. 508–600). Washington, DC: American Council on Education.

Cronbach, L.J. (1951). Coefficient alpha and the internal structure of tests. *Psychometrika, 16*, 297–334.

Ebel, R.L. (1972). *Essentials of educational measurement* (2nd ed.). Englewood Cliffs, NJ: Prentice-Hall.

Ebel, R.L. (1983). The practical validation of tests of ability. *Educational Measurement: Issues and Practices, 2*, 7–10.

Ebel, R.L., & Frisbie, D.A. (1986). *Essentials of educational measurement* (4th ed.). Englewood Cliffs, NJ: Prentice-Hall.

Fitzpatrick, A.R. (1983). The meaning of content validity. *Applied Psychological Measurement, 7*, 3–13.

Kuder, G.F., & Richardson, M.W. (1937). The theory of the estimation of test reliability. *Psychometrika, 2*, 151–160.

Marshall, J.C., & Hales, L.W. (1971). *Classroom test construction*. Reading, MA: Addison-Wesley.

Mood, D.P. (1971). Test of physical fitness knowledge: Construction, administration and norms. *Research Quarterly, 42*, 423–429.

Nedelsky, L. (1954). Absolute grading standards for objective tests. *Educational and Psychological Measurement, 14*, 3–19.

Supplementary Readings

Berk, R.A. (Ed.) (1984). *A guide to criterion-referenced test construction*. Baltimore: Johns Hopkins University Press.

Cronbach, L.J. (1984). *Essentials of psychological testing* (4th ed.). New York: Harper and Row.

Hopkins, C.D., & Antes, R.L. (1985). *Classroom measurement and evaluation* (2nd ed.). Itasca, IL: F.E. Peacock.

Kane, T., & Brennan, R. (1980). Agreement coefficients as indices of dependability for domain-referenced tests. *Applied Psychological Measurement, 4,* 105–126.

Linn, R.L. (1983). Testing and instruction: Links and distinctions. *Journal of Educational Measurement, 20,* 179–189.

Mehrens, W.A., & Lehmann, I.J. (1984). *Measurement and evaluation in education and psychology* (3rd ed.). New York: Holt, Rinehart and Winston.

Nitko, A.J. (1983). *Educational tests and measurement: An introduction.* New York: Harcourt Brace Jovanovich.

Safrit, M.J. (1986). *Introduction to measurement in physical education and exercise science.* St. Louis: Times Mirror/Mosby.

Shepard, L. (1980). Technical issues in minimum competency testing. *Review of Research in Education, 8,* 30–82.

CHAPTER 13

Measurement Methodology for Affective Tests

Jack K. Nelson
Louisiana State University

Affective behavior refers to emotional behavior. The term **affect** is a general class name for feelings, emotions, mood, and temperament (Payne, 1980). The affective domain is not a unitary concept, and terms such as attitudes, interests, and values are commonly used to describe various aspects of the domain. Many affective behaviors have been measured and analyzed in physical education and exercise science.

Types of Affective Behavior

The affective behavior that has been studied most frequently is **attitude**. An attitude consists of three components: (a) an affective component, one's feelings about the attitude object (e.g., a program, practice, group, person, or institution); (b) a cognitive component, one's knowledge or belief about the attitude object; and (c) a behavioral component, the disposition of a person to act toward the attitude object in a certain way (Borg & Gall, 1983). Attitudes are generally measured by **self-reports**. A self-report can be in the form of a questionnaire, inventory, or interview used to obtain information about the beliefs, opinions, or behavior of respondents.

Interests are likes and dislikes for specific programs, types of physical activity, and other topics. Questionnaires are used to assess interests. **Self-concept** represents the feelings or cognitions about oneself in dimensions such as personal, social, critical, and physical. **Body-image** is the physical dimension of self-concept that deals with one's perceptions of his or her body. Although self-concept can be measured by projective techniques, such as picture or story interpretation, in physical education both self-concept and body-image are usually measured by self-reports.

Sportsmanship encompasses many aspects of sports participation, including respect for rules, ethical practices, acceptance of defeat, sublimating one's personal interests for the good of the team, and teamwork. Sportsmanship is usually measured by a questionnaire that presents selected sport situations. It also can be measured by self-reports and by ratings by others. *Social behavior* refers to a myriad of traits such as leadership, self-control, confidence, maturity, sociability, and cooperation. Ratings by the teacher are the primary means of measuring social behavior in a school setting.

Perceived exertion is a subjective evaluation of the strenuousness of an exercise at any given time during a workout or physical performance test. A **rating scale** of numbers matched with verbal descriptors is used to measure perceived exertion. *Anxiety* is a subjective feeling of stress or fear. The general, enduring form that is part of one's personality is called **trait anxiety**. The temporary form of anxiety that reflects one's reaction to a perceived threatening situation is **state anxiety**. Anxiety is generally measured by self-reports. *Personality traits* include anxiety, emotional stability, extroversion-introversion, practical-imaginative, autonomy, dominance, and ego strength, to name but a few. Personality can be measured in several ways, with some methods requiring individual testing by highly trained psychologists. Written tests are used predominantly in physical education and exercise science research studies.

Uses of Affective Measures in Physical Education and Exercise Science

The physical educator, the coach, the exercise specialist, and the researcher all have special interests in the measurement of affective behaviors because of the perceived relationship and influence of the behaviors in sports performance, exercise, and skill acquisition.

In physical education. A major objective of physical education involves affective behavior. The stated goals of physical education usually include the development of affective behaviors such as attitudes, sportsmanship, leadership, self-concept, and desirable social behavior. It follows that the physical educator would be interested in assessing these behaviors. Affective measures generally are not appropriate for determining grades, because the intent of the items in most self-reports is quite obvious. Ratings of behavior by the teacher are frequently used. Unfortunately these ratings are often not performed as systematically and objectively as they should be. The teacher can, however, obtain valuable information about the students' interests and attitudes concerning the program and quality of instruction through affective measurement.

In athletics. Coaches are especially concerned with emotional and psychological traits that appear to have an important impact on athletic performance. The measurement of these traits can aid the coach in screening and selecting players and in developing effective strategies for working with them. The use of affective measurement in sports is mostly confined to college and professional levels.

In exercise programs. The exercise specialist knows that the immediate and long-range success of any exercise program hinges on the motivation and attitude of the participants. Moreover, measured perceptions of the intensity and strain of exercise can be a valuable tool in fitness testing and in monitoring exercise programs. Three of the more common uses of psychophysical ratings, according to Baumgartner and Jackson (1987), are: (a) in exercise testing to judge exercise intensity when administering graded exercise tests; (b) in exercise prescription to help select the proper intensity for exercise and to provide supplementary heart rate estimates; and (c) in the quantification of energy expenditure, especially in activities such as aerobic dance or sports, where external work cannot be quantified.

In research. Research interests in affective measurement are numerous and diverse, including the differentiation among athletes of different types of sports on certain personality traits; the influence of physical education programs on self-concept; comparisons of athletes and nonathletes on sportsmanship; the relationship of attitude and behavior in various populations; the effects of imposed stress on state anxiety and performance; and the relative influence of different physiological parameters on ratings of perceived exertion. The quality of these studies depends on valid and reliable measurement of the affective behaviors in question.

Strengths and Weaknesses of Affective Measures

Strengths

Measurement of affective behavior has had a long history in physical education and exercise science. Moreover, affective measures have been used in a variety of ways and in diverse settings. Although critiques of affective measures typically focus on weaknesses and limitations of the instruments, there are certain recognized strengths.

Reliability and validity of instruments. Affective measures in physical education and exercise science generally have acceptable reliability estimates, considering the intangible nature of the dimensions being measured. Furthermore, many authors have used the rigorous stability-over-time method for establishing reliability. The more recent tests have been based on a theoretical framework, and construct validity procedures have been employed. Factor analysis has been used to confirm researchers' hypotheses concerning the dimensions of an affect.

Application of information. When used intelligently and conservatively, many affective measures can provide valuable information about the feelings of the respondents. For example, the rating of perceived exertion (Borg, 1962) is a simple and accurate measure that has been found to have both applied and theoretical validity. Even though affective measures are not recognized as being appropriate for grading purposes in a school setting, they can be useful for formative evaluation. Most of the tests to date provide more information about group status than about the individual. Such information can prompt needed changes in programs and instruction in both physical education and exercise science.

Weaknesses

As with any measure, it is important to be aware of the limitations and to exercise good judgment in the use and interpretation of affective measures. Several weaknesses have been identified.

Truthfulness of responses. An inherent weakness of many of the instruments is that they are self-reports. The tester can never be certain the responses are accurate. The subject's willingness to tell the truth is always a limitation. Sometimes subjects do not want to admit certain feelings, even to themselves. Instruments often contain what may be called *honesty items*, or a *lie scale* or *carelessness index*. Examples of these items are:

> "I have never deliberately told a lie."
> "In all my playing experience in sports I have never had a bad day."
> "I have never been angry."

If a subject answers "True" to such items, that person's responses are discarded.

Several response sets have been studied. One is acquiescence, or the tendency to respond "Agree" or "True" regardless of the item's content. Another is social desirability, i.e., the subject's responses are motivated by what is perceived to be the socially accepted way to behave or feel. A third set is deviant responses, characterized by a deliberate portrayal of oneself as deviant or *bad*. A good rapport between the tester and the examinees is helpful in eliciting accurate responses.

Another source of concern in affective measurement is that feelings change and can be easily influenced by situations and events. Measurements taken at one time need to be evaluated with this possibility in mind. Alternatively, repeated measures are susceptible to the phenomenon of **reactivity**, wherein the subject is sensitized to the variables being measured and actually experiences a change in feelings from one test administration to another.

As with any questionnaire or inventory, the wording of the items and the format used for the responses are significant variables relative to the validity of the measure. The age, vocabulary, and cultural background of the subjects are also important considerations.

Limitations of ratings. Ratings by teachers are subject to a host of measurement errors. One of the most critical factors is whether an adequate number of observations is made to establish acceptable reliability. In some types of behavior, such as sportsmanship, the question of equal and ample opportunity to exhibit this behavior must be carefully resolved. There is also the danger of preconceived judgments about examinees, such as the **halo effect**, where a student's reputation or a teacher's prior impression of a student (good or bad) interferes with objective judgment.

Misuse of instrument. In addition to the limitations of various affective measurement techniques, including the accuracy of responses, there is the danger of improper use of the instrument. A common mistake by novice researchers is to use a trait measure to assess the effects of an experimental treatment. By definition, a trait is an enduring or permanent characteristic. It is not supposed to change. If it does, one can only assume measurement error has produced the change, the measure of the trait is invalid, or the trait is not well defined.

Many ambitious studies of personality have been undertaken by researchers in physical education and exercise science who lack the background and training to interpret the findings. In recent years, concern for the rights of subjects has justifiably restricted a number of studies involving personality traits. Asking subjects to respond to some types of items in personality inventories, for example, can constitute an invasion of privacy.

Lack of theoretical basis. Finally, a major criticism of affective measures in physical education and exercise science has been the lack of a theoretical framework in which to construct and validate the instrument. A large majority of the measures have simply claimed face validity for the items. Moreover, developers of many affective instruments have assumed the existence of only one dimension of a concept or attitude object, when several dimensions may be represented. Consequently, people with quite different attitudes may yield similar total scores. For example, a subject might have a favorable attitude toward exercise solely for its contribution to weight control; another subject might not value exercise for this purpose, but rather for its cathartic effect; and still another might view exercise as worthwhile only for its contribution to health. Yet all three may mark the same response (for different reasons) to a general statement about the value of exercise.

Validity and Reliability of Affective Measures

Researchers in the affective domain are faced with special problems with regard to the validity and reliability of their measuring instruments. Affective behavior consists of attitudes, values, interests, and perceptions. These dimensions are intangible and usually must be measured by asking examinees how they feel about an attitude object, how they normally behave in a situation, or how they have observed others to behave. Obviously there may be real differences between the responses and the actual feelings of the examinees. In addition, many factors influence a person's opinions, so that responses may fluctuate depending on the situation, circumstances, and one's state of mind at the time of the measurement. Despite the fact that some types of affective measures have unique problems of validity and reliability, there are sufficient similarities in procedures to warrant some generalizations about these facets of test construction.

Validity

Refer to chapter 2 for an in-depth discussion of the concept of validity and the different ways of establishing validity.

Content validity. A criticism often leveled at affective measures in physical education and exercise science is that the instruments have not been validated scientifically. Indeed, the most common (and inappropriate) approach to validation over the years has been that of *face validity.* If a statement appeared to be pertinent to a particular concept, it was assumed to be valid. Frequently the judgments of several persons deemed to be knowledgeable about the concept have been used to verify the validity of the description of the behavioral domain, a process more closely aligned to *content validity.*

A classic example of using expert judges to construct an attitude scale was the work of Louis Thurstone, a pioneer in the systematic measurement of attitude. Thurstone was concerned mainly with the measurement and comparison of psychological stimuli. He reasoned that human judgment could be used to determine comparative weightings for psychological stimuli, just as judges could rank order physical objects from lightest to heaviest. Thus, if a number of individuals were asked to judge a stimulus on some criterion, the most frequently occurring judgment could be determined, and different stimuli could then be compared on their relative modal discriminal score (McIver & Carmines, 1981).

Criterion-related validity. In chapter 2, a criterion was described as an external variable(s) considered to be a direct measure of the behavior or characteristic being tested. Criterion-related validity has had limited use in affective measurement, because few relevant criterion variables exist. For example, in attempting to measure self-concept, what would be a suitable criterion? Which type of behavior do people with high or low self-concept exhibit that could be used to validate a test of this trait? Occasionally, a test is correlated with some standardized test(s) that presumably measures the behavior in question. For example, in validating the State Trait Anxiety Inventory (STAI) A-Trait anxiety scale, the authors (Spielberger, Gorsuch, & Lushene, 1970) determined concurrent validity by correlating the scale with the IPAT Anxiety Scale, the Taylor

Manifest Anxiety Scale, and the Affect Adjective Checklist. Ordinarily, if a valid instrument already exists, the test developer's primary purpose is to develop another measure that is less time-consuming, less expensive, and easier to administer and score. Obviously the test will not be useful unless it correlates significantly with the criterion. There is always the possibility that the test is better (more valid) than the criterion, but this cannot be established through concurrent validity procedures.

Construct validity. Construct validity is generally accepted as the method of choice for validating an affective measure. As explained in chapter 2, construct validity focuses on the extent to which a measure performs in accordance with theoretical expectations. A theoretical framework must be identified concerning the behavior or concept in order to generate predictions, which are followed by empirical tests involving measures of this behavior or concept.

Referring again to the STAI, empirical evidence of construct validity was obtained by administering the STAI A-State scale at (a) the beginning of a testing session, (b) immediately after a 10-min relaxation training session, (c) during a difficult exam in which subjects were interrupted every 10 min, and (d) immediately following a gory, stressful movie. The ability of the individual STAI A-State items to discriminate between these conditions, which reflected different degrees and kinds of stress, demonstrated construct validity for a new test theory concept, that of state anxiety (Spielberger et al., 1970).

The comparison of test scores of groups of known (or assumed) affective behavior differences is a popular approach to construct validation. Construct validity for both the Attitude Toward Physical Activity (ATPA) (Kenyon, 1968a, 1968b) and the Children's Attitude Toward Physical Activity (CATPA) (Simon & Smoll, 1974) has been provided by comparisons of attitude scores between sport groups, gender and age groups, and athletes and nonathletes. In this approach, it is hypothesized that groups will differ on certain dimensions of attitude toward physical activity. Similarly, construct validity was demonstrated for the Sport Competition Anxiety Test (SCAT) by comparing groups (formed on the basis of their SCAT scores) based on their responses to manipulated success-failure situations (Martens, 1977). Evidence of construct validity by the group-difference method was reported by Sonstroem (1978) in a study in which high- and low-fit boys were found to differ significantly on both Estimation and Attraction items in the Physical Estimation and Attraction Scale (PEAS).

Other approaches used in establishing construct validity include *convergent validity* and *discriminant validity* procedures. Convergent validity involves correlation between measures of the same construct. Martens (1977) found moderate correlations between the SCAT and general anxiety instruments, thus demonstrating convergent validity. In discriminant validity, the assumption is that the measure in question should *not* correlate with measures of different constructs. For example, a negative correlation was found between the SCAT and an internal-external control scale for children, indicating that high SCAT persons tended to be more external, which agreed with the hypothesized construct of competitive anxiety. Discriminant validity was further demonstrated by a low correlation between SCAT scores and an achievement motivation scale. This was also expected, because persons scoring low in achievement motivation are both high in the fear of failure and low in the motive to achieve success. Thus, high SCAT scores could be associated with either low or high scores in both dimensions of achievement motivation; consequently a very low correlation was obtained.

Stronger evidence of construct validity can be obtained if subsequent analyses reveal successful predictions involving different theoretically related variables. Thus, construct validity is not established by confirming a single prediction on different occasions or confirming several predictions in a single study. Ideally the developer of an affective measurement instrument attempts to establish a pattern of consistent results from different studies by different researchers employing various theoretical models.

Factor analysis. Factor analysis can be used in assessing the validity of affective measures. Refer to chapter 8 for a discussion of factor analysis. To be used properly, it must be interpreted within a theoretical framework. Without theoretical guidance, it can result in misleading conclusions (Nunnally, 1978). In the construction of the PEAS, Sonstroem (1974) used factor analysis to examine the dimensions of the inventory and test the separation of the Estimation and Attraction statements. Subsequently, Safrit, Wood, and Dishman (1985) used factor analysis in the process of revising and shortening the PEAS for its use with men and women.

It might be argued that factor analysis establishes primarily content validity by confirming or refuting the existence of certain dimensions or subdomains. However, this technique also may be viewed as a tool of theoretical analysis for demonstrating evidence of construct validity. The key word is *tool*. It should not be used as a replacement for theoretical analysis.

Reliability

A comprehensive coverage of reliability is provided in chapter 3. Moreover, the various procedures for establishing reliability of knowledge tests, which are also applicable to affective measures, are described in chapter 12. Hence, the strengths and weaknesses of the different methods will be reviewed only briefly here.

Stability over time. The stability-over-time approach is an intuitively attractive method for establishing reliability. However, there are some problems in using this method for affective measurement instruments. When a test is given on different occasions, many small variations in the testing situation can produce inconsistencies, such as in the way instructions are read and in the lighting, noise, and condition of the room. In addition, there are mood fluctuations, motivation, fatigue, and other variables involving the subjects. There are also *memory* effects, which can operate in different ways depending on the type of instrument and disposition of the subject. Usually memory effects cause an inflated reliability estimate, because the subjects remember their previous responses and answer items the same way.

A *reactive* effect is another weakness of the stability-over-time method. The initial test can sensitize a subject, producing a change in affective behavior. For example, as a result of taking a test on exercise and weight control, the subject might begin to think and read about the benefits of exercise in weight control and develop a more positive attitude toward exercise. Reactivity tends to reduce the size of the reliability estimate.

An event between the two test administrations might also affect a person's responses. A newspaper article on an athletic recruiting scandal, for example, may alter a person's views toward the value of athletics. If the test was readministered on the same day, reactivity and intervening events would not be a problem. Reliability estimates almost always decrease as the interval of time between test administrations increases.

Parallel forms. In the parallel-form method, the subject takes two forms of a test designed to measure the same attribute. Reliability is established by correlating scores on the two forms. The recommended time interval between testing is generally 2 weeks. The main advantage of the parallel-form method is that the memory effect is drastically reduced. The parallel-form method is more appropriate when the phenomenon being measured is a relatively enduring trait or behavior. One of the main limitations with this method is the difficulty of constructing two truly parallel instruments.

Split halves. The split-halves method of reliability has been used with a number of affective measures. This method does not require two test administrations; therefore, the primary weaknesses of the test-retest and alternate-forms methods are avoided. But this method is weaker from a theoretical basis and yields a spuriously high reliability estimate. Although the odd-even method of separating the test into halves is frequently used, there are numerous ways of splitting a test. For a 10-item scale, for example, there are 125 different possible splits. It is likely that different reliability estimates will be obtained, depending on how the test is divided. An assumption underlying this method is that no systematic differences exist between two halves of the test. The Spearman-Brown prophecy formula is used to statistically correct the estimate.

Kuder-Richardson. The Kuder-Richardson (KR) formulas for rational equivalence also provide estimates of internal consistency. It is the only widely used technique that does not require the calculation of a correlation coefficient. It requires only a single administration of the test. The two equations most widely used are KR20 and KR21. (See chapter 12, equations 12.5 and 12.6.) *Hoyt's analysis of variance* procedure is occasionally used. It provides the same results as KR20.

Cronbach's alpha. Cronbach's alpha is the most popular of several internal-consistency methods of assessing reliability that do not require repeating or splitting test items. (See Equation 12.7.) The coefficient alpha provides a conservative estimate of an instrument's reliability. Alpha is versatile in that it can be used with items having several possible answers, each with a different weight.

Measurement Formats in the Assessment of Affective Behavior

A variety of formats are used in the measurement of affective behavior. A logical sequence of steps in the construction of an instrument has been to carefully define the type of affect and then determine what subcategories of behavior should be included and what their relative weightings should be. In accomplishing this task, the test developer must decide what format to use. Several formats and scaling procedures will be discussed.

Open vs. Closed Questions

There are two general categories of formats used in measuring responses to written tests: **open items** and fixed or **closed items**. An open question asks respondents to express themselves in their own words rather than to select an answer from a fixed set of possibilities. Closed items include checklists, rating scales, and rankings. Since the beginning of social science research, there have been arguments over the relative merits of open and closed modes of inquiry. The arguments are largely based on opinion, common sense, and anecdotal experiences (Schuman & Presser, 1981). Experiments are rare in which open and closed versions of the same questions are compared.

The main arguments supporting open items are that closed items fail to provide an appropriate set of meaningful choices for the respondent, and that respondents are apt to be influenced by the specific fixed alternatives given. The open form can more appropriately assess salience of the question. The avoidance of social-desirability effects is supposedly better achieved with open items. While many persons would agree with these arguments intuitively, there are several points to consider in the formulation of open items to keep them open and still germane to the subject at hand. First, open items are not always as open as they seem. There are often subtle constraints in the inadvertent phrasing of open questions. But without adequate direction, the respondents may wander outside of the desired frame of reference. The educational level of the respondents can also be a factor in their understanding the questions and adequately expressing their beliefs and attitudes.

Advocates of the fixed or closed item contend that it separates types of responses that are often indistinguishable in open coding. Despite the presumed advantages of open items regarding such factors as salience and avoiding social-desirability effects, there seem to be even greater disadvantages in open items, i.e., vagueness of expression by respondents and misunderstanding by coders (Schuman & Presser, 1981). All of this is avoided in closed items, where the respondents in effect are asked to code themselves. The closed item restricts responses to those pertinent to the aim of the question and produces data in a form that is much easier to code and analyze than the open form.

Despite the years of controversy over open versus closed items, most instruments designed to assess affective behavior use the closed form. A sound suggestion in the construction of an inventory is to first use open items on a large sample of the target population and then use these responses to formulate closed alternatives that reflect the substance and wording of the open responses. This suggestion is not often followed, or, if it is, it often involves a very small and unrepresentative sample. Another option is to use open items to follow up some closed items to better understand why people answer as they do (Schuman, 1966). A brief description of some of the measures used in assessing affective behavior is given below.

Forced Choice-Two Alternative Items

Items to which respondents must choose between two answers (e.g., agree or disagree, yes or no, true or false) have frequently been used in affective measurement. These are known as forced choice-two alternative items. For example:

"I enjoy strenuous physical activity." (True or False)
"There is too much emphasis on athletics in the public schools." (Agree or Disagree)

An obvious advantage of such items is that they provide a rapid means of obtaining information. The items are easy to score, and they avoid the "middle of the road" position that may invite evasion. Conversely, a primary argument against these forced-choice items is that they do not allow a middle alternative. The question of acquiescence is also frequently raised with agree-disagree items. *Acquiescence* refers to a presumed tendency for people to agree with attitude statements. The term *presumed* is used to point out that not everyone agrees it exists. Campbell, Siegman, and Rees (1967) acknowledge that although acquiescence may affect responses, the content of the question is the primary factor.

Scaling Procedures

Scales are used to measure responses concerning stimuli, persons, or both. *Stimuli scaling* is sometimes used when people are expected to judge the strength of stimuli, such as weights of objects, loudness of sound, or brightness of light. Ratings of perceived exertion would probably fall under this category.

People scaling is the most common model in attitude assessment. Individuals respond to statements about a topic by indicating a degree of agreement or disagreement. The **Likert scale** method is an example of this.

A third approach is to scale both the stimuli and the person. The subject is expected to respond to the stimulus on the basis of the position of the stimulus relative to his or her own position. The Guttman scale is an example of this approach. These models are often used in political science surveys to determine the degree to which congressmen (or the public) vote on certain issues in relation to their party or liberal-conservative position.

The Likert scale. As mentioned previously, Likert scaling is person-centered. In this model all systematic variation in the responses to the stimuli is attributed to differences among the respondents. The stimuli are considered replications of one another (McIver & Carmines, 1981).

Typically a Likert scale has a set of items consisting of approximately an equal number of favorable and unfavorable statements. Subjects are asked to select one of five responses to each statement: strongly agree, agree, undecided, disagree, or strongly disagree. For example:

"Exercise is helpful in relieving emotional tension."

Strongly Agree	Agree	Undecided	Disagree	Strongly Disagree
5	4	3	2	1

The scoring is summative, in that the highest scores reflect the most favorable attitudes toward the topic. For negatively worded items, the score values are reversed:

"Exercise is of little value in relieving emotional tension."

Strongly Agree	Agree	Undecided	Disagree	Strongly Disagree
1	2	3	4	5

Several modifications of the Likert scale are used in affective measurement instruments. Sometimes the scale is expanded to 7 categories by adding "very strongly agree" and "very strongly disagree" to the ends. Nunnally (1978) suggests a 7-point (or degree) scale that lists the extreme statements at each end and then uses numbers in between, instead of word categories. For example:

"Exercise is helpful in relieving emotional tension."

Completely Disagree ___ ___ ___ ___ ___ ___ ___ Completely Agree
 1   2   3   4   5   6   7

A person who marks 5, for example, displays a positive attitude. A negative statement is scored by subtracting the selected score from the total number plus 1. To illustrate, in the above 7-point scale, if a person marked "5" to this statement:

"Exercise is of little value in relieving emotional stress."

Completely Disagree ___ ___ ___ ___ ___ ___ ___ Completely Agree
 1   2   3   4   5   6   7

---

the score would be $(7 + 1) - 5$, or $8 - 5 = 3$, which reflects a negative attitude. If a person marked 2 for the above question, the adjusted score would be $8 - 2 = 6$, which shows a positive attitude toward the benefits of exercise.

Order of categories. There has been speculation and subsequent research on whether the order of the category responses is a factor in scaled items. Is there a **primacy** or

recency effect? This refers to a systematic tendency of the respondents to choose the first or last alternative in a set. Some studies have found an order effect, regardless of whether the favorable alternative is first or last (Belson, 1966). However, the problem does not appear to be too serious, especially when the examinee is given adequate time to study the items.

Middle choice. Another source of possible measurement error concerns the middle choice in a response scale. Some investigations have contended that the middle alternative is unnecessary, because almost everyone really leans in one direction or the other. Moreover, it invites evasiveness. Others have argued that frequently there is a logical middle position, and that one rarely behaves or believes in an "all or none" manner. Examine the following statements:

"Vigorous exercise does more harm than good."
(A) True   (B) Uncertain   (C) False
"I prefer playing team sports to individual sports."
(A) Always   (B) Sometimes   (C) Never

Two hypotheses are implied when we use or omit the middle position. One, most of the people who choose the middle position lean toward one or the other polar positions, even though the degree of lean is slight. If so, the middle choice could be omitted. Two, people who choose the middle position may be expressing their opinions accurately. If the middle item is omitted and the subjects are forced to pick one of the polar alternatives, the response will be affected by measurement error.

The number of studies that have addressed the issue of middle position is rather small, and the results inconsistent. Schuman and Presser (1981) conducted several studies in which they added the middle position to agree-disagree items; they also experimented with providing more alternatives between the polar positions and the middle point. As might be expected, they found significant increases (10–20%) of respondents choosing the middle position when it was added. They also found that the addition of more response categories between the poles and the middle elicited responses, but the shift seemed to be more from the polar alternatives than from the middle—indicating that people really do have a middle position. A question of critical importance that has not been resolved is whether the decision to omit or use the middle position has consequences for the conclusions that are drawn from the results.

Semantic-differential scales. The **semantic-differential scale** consists of bipolar adjectives describing an attitude object, such as an activity, person, experience, or situation. The scale, which is a combination of an adjective checklist and rating scale, was developed by Charles Osgood and associates (Osgood, Suci, & Tannenbaum, 1957; Snider & Osgood, 1969). In this format, a single concept is rated by a number of 7-point scales. At the ends of each scale are adjectives or short phrases that are opposites, such as competent-incompetent, unhappy-happy, and lively-quiet.

The semantic-differential scale is intended to measure three dimensions of a concept: evaluation, activity, and potency. The *evaluation dimension* may be described by adjective pairs such as appropriate-inappropriate, fair-unfair, and clear-confusing. *Activity* is measured by action-adjective pairs like lively-quiet, dynamic-static, and fast-slow. The *potency dimension* refers to strength of the concept and is represented by adjective pairs such as powerful-feeble, warmhearted-coldhearted, and sturdy-fragile.

When setting up a semantic-differential scale, the concepts that pertain to the attitude object are identified. Next, adjective pairs relevant to each concept are selected. The age and comprehension level of the subjects must be considered in choosing the adjective pairs. Each dimension (evaluation, activity, potency) should have at least three adjective pairs for reliability purposes. Another guideline is to randomly switch location of the positive and negative adjectives.

Scoring is handled the same way a Likert scale is, i.e., the highest numbers are given to the positive-adjective end of the scale. The numbering of the 7-point scale is reversed when the negative adjective is on the left side.

Magnitude scaling. In the previous sections, different forms for scaling the direction and strength of people's feelings were presented, along with some of their limitations. Lodge (1981) summarized the major weaknesses of category scales as follows: (a) Information is lost, because the categories do not allow fine enough discrimination between judgments. In other words, there may be differences in respondents' strength of belief or preferences within a given category that are not able to be measured; (b) The designer of the measuring instrument inadvertently affects the responses by offering a fixed number of categories, whether few or numerous. Thus, sometimes judgments are constrained by too few categories, while at other times the range of categories is too expansive for the range of responses; and (c) The category scales are ordinal measures, and some critics contend this limits the type of statistical methods that can be used in describing, predicting, and modeling relationships.

The consequences of the weaknesses of category scaling in the measurement of people's beliefs and preferences may be far reaching. For example, the low relationships consistently found between attitudes and behavior may be a function of measurement deficiencies as much or more so than weaknesses in theoretical assumptions (Lodge, 1981). As an answer to the limitations of category scaling, Lodge proposes **magnitude scaling**. This scaling procedure parallels the methodology that has been developed for the ratio scaling of such sensations as brightness of light, loudness of sound, exertion of force, odors, tastes, and other sensory dimensions.

For example, in scaling the magnitude of the loudness of sound, the first sound acts as the reference and a number is arbitrarily assigned to it. Subsequent sounds are given numbers that reflect how much louder or softer they are in comparison.

It has been shown that people are able to reliably quantify the degrees of sensations. Moreover, the correlations between different forms of psychophysical sensation measurements are remarkably high (Lodge, 1981). These scales are ratio measures, which have all three features of the real number series: order, distance, and origin or reference base.

The general procedure for magnitude scaling of social opinions, such as an attitude assessment instrument, is to first use a calibration task (such as line production, in which the subject is asked to draw lines relative to a reference line) to express the strength of impressions. The purposes of this task are to supply instruction in making magnitude judgments, so that the subjects will not make ordinal judgments, and to provide a means to estimate and correct for any bias in response modalities.

Following the calibration task, the subjects are given words and phrases that essentially substitute for lines and numbers in the calibrating instructions, e.g., *more approval* and *less approval* for longer and shorter line lengths and numbers. A word such as *so-so* serves as the reference. By such procedures, cross-modality validation can be accomplished.

An early study that has had a considerable impact on the efficacy of magnitude scaling assessed the social judgments concerning juvenile delinquency (Sellin & Wolfgang, 1964). Juvenile Court judges, parole officers, and college students were asked to assign numbers expressing their opinions of the seriousness of certain crimes. The instructions for this social scaling task were similar to those for estimating the sensory stimuli (e.g., sound intensity, line lengths) mentioned above. First the reference situation was presented: a person stole a bicycle that was parked on a street. An arbitrary score of 10 was given for its seriousness. Subsequently, all other situations including trespassing, theft of various sums of money, arson, rape, and murder were judged in relation to the bicycle-theft situation. If the subjects considered the crime to be 10 times more serious, it was given a number of 100. In this process there is no upper limit, and any number can be used as long as it shows how serious the subject thinks the situation is. Sellin and Wolfgang (1964) reported a remarkable degree of consensus among experts in the criminal justice system and among students. This study has been replicated many times. Figlio (cited in Lodge, 1981) used these procedures in surveying 54,000 people in the United States Bureau of Census Crime Victimization Study of more than 200 descriptions of criminal offenses.

One of the most promising approaches in magnitude scaling involves the use of multiple-response measures within linear structural relationships (LISREL) models (Bentler, 1980). Studies in this area have shown approximately a 15% increase in explained variance for magnitude over categorical measures (Saris, 1980).

Other Formats

There are other formats for measuring affective behavior. The choice of which type to use depends on the situation, the nature of the subjects, and the kind of information that is desired. The rating scale and the questionnaire have often been used in the measurement of affective behavior.

Rating scales. In some types of affective measurement, such as evaluating social behavior, the individual is rated on a specified behavior. The ratings are usually on the frequency or degree to which the behavior is displayed. For example, to the behavior description, "Student displays leadership in physical education," the following rating scale might be used:

Never	Seldom	Occasionally	Frequently	Very Often
1	2	3	4	5

There is usually also a category of "No opportunity to observe." A similar scale is exemplified by the Cowell Social Adjustment Index (Cowell, 1958):

"Self-confident and self-reliant, tends to take success for granted, strong initiative, prefers to lead."

Markedly	Somewhat	Only Slightly	Not At All
+3	+2	+1	0

Typically a high rating denotes desirable behavior.

Questionnaire. Affective behavior can also be measured by a questionnaire. Subjects may be polled on their beliefs, interests, opinions, and values by a series of questions. These are self-report instruments, and the responses may be a yes-no, a brief statement, or a category-of-response scale. For example, some questions and modes of responses that might be included in a social-adjustment questionnaire are:

"Do you make friends easily?" (Yes, No)
"How many teachers have you disliked very much?" (a) none (b) 1 to 3 (c) 4 to 6 (d) 7 to 10 (e) over 10
"Which would you prefer (a) to be very popular but not to have any very close friends, or (b) to have only a few close friends?"

The scoring of questionnaires may be a simple tabulation of score values, conversion to percentages, or a more complex weighting system in which certain responses reflect certain degrees of some trait, behavior, or feeling.

Some Affective Measures in Physical Education and Exercise Science

Safrit (1981) observed that although there have been numerous tests of affective behavior constructed in our field, only a few have been developed using well-defined, scientific methodology, such as that described by the American Psychological Association (1985). Many of the instruments were developed years ago, when standards were not so exact. Examples of affective measures that represent sound test construction are summarized in the following pages. These instruments have been developed within theoretical models and have been subjected to construct validity research procedures.

Attitude Toward Physical Activity (ATPA) Inventory

Kenyon (1968a, 1968b) developed an inventory based on a theoretical model that attitude toward physical activity is multidimensional and relatively stable. The ATPA items relate to both active (participating) and passive (watching others) involvement in physical activity. The ATPA assesses six dimensions of attitude toward physical activity: as a social experience, for health and fitness, as the pursuit of vertigo, as an aesthetic experience, as catharsis, and as an ascetic experience.

The ATPA is applicable for high school and adult age levels. There are separate test forms for males and females with 59 and 54 items, respectively. Each of the six scales is scored separately. Kenyon verified the content validity of the six dimensions with factor analysis and elicited expert opinion to verify the active-passive involvement of the items. Construct validity has been demonstrated by studies of group differences, such as between athletes and nonathletes, males and females. Reliability coefficients of within-day and stability-over-time estimates for males and females have been acceptable for all six dimensions, ranging from .78 to .91.

Two versions of the ATPA are available—semantic-differential and Likert. The Likert version has a 7-point response scale: very strongly agree, strongly agree, agree, undecided, disagree, strongly disagree, and very strongly disagree. Items are worded both positively and negatively. A sample of a positively worded item (from the social experience dimension) is:

> "The best way to become more socially desirable is to participate in group physical activities."

A sample of a negatively worded item (from the health and fitness dimension) is:

> "Being strong and highly fit is not the most important thing in my life."

The entire instrument is presented in Baumgartner and Jackson (1982) and in Safrit (1981).

Children's Attitude Toward Physical Activity (CATPA)

A children's version of the ATPA was constructed by Simon and Smoll (1974). This instrument, called the *Children's Attitude Toward Physical Activity (CATPA)*, was designed to measure the six dimensions of physical activity identified by Kenyon. Patterned after the ATPA's semantic-differential version, the CATPA was proposed as being logically valid in that it subscribed to the same theoretical model as the ATPA. The instrument has been subjected to continuous analysis and application.

Schutz and Smoll (1977) established concurrent validity of the CATPA with the ATPA. Internal-consistency reliability coefficients are high (.80 to .89); test-retest coefficients are considerably lower. The median coefficient for a 2-week interval was .71, and the median for a 9-week interval was .67. The authors stress that the CATPA should be used in assessing group attitudes rather than individuals.

In an extensive study, Wood (cited in Schutz, Smoll, Carre, & Mosher, 1985) evaluated the psychometric properties of the CATPA and, for the most part, reaffirmed its internal-consistency characteristics and the six-factor structure. On the basis of this study, the CATPA's semantic-differential scales were reduced from eight to five bipolar adjective pairs. The Health and Fitness subdomain was shown to consist of two factors identified as *value* and *enjoyment*. The Social subdomain was also split into two dimensions: "Taking part in physical activities which give you a chance to meet new people" (Social growth), and "Taking part in physical activities which give you a chance to be with your friends" (Social continuation).

Schutz et al. (1985) modified and shortened the CATPA and introduced a new CATPA inventory for 3rd-grade children. In the grade-3 form, each of the five factors are represented by only one questionnaire item, in which "happy faces" are used rather than semantic-differential scales. Hence, it essentially only uses the adjective pair happy-sad. The Catharsis and Ascetic subdomains were eliminated for this age group, and all the subdomain descriptions are presented in question format. For example, under the Vertigo subdomain is the question:

"How do you feel about taking part in exciting physical activities that could be dangerous because you move very fast and must change direction quickly?"

Instructions for administration and norms for both CATPA instruments are presented by Schutz et al. (1985).

Physical Estimation and Attraction Scales (PEAS)

The theoretical model underlying the Physical Estimation and Attraction Scales, by Sonstroem (1974), proposes that participation in physical activity is influenced not only by interest in vigorous activity but also by the estimation of one's own physical fitness, ability, and potential for success in motor performance. Sonstroem's PEAS model differs somewhat from Kenyon's ATPA theoretical framework in that the attraction and estimation components of attitude toward activity are not considered stable. They can be modified as a result of situations and experiences.

The original validity and reliability research was conducted using boys, grades 8 through 12, as subjects. Factor analysis revealed that the estimation and attraction items represented clearly distinct components. In subsequent studies, the estimation scale was found to correlate with self-concept, as measured by the Tennessee Self-Concept Scale (Sonstroem, 1976). Attraction scores were correlated with fitness activities and sports participation (Sonstroem, 1978). Reliability estimates have been very high with both internal consistency (estimation = .87, attraction = .89) and stability over time (estimation = .92, attraction = .94).

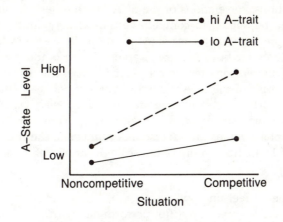

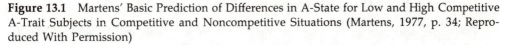

Figure 13.1   Martens' Basic Prediction of Differences in A-State for Low and High Competitive A-Trait Subjects in Competitive and Noncompetitive Situations (Martens, 1977, p. 34; Reproduced With Permission)

The PEAS consists of 100 items: 33 measure physical estimation, 56 measure attraction, and 11 are considered neutral and are not scored. The neutral items are included to attempt to mask the nature of the test. There are also two unscored items related to the social aspects of participation in sports and physical activity. The responses are all true-false. Separate scores are computed for the estimation and attraction items. A sample *neutral* item is:

"I would rather see a play than a movie."

A sample *estimation* item is:

"I lack confidence in performing physical activities."

A sample *attraction* item is:

"I would rather run in a track meet than play badminton."

The 100-item scale may be found in Baumgartner and Jackson (1982) and Safrit (1981). Safrit, Wood, and Dishman (1985) revised the PEAS scale for men and women. The revised scale contains only 23 items for men and 25 items for women. The adult scales are presented in Baumgartner and Jackson (1987).

Sport Competition Anxiety Test (SCAT)

Martens (1977) developed the SCAT as a research tool to assess competitive trait anxiety, which Martens considers a construct that describes an individual's tendency to perceive competitive situations as threatening and to respond to the particular situation. The reaction to the situation is *state anxiety*. The instrument was developed within a theoretical framework of anxiety in the competitive situation (see Figure 13.1).

Construct validity was approached from several dimensions, including comparisons of SCAT test scores of persons who exhibited high and low state anxiety levels in competitive situations; correlations of the SCAT with other personality constructs that were presumed to be related to competitive trait anxiety; and correlations with constructs that were presumed to be unrelated to competitive anxiety. Same-day test-retest reliability coefficients for boys and girls, grades 5 and 6 and grades 8 and 9, ranged from .85 to .93. Different-day test-retest reliability coefficients ranged from .61 to .89.

There are two forms of the SCAT: one for children between 10 and 15 years of age, and one for adults. The response categories are *hardly ever, sometimes,* and *often.* The scoring is 1, 2, 3. A high score indicates high anxiety. Thus, for some items that reflect low anxiety, the point values are reversed. A number of the items are not scored but are included to hide the true nature of the scale. Examples of items (from the children's form) are:

"Before I compete I feel uneasy."
"Before I compete I worry about not performing well."
"Before I compete I am calm." (scoring is reversed)

The scales and normative data for the SCAT are available in Martens (1977). The children's form of the SCAT is reproduced in Safrit (1986).

Ratings of Perceived Exertion (RPE)

Borg (1962) constructed a scale to measure an individual's perceived efforts during exercise. The underlying rationale for the scale is that the many physiological indicators of exertion (e.g., heart rate, respiration, oxygen consumption, blood and muscle lactate accumulation, muscular and joint aches and pains) are combined and integrated into a *whole* or *gestalt* of subjective feeling of physical effort (Borg, 1982). This feeling of perceived exertion was quantified by Borg into a scale with numbers ranging from 6 to 20 (see Figure 13.2). Borg proposed the numbers to coincide roughly with heart rates from 60 to 200 beats per minute (bpm).

In addition to the numbers, there are word descriptors in categories ranging from *very, very light* to *very, very hard* to help the subject in the subjective ratings of effort. For example, moderate exertions paralleling heart rates of around 130 to 150 bpm (numerical values of 13 to 15) have verbal cues of *somewhat hard* to *hard.*

The scale has been validated in numerous studies demonstrating that ratings are reliably related to physiological indicators of exercise intensity, such as heart rate, oxygen consumption, and lactic acid build-up (Borg, 1982). The RPE scale has great practical and research applications in exercise testing, performance, and exercise prescription.

Borg has developed another scale with ratio properties to account for the fact that ratings of exertion and physiological responses are not totally linear (Baumgartner & Jackson, 1987). The scale has ratings from 0 to 10, with verbal descriptors of *extremely weak* (just noticeable) to *extremely strong* (almost maximum). Ratings between 4 and 7 reflect exercise intensities of about 50% to 85% of aerobic capacity. Fractional ratings and ratings above 10 may be used to represent estimates of exertion as accurately as

6

7 Very, very light

8

9 Very light

10

11 Fairly light

12

13 Somewhat hard

14

15 Hard

16

17 Very hard

18

19 Very, very hard

20

Figure 13.2   Ratings of Perceived Exertion (RPE) Scale (Borg, 1982, Reproduced With Permission)

possible. Both RPE scales, along with instructions, are presented in Baumgartner and Jackson (1987).

Other Affective Measures

Numerous affective measurement instruments have been developed for use in physical education and exercise science. It is beyond the scope of this text to attempt to provide sample coverage. In addition to the measurement and evaluation texts already cited in this chapter, refer to Barrow and McGee (1983), Johnson and Nelson (1987), Kirkendall, Gruber, and Johnson (1980), and Neilson and Jensen (1972) for descriptions of tests of self-concept, sportsmanship, leadership, social behavior and adjustment, body-image, stress, and sociometry.

Conclusion

It is difficult to predict the direction of future measurement efforts in the affective domain. Research interests are often cyclical, and presently there is very little work being done in affective measurement in physical education and exercise science.

In a series of articles on measurement and evaluation in the *Journal of Physical Education, Recreation and Dance* (Wiese & Shick, 1982), nearly all of the authors supported the need for and use of affective measurement but recognized the inadequacies of the present measures. Although no specific recommendations for future directions in measurement were given, Griffin (1982) argued that teachers need more practical, action-oriented ways to evaluate affective learning instead of the written tests now available. In a later article, Frye (1983) acknowledged the points made by the authors in the 1982 series and endorsed an alternate approach: to use formal written instruments to assess group interests and attitudes to aid in program evaluation and to use informal observation and guidance for individual evaluation. Perhaps future efforts will focus on more accurate ways of observing behaviors.

There is considerable work being done in observational research concerning the interaction of the teacher and the student. Although this research basically relates to cognitive and psychomotor behaviors, it may soon spread into the affective domain. Studies in which students are interviewed following (or before) some lesson segment with regard to their thought processes could just as well include an affective dimension. The increasingly sophisticated use of video observation in research may lend itself to the observation of various types of behavior. In fact, little work has been done in the rating of social behavior in physical education for about 50 years. Modern technology and innovative research strategies could stimulate renewed interest in this area.

An affective measure that has been studied actively for a number of years is *perceived exertion*. The demonstrated validity of such ratings and their practical applications should prompt continued research efforts on this instrument. The phenomenon of mental imagery is becoming increasingly topical among athletes in some sports, e.g., weightlifting. Attempts to measure aspects of this dimension may be forthcoming. For example, Tew (1987, 1988) has developed an instrument designed to identify aptitude for mental imagery.

One can accurately predict that to be publishable, affective measurement endeavors in the future will have to conform to rigorous test-construction procedures. New measures can be expected to have a sound theoretical base, with construct validity demonstrated in a variety of ways involving different theoretically related variables.

In recent years, research efforts in cognitive and affective test theory in education and psychology have focused on item response theory (IRT) and adaptive testing (see chapter 11). Another term for IRT is **latent trait theory** and another term for adaptive testing is **tailored testing**. IRT research suggests that the traditional Likert-type opinion scales and attitude instruments can be replaced by rating scales that utilize polychotomous graded responses to questions (Spray, 1987). IRT enables testers to validate test inferences at the item level rather than the test level. Thus, the measurements are not confined to the specifics of the test and test situation (Hambleton & van der Linden,

1982). Adaptive testing in the affective domain uses IRT procedures to match a respondent with a test, item by item. Tew (1988) used IRT in the construction of a sport-specific test of mental imagery.

One of the drawbacks of IRT is the large sample sizes needed for accurate estimates of item parameters. Wood (1987) foresees researchers developing and packaging test-item banks that could then be used by practitioners. In light of the widespread interest in IRT and adaptive testing in other disciplines, coupled with advances in methodology and increased availability of microcomputer software for the administration and scoring of items, it is highly likely that researchers in physical education and exercise science will soon apply these techniques to affective measurements. As all areas of research in physical education and exercise science become more refined, progress will continue to be made in the development of more valid and functional measures of affective behavior.

References

American Psychological Association. (1985). *Standards for educational and psychological tests*. Washington, DC: Author.

Barrow, H.M., & McGee, R. (1983). *A practical approach to measurement in physical education* (3rd ed.). Philadelphia: Lea & Febiger.

Baumgartner, T.A., & Jackson, A.S. (1982). *Measurement for evaluation in physical education* (2nd ed.). Dubuque, IA: Wm. C. Brown.

Baumgartner, T.A., & Jackson, A.S. (1987). *Measurement for evaluation in physical education* (3rd ed.). Dubuque, IA: Wm. C. Brown.

Belson, W.A. (1966). The effects of reversing the presentation order of verbal rating scales. *Journal of Advertising Research, 6*, 30–37.

Bentler, P.M. (1980). Multivariate analysis with latent variables: Causal modeling. *Annual Review of Psychology, 31*, 419–456.

Borg, G.A. (1962). *Physical performance and perceived exertion*. Lund, Sweden: Gleerup.

Borg, G. A. (1982). Psychophysical bases of perceived exertion. *Medicine and Science in Sports and Exercise, 14*, 377–381.

Borg, W.R., & Gall, M.D. (1983). *Educational research* (4th ed.). New York: Longman.

Campbell, D.T., Siegman, C.R., & Rees, M.B. (1967). Direction-of-wording effects in the relationship between scales. *Psychological Bulletin, 68*, 292–303.

Cowell, C.C. (1958). Validating an index of social adjustment for high school use. *Research Quarterly, 29*, 7–18.

Frye, P.A. (1983). Measurement of psychosocial aspects of physical education. *Journal of Physical Education, Recreation and Dance, 54*(8), 26–27.

Griffin, P.S. (1982). Second thoughts on affective evaluation. *Journal of Physical Education, Recreation and Dance, 53*(2), 25, 86.

Hambleton, R.K., & van der Linden, W.J. (1982). Advances in item response theory and applications: An introduction. *Applied Psychological Measurement, 6*, 373–378.

Johnson, B.L., & Nelson, J.K. (1987). *Practical measurements for evaluation in physical education* (4th ed.). New York: Macmillan.

Kenyon, G.S. (1968a). A conceptual model for characterizing physical activity. *Research Quarterly, 39,* 96–105.

Kenyon, G.S. (1968b). Six scales for assessing attitude toward physical activity. *Research Quarterly, 39,* 566–574.

Kirkendall, D.R., Gruber, J.J., & Johnson, R.E. (1980). *Measurement and evaluation for physical educators.* Dubuque, IA: Wm. C. Brown.

Lodge, M. (1981). *Magnitude scaling: Quantitative measurement of opinions.* Beverly Hills, CA: Sage.

Martens, R. (1977). *Sport Competition Anxiety Test.* Champaign, IL: Human Kinetics.

McIver, J.P., & Carmines, E.G. (1981). *Unidimensional scaling.* Beverly Hills, CA: Sage.

Neilson, N.P., & Jensen, C.R. (1972). *Measurement and statistics in physical education.* Belmont, CA: Wadsworth.

Nunnally, J.C. (1978). *Psychometric theory.* New York: McGraw-Hill.

Osgood, C.E., Suci, G.J., & Tannenbaum, P.H. (1957). *The measurement of meaning.* Urbana, IL: University of Illinois Press.

Payne, D.A. (Ed.) (1980). *Recent developments in affective measurement.* Washington DC: Jossey-Bass.

Safrit, M.J. (1981). *Evaluation in physical education.* Englewood Cliffs, NJ: Prentice-Hall.

Safrit, M.J. (1986). *Introduction to measurement in physical education and exercise science.* St. Louis: Times Mirror/Mosby.

Safrit, M.J., Wood, T.M., & Dishman, R.K. (1985). The factorial validity of the Physical Estimation and Attraction Scales for Adults. *Journal of Sports Psychology, 7,* 166–190.

Saris, W. (1980). Linear structural relationships. *Quality and Quantity, 14,* 205–224.

Schuman, H. (1966). The random probe: A technique for evaluating the validity of closed questions. *American Sociological Review, 21,* 218–222.

Schuman, H., & Presser, S. (1981). *Questions and answers in attitude surveys.* New York: Academic Press.

Schutz, R.W., & Smoll, F.L. (1977). Equivalence of two inventories for assessing attitudes toward physical activity. *Psychological Reports, 40,* 1031–1034.

Schutz, R.W., Smoll, F.L., Carre, F.A., & Mosher, R.E. (1985). Inventories and norms for children's attitudes toward physical activity. *Research Quarterly for Exercise and Sport, 56,* 256–265.

Sellin, J.T., & Wolfgang, M.E. (1964). *The measurement of delinquency.* New York: John Wiley.

Simon, J.A., & Smoll, F.L. (1974). An instrument for assessing children's attitude toward physical activity. *Research Quarterly, 45,* 407–415.

Snider, J.G., & Osgood, C.E. (1969). *Semantic differential technique.* Chicago: Aldine.

Sonstroem, R.J. (1974). Attitude testing examining certain psychological correlates of physical activity. *Research Quarterly, 45,* 93–103.

Sonstroem, R.J. (1976). The validity of self-perceptions regarding physical and athletic ability. *Medicine and Science in Sports, 8,* 126–132.

Sonstroem, R.J. (1978). Physical estimation and attraction scales: Rationale and research. *Medicine and Science in Sports, 10,* 97–102.

Spielberger, C.D., Gorsuch, R.L., & Lushene, R.E. (1970). *STAI manual.* Palo Alto, CA: Consulting Psychologists Press.

Spray, J.A. (1987). Recent developments in measurement and possible applications to the measurement of psychomotor behavior. *Research Quarterly for Exercise and Sport, 58,* 203–209.

Tew, J. (1987). Item calibration procedures for a questionnaire on mental imagery. In J.K. Nelson (Ed.), *Proceedings of the fifth measurement and evaluation symposium* (p. 87). Baton Rouge, LA: Louisiana State University Press.

Tew, J. (1988). *Construction of a sport specific mental imagery assessment instrument using item response and classical test theory methodology.* Unpublished doctoral dissertation, Louisiana State University, Baton Rouge.

Wiese, C.E., & Shick, J. (Eds.) (1982). Affective measurement in physical education: Doing well and feeling good. *Journal of Physical Education, Recreation and Dance, 53*(2), 15–25, 86.

Wood, T.M. (1987). Putting item response theory into perspective. *Research Quarterly for Exercise and Sport, 58,* 216–220.

Supplementary Readings

Anastasi, A. (1982). *Psychological testing* (5th ed.). New York: Macmillan. Chapter 17.

Ebel, R.L., & Frisbie, D.A. (1986). *Essentials of educational measurement.* Englewood Cliffs, NJ: Prentice-Hall. Chapter 18.

Kubiszyn, T., & Borich, G. (1987). *Educational testing and measurement* (2nd ed.). Glenview, IL: Scott, Foresman & Co. Chapter 10.

Schuman, H., & Presser, S. (1981). *Questions and answers in attitude surveys.* New York: Academic Press.

Wiese, C.F., & Schick, J. (Eds.) (1982). Affective measurement in physical education: Doing fine and feeling good. *Journal of Physical Education, Recreation and Dance, 53*(2), 15–25, 86.

14

Testing and Grading in the Psychomotor Domain

Larry D. Hensley
University of Northern Iowa

and Whitfield B. East
East Tennessee State University

Measurement and evaluation contribute in many ways to the discipline of physical education. One of the most significant contributions is to the instructional process. A primary goal of the trained physical educator is to facilitate the acquisition of movement skills, i.e., to help students learn to move and move to learn. Since skill learning is most often measured as a function of skill performance, direct measures of pre- and post-instructional performance offer the most objective measures of learning. To determine the extent to which learning has occurred, physical educators need measures that adequately discriminate among ability levels. Establishing this evidence of learning is an ongoing process, the results of which may be used to evaluate programming, instruction, and achievement.

In simple terms, measurement and evaluation tie the process of learning to the product of performance. Without the valid and reliable feedback provided by measurement and evaluation, the system cannot function properly. Exploring the various applications of measurement to the world of movement should benefit both the physical educator and the exercise scientist.

Testing in the Psychomotor Domain

Historically, measurement in the psychomotor domain has progressed through a number of eras since the early 1900s. Tests have been constructed that purport to measure athletic ability, physical fitness, motor educability, general motor ability, motor fitness, sport skills, and so forth. The variety of psychomotor qualities included within these terms represents a vast repertoire of potential test items. Unfortunately considerable confusion exists regarding the definition of these terms, and there is little agreement as to which psychomotor qualities should be included in test batteries designed to measure these constructs. Definitions for these terms vary from one author to another. No attempt will be made to derive a consensus definition for each of these terms. The intent is simply to inform the reader of the general lack of agreement that exists within the profession.

The principles of measurement and evaluation are often applied to a variety of movement abilities and skills. The four areas of movement most commonly measured today are: (a) developmental skills, (b) motor abilities, (c) physical fitness, and (d) sports skills. Physical fitness and motor abilities represent human characteristics that to a large extent delimit movement. Although unmeasurable as a single construct, the underlying components of both physical fitness and motor ability are measurable and are often thought of as desirable qualities of human movement and performance. The components of **physical fitness**, specifically **health-related fitness**, typically include muscular strength and endurance, cardiovascular endurance, flexibility, and body composition. In addition, the components of motor ability may also include power, speed, agility, coordination, balance, and perhaps kinesthesis. Developmental skills are those movements that Gallahue (1976) described as fundamental movement patterns (e.g., *locomotor*: running, leaping, hopping; *stability*: body awareness; and *manipulation*: throwing, kicking, catching, striking). Sport skills are those movements specific to performance in a sport (e.g., tennis, golf, basketball, etc.). Although it is vital that valid and reliable measurement techniques be available to assess the movement skills in each of these areas, a comprehensive discussion of the tests and measurement techniques applicable for each of these areas is beyond the scope of this chapter. Instead, we will focus on a few significant trends in psychomotor testing that pertain to measuring motor abilities, physical fitness, and sports skills.

Testing Motor Ability

Traditionally, physical educators have surmised that there must be a general trait or ability that enables an individual to perform motor tasks. This concept has been taken to mean an all-around ability in the psychomotor domain. Typically this general ability has been thought to be an integrated composite of such specific traits as strength, coordination, endurance, agility, balance, power, speed, flexibility, and so forth. Conversely, the ability to perform a specific motor task in a particular performance area was considered to be a sport skill, or what Fleishman (1964) termed a *psychomotor skill*. Although there has never been a consensus regarding the essential components of this general physical ability, numerous test batteries were developed during the first half of this century that purported to measure this human trait, commonly referred to as **general motor ability**. As defined by Barrow and McGee (1964), general motor ability was "the present acquired and innate ability to perform motor skills of a general or fundamental nature."

Early researchers used logic and arbitrary selection to identify the components to be measured by a general motor ability test battery; more recently the use of factor analytic procedures enabled researchers to empirically identify these components or traits. In the later 1940s and 1950s, measures of general motor ability abounded. Researchers developed battery after battery to measure general motor ability, culminating in 1954, when Barrow published the Barrow Motor Ability Test. This particular battery was used extensively throughout the country for a variety of purposes. As an example of the scope of this test's use, the University of North Carolina at Chapel Hill used the Barrow Motor Ability Test for freshmen physical education competency examinations until 1971. The assessment of general motor ability was a significant part of most physical education curricula. Tests of general motor ability would often include a variety of individual test items, as is illustrated by the examples shown in Table 14.1. Scores on these individual tests were then combined into a single score that supposedly represented a general motor ability factor. Reliability on such test batteries was generally high, because the individual test items that comprised the battery were very reliable. Validity was typically determined by administering a large number of test items to a group of subjects and then selecting a smaller subset of test items (the actual test battery) that was highly correlated with the composite index of the larger test. The underlying assumption of this validation approach for generality testing was that general ability could be predicted from the results of a limited number of test items. This validation approach was later determined to be questionable, because the criterion score used for validation purposes (the composite score for the larger set of test items) actually included the predictor variables in its computation. Thus, a spuriously high correlation coefficient was almost guaranteed. There was also no evidence to indicate that the criterion score based on the larger set of test items actually measured general motor ability.

In the late 1950s and 1960s there was a dramatic shift in attitude toward measuring motor ability sparked by the work of Henry (1958) and others. Henry proposed a theory of motor performance and learning called the **memory-drum theory.** This theory postulated that motor skills were executed in a somewhat automatic, sequential fashion. Once the movement was elicited, the *memory-drum* would control the movement along a predictable and replicable path. Although this theory was proposed to describe the acquisition and execution of motor skills, the tenets of the theory were

Table 14.1   General Motor Ability Test Batteries

BARROW MOTOR ABILITY TEST (1954)
1. Standing long jump
2. Zigzag run
3. Softball throw for distance
4. Wall pass
5. Medicine ball put
6. 60-yard dash

SCOTT MOTOR ABILITY TEST (1939, 1943)
1. Basketball throw for distance
2. Four-second dash
3. Wall pass
4. Standing long jump
5. Obstacle race

LARSON MOTOR ABILITY TEST (1940)
1. Dodging run
2. Bar snap
3. Chinning
4. Dips
5. Vertical jump

---

soon applied to the assessment of general motor abilities. Basically this research evidence indicated that motor ability is task-specific and not generalizable to many tasks. Thus, an individual who scores well on a general motor ability test or who is considered to be an all-around athlete possesses many specific motor abilities rather than a great amount of general motor ability. As a result of the formulation of this specificity theory, the concept of general motor ability lost popularity, leading to a demise in the use of these tests.

During the early 1960s there followed a plethora of research designed to support the specificity of motor behavior theory. Battinelli (1984) and Baumgartner and Jackson (1987) reviewed a variety of these studies. Two classic examples of this type of research were reported by Singer (1966) and Smith (1969). Singer used a wall-volley measure for arms and legs to assess the generality of coordination measures. The resultant correlation coefficients were low (.146 to .539), accounting for only a small percentage of common variance. Singer concluded that there was strong evidence of specificity in limb performance, thus adding support to the theory of specificity. Smith obtained similar spurious relationships between arm strength and speed of movement for various degrees of elbow flexion. He concluded that the results supported the theory of specificity, in that differences in limb speed were independent of arm strength associated with a particular limb and joint.

Many correlational studies were conducted to compare the relationships between various specific measures of motor performance. Low correlation coefficients were consistently obtained, and the results were used to repudiate much of the work on general motor ability. A major problem in the application of these findings was a misunderstanding of the purpose of motor ability testing. The conclusions by Singer, Henry, Smith, and many others were directed at the practice of generalizing motor performance across a range of specific skills and the assertion that measuring these abilities somehow provided a general indication of one's ability. General motor behaviorists may have erred by concluding that the function of motor ability assessments was to provide information that could be generalized in a measurable way across a broad spectrum of sports skills. The advocates of motor specificity may have extended their conclusions beyond the bounds of repudiating the assertions of general motor ability.

Although measures of motor ability may not be generalizable to specific sports, it may be reasonable to assume that these qualities contribute in some generalizable way to a repertoire of fundamental movement patterns and motor skills (Battinelli, 1984). Battinelli suggested that general components of motor ability are the physical supports providing the foundation on which future specific movements can be built. Barrow and McGee (1964) even stated that "motor ability is made up of factors which are basic to all movements" (p. 122). The work of Fleishman (1964) also provided evidence to suggest there are certain basic physical abilities common to many psychomotor tasks. He suggested that both the rate of learning, or skill acquisition, and the final level of achievement is dependent on one's level of achievement of the basic physical abilities.

Clearly the concept of specificity, as contrasted with general motor ability in motor skill acquisition and performance, must be recognized. Although the research evidence suggests it may be inappropriate to use motor ability tests as a predictor of some illusive general motor ability, physical educators should not simply discard motor ability tests. Rather, as suggested by Johnson and Nelson (1986), physical educators should make decisions concerning the efficacy of motor ability tests on the basis of their particular programmatic goals, needs, and testing purposes.

Testing Physical Fitness

Physical fitness has long been recognized as one of the foremost goals of physical education. Thus, it is not surprising that the professional literature abounds with physical fitness tests. What is surprising, however, is the lack of a universally accepted definition of physical fitness. Historically, physical fitness was generally viewed in broad terms, combining aspects of both physiological function and motor ability (Baumgartner & Jackson, 1987). A typical physical fitness test battery would include test items to measure such qualities as muscular strength, muscular endurance, and cardio-respiratory endurance, along with balance, flexibility, speed, power, and agility. As defined by the President's Council on Physical Fitness and Sports, physical fitness is "the ability to carry out daily tasks with vigor and alertness, without undue fatigue, and with ample energy to enjoy leisure-time pursuits and to meet unforeseen emergencies" (Clarke,

1971, p. 1). This rather general definition did little to differentiate between those qualities associated with physiological function and those associated with motor performance, although there may have been an implicit connection to healthy living.

Recent research evidence has established a link between physical activity and functional health. This basic relationship between exercise and health has led to a more focused view of physical fitness, one that distinguishes between health-related fitness and performance-related fitness (primarily associated with athletic ability). In a discussion of these new concepts of physical fitness, Falls (1980) indicated that health-related fitness was associated with the physiological and psychological functioning that was thought to offer the individual some degree of protection against degenerative diseases, such as coronary heart disease, obesity, and musculoskeletal disorders. Since the available physical fitness test batteries did not properly reflect the relationship between physical activity and health, newer test batteries have been developed that subscribe to the definition of health-related fitness. The American Alliance for Health, Physical Education, Recreation and Dance (AAHPERD) has assumed leadership for the development of new fitness tests that emphasize the relationship between physical activity and health, and has published the Health-Related Physical Fitness Test (1980) and, more recently, the Physical Best (AAHPERD, 1988). The Physical Best Program is a comprehensive educational and assessment program that places major emphasis on health-related fitness: aerobic capacity, body composition, flexibility, and muscular strength and endurance.

With the current emphasis on health-related fitness, less attention has been focused on performance-related or athletic fitness, although it is still appropriate for some purposes in sports and physical education. In his discussion of modern concepts of physical fitness, Falls (1980) described performance-related fitness as including those qualities of function that provide the individual with the ability to participate in sports activities with greater power, strength, endurance, and so forth. Performance-related fitness is perceived by some to be similar to motor fitness, a term whose origin has been traced to World War II. According to Clarke and Clarke (1987) motor fitness is a limited aspect of general motor ability, yet it is broader than physical fitness and includes the following components: muscular strength, muscular endurance, circulatory-respiratory endurance, power, agility, speed, and flexibility. According to these descriptions, performance-related fitness and motor fitness are referring to the same thing and can be used interchangeably. Recognizing this similarity and the confusion that surrounded fitness testing, Clarke and Clarke proposed that motor *performance* be used rather than motor *fitness* to designate this type of testing. Since basic physical abilities as described earlier in this chapter are being measured, we would propose that motor ability testing might even be a better choice of terms. Regardless of the term used, numerous test batteries, such as the AAHPERD Youth Fitness Test (1976), have been published that purport to measure some of these qualities.

Considerable confusion exists today among practitioners, who are being confronted with many different types of physical fitness tests. Almost every fitness test has a different national agency endorsing its use, and some of the tests contain items that seem to measure both health-related and performance-related fitness. Under these difficult circumstances, it is easy to understand why one would become confused and lose interest in any type of fitness testing. It is our opinion that the critical issue facing physical educators today is not whether health-related fitness is better than performance-related fitness, or vice versa; rather it is to recognize the important distinction between the two and to select the appropriate test battery based on the purposes and needs of one's program.

Testing Sport Skills

Historically, sport skill testing has received significant attention from physical educators. In fact, hundreds of tests purporting to measure various sport skills have been developed and published since the early 1900s. Skill tests have traditionally been either a target or accuracy test, a speed-type test, a power test, a repetition or volley test, or the actual performance itself, such as bowling, golf, or archery. One positive outcome of the demise of testing for general motor ability was the increased attention placed on physical fitness and sport skill testing. As the fitness craze grew, so did the attempts to establish valid and reliable measures. The Texas Physical Fitness Test (1973), the Health-Related Physical Fitness Test (AAHPERD, 1980), and measures of body composition and cardiovascular endurance evolved from the research of the 1960s and 1970s. Similar contributions were also made in the measurement and evaluation of sport skills.

The development of sport skill tests generally involves four phases: (a) select the attributes to be measured, (b) establish measures that will assess the appropriate attributes, (c) determine the reliability and establish an appropriate measurement schedule, and (d) estimate the validity of each measure. When constructing a sport skill test, it is important to consider the characteristics of a good measure. Most measurement specialists maintain that reliability, validity, and selected administrative characteristics (e.g., ease of setup, equipment, number of testers, and time) are major delimiters of a good measure. However, the measure should also be gamelike, discriminate among ability levels, measure only a single attribute, and be independent of the ability of others. The development of sport skill tests has changed dramatically over the past 20–30 years. With the use of high-speed computers, multi-item batteries can be developed that assess the extent of complete skill development. Rather than discussing test development from a conceptual viewpoint, it may be more appropriate to first focus on a few examples of sport skill tests that have been published recently.

Perhaps the simplest approach to test development was utilized by Hensley, East, and Stillwell (1979) to develop a racquetball skills test. The attributes selected for this test battery were measures of the forehand and backhand stroke. The dependent measure was simply the number of repetitions or volleys during a given time period. Once the test was developed and data were collected, estimation of the reliability and validity of the skill measures was straightforward. For the racquetball skills test, a stability reliability coefficient was computed for the sum of two trials over two days. The intraclass R stability coefficients were found to be acceptable (.76 to .86). Evidence of concurrent validity was established by determining the relationship between a criterion measure (instructors' ratings) and the observed scores from the skills test. Although the reported validity coefficients were relatively high (.79 for women and .86 for men), the use of instructors' ratings as the criterion score represented a limitation. The results would have been more compelling if another measure, such as tournament ratings or a *known-groups* approach, had been utilized.

A step up in test construction complexity was evidenced in the Green Golf Skills Test (Green, East, & Hensley, 1987). Attributes were selected based on a conceptual analysis of the game of golf. The skill measures were developed and then analyzed using a multiple linear regression model to determine the relative contribution of each measure to golf playing ability. By using the regression model with several predictor measures, the size of the validity coefficient may be significantly increased. Thus this approach to test development is likely to approximate a more general measure of sport skill. The components identified for the test battery were the short putt, long putt, chip shot, pitch shot, middle-distance shot, and the drive. Golfing ability was measured by the score for 36 holes of golf. The regression analysis approach to skill test development served two functions. First, it functioned as a method of establishing a concurrent validity coefficient for the test battery. Second, it delimited the skill components to those that accounted for the greatest proportion of explained variance. The use of a multiple regression approach also provided a certain degree of flexibility to potential test users by enabling them to select subtests of the complete battery. As a result of limitations such as time, equipment, and personnel, an instructor may select a combination of test items that is best suited to a specific situation. In such cases, the multiple R still provides evidence of the validity for this combination of test items. For the Green Golf Test, the highest simple correlation between any single test item and the 36-hole criterion score was .66. However, various combinations of test items yielded validity coefficients as follows: .72 for middle-distance and pitch shot, .76 for middle-distance shot, pitch shot, and long putt, and .77 for the middle-distance shot, chip shot, pitch shot, and long putt.

An additional point should be discussed that concerns the use of the 36 holes of golf as the criterion measure for the establishment of concurrent validity. Many times, participation or performance in a sport may not be indicative of a person's overall skill in that sport. Two examples are golf and bowling. Often 18 holes of golf or 1 game in bowling may be utilized as a criterion measure of skill for that sport. This may be fallacious, because during any given round of golf or game of bowling not every skill situation may arise. Consider, for example, the bunker shot. Student A may play 18 holes of golf, avoiding the bunkers, and shoot an 80. The next day the same student may play the same course and hit 3 bunkers. Because of a lack of bunker skills the golfer scored 90 on day 2. This illustrates the importance of (a) using a valid and reliable skill test that measures all possible skill components and (b) carefully selecting the criterion measure.

A more complex model for developing a sport skill test was used by Hopkins, Shick, and Plack (1984) in the development of the AAHPERD Basketball Skills Test. For this battery, a factor analysis model was used to identify those measures of basketball playing ability that largely explained the basketball construct. Such a model incorporates both logical and statistical considerations of validity. Many measures of dribbling, shooting, defense, passing, and other components of basketball playing ability were analyzed initially. Using factor analytic procedures, four factors were established, and measures with the highest factor loadings were selected for the test battery. For each of the four measures (shooting, control-dribble, speed-passing, and defensive movement), concurrent validity coefficients and intraclass R reliability coefficients were computed. Although validity coefficients of individual measures ranged from .40 to .95, the validity for the complete battery was reasonably high, ranging from .65 to .95. The factor analysis model provides a more comprehensive method of establishing the appropriate attributes of sport skills constructs.

Limitations of skills testing. Unfortunately, the multitude of existing skills tests lie dormant. Many of these suffer from questionable validity, but most do not lend themselves to use in the mass-testing situation likely to occur in the typical physical education class. Over the past twenty years, several events have contributed to the complexity of sports skill test development and administration. With fewer teachers, more students, and shorter class periods, the time taken to administer a skills test has become a major constraint. These problems have generally resulted in a shift away from valid and reliable product-oriented measures of sport skills to less time-consuming process-oriented, observational measures. This problem is further complicated by the increasing heterogeneity of classes created by the implementation of Title IX. It takes a dedicated and well-prepared physical educator to administer, without help, the AAHPERD Basketball Skills Test to a class of 50 9th-graders. A short overview of the status of research in sports skill testing and efforts to alleviate several problems was provided by Disch (1986) and may provide additional insight for those interested in this topic.

Possible solutions to this growing problem should be explored. First, test construction should take into account restrictive factors that directly affect utilization of a given test. Skill tests must incorporate setup, testing, and scoring procedures that will enable them to become administratively feasible in a typical physical education class. The Green Golf Test (Green et al., 1987) provides a good example of a contemporary test in which the administrative procedures facilitate its use.

A second alternative to the time dilemma is to develop a parent support club. Such clubs have been used successfully in Logon County, West Virginia, and one is currently being developed in Upper East Tennessee. A club would consist of parents who can serve as volunteer test administrators for sport skill assessments (or any other type of assessment). Parents would be trained as needed to assist the physical educator with test administration. There are several advantages of such a program: (a) the instructor gains much needed help, (b) there tend to be fewer behavior problems with parents in the classroom or gymnasium, and (c) parents become more familiar with a quality physical education program. Thus, the support club can provide "people power" that allows the instructor to conduct a quality program by administering appropriate measures of movement skills.

An alternative approach to dealing with the problems associated with skills testing may be through the use of a trials-to-criterion testing approach (Spray, 1983; Spray, Sorenson, & Hooper, 1985; Shifflett, 1985). This method of testing involves the use of sequential trials of some task until a prespecified number of successes is attained by the examinee. An examinee's test score is the number of trials needed to attain the prespecified success level or criterion score. For example, if the main goal of a tennis serve is to hit the ball into the appropriate section of the court, then one might specify that 5 serves in the proper court would constitute the desired criterion to achieve. One student might require 10 trials to achieve the goal, another 8 trials, and yet another might require only 5 trials. Such a testing approach would probably require setting an upper limit on the number of trials, but at the same time it provides excellent practice opportunities for the skill. This technique is best for the target-type tasks common in many sports, and it may be adapted across skill levels.

Another innovative approach to test development that has direct applications to skills testing is the use of a validity generalization model. Through such an approach it is possible to collect data on a test from divergent groups, often using convenience samples, and then combine the validity and reliability coefficients across groups to determine the generalizability of validity and reliability information (Patterson, 1986; Safrit, Costa, & Hooper, 1986). This technique adds considerable flexibility to the task of test development. (See chapter 5 for a more complete discussion of validity generalization.)

A series of articles in the September 1987 *Research Quarterly for Exercise and Sport* pointed out that many of the current testing practices in physical education are less than satisfactory, and further suggested that item response theory (IRT) and adaptive testing might be an alternative approach to testing in our field (Spray, 1987; Disch, 1987; Safrit, 1987; Wood, 1987). The possibilities that IRT holds for sport skills testing is particularly exciting. Traditionally, using classical test theory (CTT), skills tests have been designed that measure certain skill components that have been determined to be necessary to perform a certain sport. Taken together, these components are then thought to reflect a person's ability to perform the sport. Such tests have focused largely on the *product* of the movement rather than on the *process* of the movement. Product measurements generally facilitate the recording of a quantitative score, are deemed more objective than process measurements, and may possess higher reliability and validity. However, as Disch (1987) pointed out, the subjective ratings by an expert during actual game performance may be more *practically valid* than the traditionally developed skills test. That is, the ratings of an expert observer may more accurately reflect the integration of component skills required in an actual game situation.

A traditional sport skill test generally considers a sport skill as an isolated component, with little concern as to how this skill is integrated with other skills in a game. Spray (1987) also suggests that traditional tests may be *test-bound* and *population-bound* so that changing any one of several circumstances (e.g., the test situation, the intended use, or the intended population) is likely to change the validity and reliability as well. Through the use of IRT and adaptive testing, it may be possible to more efficiently measure sport skills and the underlying latent traits of sport performance that have heretofore been reserved for experts' ratings. (See chapter 11 for more information on this topic.)

The limitations of assessing movement skills are considerable and present many challenges for the instructor and for the measurement and evaluation specialist. By being more innovative in test construction, using available technology, and utilizing support groups for assistance, it is possible to conduct valid and reliable assessments of movement skills.

Sport profiles. Once a valid and reliable sport skills test has been administered, the instructor has only begun the process of making a final determination or judgment about the value of that performance. The evaluation process often breaks down at this crucial point. Instructors are often bewildered by the wide variety of scores in varying units of measurement. Some teachers administer, in a very professional manner, excellent tests only to apply a relatively meaningless alphabetic scale to the resultant measures, because they were unable to combine the various scores within the battery. This becomes an even more difficult task when subsequent instructional units are combined.

A variety of student attributes are frequently examined for evaluation purposes in the typical physical education class. Some of the more commonly measured attributes are: attendance; participation; knowledge of rules, strategies, and principles; skill performance and achievement; attitude; and improvement. In most assessment situations, different units of measurement and even different measurement scales are used. Combining the data into a single meaningful score is difficult and not always relevant. When it is appropriate to form a composite score, several approaches have been recommended, e.g., the weighted sums of standard scores (such as T-scores) or the development of alpha-numeric scales to standardize the data and thus permit their summation (Baumgartner & Jackson, 1987). A *sport profile*, an innovative alternative to these procedures with applications to sport skill assessment, has been described by Davis (1983) and warrants additional discussion.

A sport profile is a flexible tool for standardizing a variety of components of instructional performance. Figure 14.1 depicts a bowling profile with four components: (a) participation, (b) knowledge, (c) mechanics or skill-process, and (d) skill-product. These components may be changed or modified to meet the needs and philosophy of the instructor. Once the measurement strategies have been identified, each component is scaled to allow the transformation from real data to standardized scores. The instructor may also weight each component according to its contribution to the total performance. The end product of the sport profile is a cumulative scale-free score that may be used to assess student achievement for a single sports skill or combined with other scores to measure an entire term's performance.

The sport profile is an efficient method of handling a variety of measures associated with the evaluation of skill learning. The advantages of the profile are numerous. It allows flexibility in selecting attributes for grading. The profile provides a weighting system to support content relevance. Scales are standardized, thereby providing uniformity among instructors for assessing performance. Finally, sport profiles provide a cumulative record of student performance that may be used to justify a grade or chart progress throughout a longitudinal period. In making the difficult transition from measures of performance to measures for evaluation, the sport profile provides a simple and effective solution.

Evaluating Student Achievement in Physical Education

Perhaps the primary function of schools in this country is to facilitate learning. It is through this process that humans are generally hopeful of achieving a richer, more

WSC: PE 111
Bowling, Elementary
W.M. Davis

Unit: 01-08
Handout: 04
Revised: 1078

PROFILE OF ___Myron Webber___ ID _201-73-0491_ QUARTER _FALL '87_

FACTOR COMPONENTS	0	1	2	3	4	5	6	7	8	9	10	WT	SUB TOTAL
A. PARTICIPATION													
1. Attendance (0-9/10-11/12,13,14/15,16,17/18,19,20)	0	0	0	0	0	0	0	0	0	●	0	10	90
2. Bowling Outside of Class (0/1/2,3,4/6,8,10/12,14,16)	0	0	0	0	0	0	0	●	0	0	0	5	35
B. KNOWLEDGE													
3. Etiquette, Ball Selection	0	0	0	0	0	0	0	0	●	0	0	1	8
4. Rules, Terms	0	0	0	0	0	0	●	0	0	0	0	1	6
5. Approach, Delivery	0	0	0	0	0	0	●	0	0	0	0	1	6
6. Spot Bowling	0	0	0	0	0	0	0	0	●	0	0	1	8
7. Scoring	0	0	0	0	0	0	0	0	●	0	0	1	8
8. Competition	0	0	0	0	0	●	0	0	0	0	0	1	5
C. MECHANICS (0/1/2,3,4/5,6,7/8,9,10)													
9. Stance _7 8 9_ Too Upright	0	0	0	0	0	0	0	0	●	0	0	2	16
10. Push-away _6 6 6_ Shorter Step	0	0	0	0	0	0	●	0	0	0	0	2	12
11. Swing _5 4 5_ arm straight - forward lean	0	0	0	0	0	●	0	0	0	0	0	2	10
12. Delivery _8 5 5_ don't rush - glide.	0	0	0	0	0	●	0	0	0	0	0	2	10
13. Follow-through _9 8 7_ Finish higher - more lift	0	0	0	0	0	0	0	0	●	0	0	2	16
D. SKILL-Objective													
14. Bowling Average — In Class (0/1-100/101,113,125/126,133,140/141,150,160) _148 130 140 144 158_ (144)	0	0	0	0	0	0	0	0	●	0	0	10	80

Total Weighted Score   310

Note: From M.W. Davis, Weber State University. Reprinted by permission of author.

Figure 14.1   Bowling Sports Profile

rewarding, and effective life. An integral part of the educational process, however, is the identification of important learning outcomes that promote the desirable changes we seek in our students. Hence, the importance of identifying the appropriate learning outcomes and translating these to instructional objectives is critical to the success of the educational process. Gronlund (1981) indicated that the first step in teaching (and evaluation) is that of determining the learning outcomes to be expected from the classroom experience. According to Baumgartner and Jackson (1987), if the instructional process is to be meaningful, it is essential that (a) the instructional objectives be relevant, (b) the actual instruction be appropriately designed to meet the objectives, and (c) the evaluation procedures be reliable and valid assessments of students' achievement of the stated objectives. Broadly conceived, the measurement and evaluation process facilitates the achievement of intended learning outcomes.

Some type of evaluation is inevitable in teaching. Since virtually all school systems require the practice of giving grades, the assessment of student achievement and the subsequent awarding of grades should be one of the most frequently occurring tasks performed by a teacher. This is not to say that grading is the sole purpose or even the major purpose of the measurement and evaluation process; it is simply to suggest that grading is a requirement of most teachers in the educational system in this country. It might be suggested that a teacher could be ineffective in the classroom, at least up to a point, but it is unlikely that a teacher would escape notice for even a short time if the periodic grade reports were not turned in on time. Unfortunately, in the typical physical education class, the measurement and evaluation component may be the least understood and most abused educational function.

Status of Grading Practices in Physical Education

Evidence over the last 25–30 years suggests that little systematic evaluation is being done in physical education classes. Fox (1959) indicated that little testing was being used to evaluate the performance of students in physical education classes in Oregon public schools. Similarly, Coker (1972) reported a lack of formal testing to evaluate performance in physical education in Louisiana public schools. Both of these investigators reported that class attendance and "dressing out" were the most frequently used variables in the assessment of students in physical education classes. In a survey of student teachers in Colorado public schools, Morrow (1978) determined that evaluation was based primarily on dress and participation. More than two-thirds of the respondents indicated they had little or no opportunity to use the measurement techniques learned in their measurement and evaluation course. Imwold, Rider, and Johnson (1982) surveyed Florida public school physical education teachers and reported that slightly more than one-half of the respondents utilized skill tests to assess performance of their students, while less than 40% used knowledge tests.

In a recent survey of Iowa public school teachers, Hensley (1987) reported that only 18% used the Health-Related Physical Fitness Test and that *participation/effort* was the overwhelming choice as the most important factor used in determining a student's final grade. Only about one-third (35%) of the respondents used sport skill tests. In a survey of approximately 1,400 public school teachers in Iowa, Wyoming, Kansas, and Georgia (Hensley, Lambert, Baumgartner, & Stillwell, 1987), the authors noted some positive changes regarding the evaluation efforts in our public school physical education programs, but overall gave poor marks to current practices. For example, slightly less than 50% of the teachers reported the regular use of skill tests or written knowledge tests. Furthermore, 54% reported using the AAHPERD Youth Fitness Test, while only 19% reported using the newer AAHPERD Health-Related Physical Fitness Test (HRPFT). Similiar results on the usage rate were reported by Safrit and Wood (1986) among Illinois, Oregon, and Arizona physical education teachers. Hensley and his colleagues found that female teachers were the more frequent users of sport skill tests, written tests, and the HRPFT. Interestingly, 25% of the survey respondents indicated they did not use written tests of any type. More than half of the teachers surveyed (59%) reported that the grading practices used were determined by the individual teacher and not by the school district or the school administration. The use of letter grades to report performance in physical education was the overwhelming choice by teachers, although elementary school teachers were most likely to use alternative methods to report grades.

Compared with previous studies, Hensley et al. (1987) reported an increased use of **criterion-referenced evaluation**. Fifty-eight percent reported using a criterion-referenced approach to evaluation, while only 37% reported using a norm-referenced approach. Criterion-referenced evaluation was employed more frequently by less experienced teachers, while the more experienced teacher preferred **norm-referenced evaluations**. When asked about their use of subjective ratings to evaluate students, 33% of those surveyed indicated they used subjective ratings frequently; another 55% reported using subjective ratings occasionally. There were no differences in the use of subjective ratings between gender groups, between coaches and non-coaches, or based on years of experience.

Respondents also were asked to indicate the relative frequency with which selected factors were used in determining a student's final grade, and to identify the most important attribute used in determining the course grade. Table 14.2 illustrates the relative frequency with which selected factors were used to determine grades in physical education.

Clearly *participation* was the *most frequently used* factor in determining student grades. Furthermore, when asked to identify the *most important* factor used in determining students' final grades, *participation* was named by 46% of the respondents. The next most frequently mentioned factor was *attitude* at 16%, followed by *skill* at 11%, and *attendance* at 7%. Male teachers, coaches, and those with more experience indicated a greater use of *attendance* and *dressing out* for the determination of grades. Finally, female teachers and coaches reported using *skill tests* and *written knowledge tests* more frequently than their counterparts. *Attitude* and *effort* were cited more frequently among elementary physical education teachers. Clearly the evidence from this most recent study and those preceding it suggests that physical education teachers, in general, are basing their grades on questionable criteria and in fact are showing little evidence of using the information normally provided in the undergraduate measurement and evaluation class. One might infer from this analysis that evaluation and grading are not high priorities among most physical educators.

Table 14.2   Attributes Used in Determining Grades

Factor	Percent of Responses		
	Frequently	Occasionally	Never
Attendance	58	23	19
Attitude	76	18	7
Dressing Out	72	7	21
Effort	88	9	3
Homework	11	33	56
Improvement	68	28	4
Knowledge Tests	46	32	22
Participation	96	2	2
Potential	25	42	33
Skills-Observation	58	33	9
Skills-Test	45	36	19
Sportsmanship	75	20	5

Using Evaluation in Teaching

While most teachers are concerned about the quality of education, many view evaluation as a "necessary evil" of the educational process. Given that most certified teachers have had a measurement and evaluation class during their professional preparation, why do evaluation and grading cause such a problem?

Educational trends today clearly suggest movement toward new and greater demands on teachers in the area of testing and evaluation. Recently a number of state legislatures passed laws making schools and teachers accountable for student learning—in essence mandating testing programs to determine the quality of student learning. Furthermore, since the late 1970s educators have been embracing the idea of competency-based education, whereby the attainment of satisfactory levels of a specified behavior is required for such purposes as graduation, certification, or employment. For example, many states now mandate some type of minimum-competency testing. Consider also the requirement for lawyers to pass the bar exam; accountants, the CPA exam; or swimming pool lifeguards, the American Red Cross certifying exam. The need for good measurement and evaluation programs in our schools is becoming greater. Educators should work to improve such programs and should not abuse them.

Student evaluation has many uses in the school. The product of the evaluation process can be used to (a) provide feedback to the student regarding his or her achievement, (b) report to parents the student's status, (c) keep school personnel informed of a student's status, (d) provide a permanent record of the student's achievement, and (e) enhance the instructional process. It should be clear that the evaluation process plays a vital role in the efficacy of contemporary school programs. The simplified instructional model shown in Figure 14.2 illustrates the steps involved in the teaching process and emphasizes the interrelated nature of teaching and evaluation.

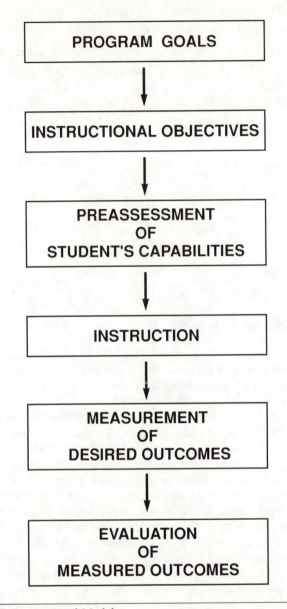

Figure 14.2   Simple Instructional Model

Evaluation is an integral component of the educational system and should not be viewed as an end in itself. This does not suggest, however, that teachers, administrators, and measurement specialists agree on the best evaluation system to use. Certainly this issue becomes somewhat philosophical, but there are certain dimensions of the issue having particular significance in physical education that deserve further discussion.

Criterion or norm-referenced standards. The interpretation or judgment that is applied to the test score constitutes the process of evaluation. Normally such judgments are made with reference to some standard. The two most widely used types of standards are criterion-referenced and norm-referenced. Criterion-referenced standards refer to the method of interpretation in which test scores or measurements are judged directly in terms of a specified criterion behavior. Students who achieve the specified standard may be labeled *masters* and those who do not labeled *nonmasters*. Norm-referenced standards, on the other hand, involve the hierarchical ordering of individuals on the basis of their test scores. That is, interpretations are made with respect to how one person's performance compares to others in some known group. (See sections II and III in this text for a more detailed discussion of norm-referenced and criterion-referenced measurement.)

Traditionally the norm-referenced approach has been applied to testing practices in physical education. Recently, however, many measurement specialists have been strongly advocating the use of criterion-referenced standards, claiming that this approach constitutes a significant improvement to the conventional norm-referenced method. Whether such claims can actually be supported remains to be seen. Most authorities recognize that each approach provides a meaningful contribution to the area of testing and evaluation. Perhaps Ebel (1979) put the dilemma in proper perspective:

> Neither form of test is superior to the other for all educational measurement needs. Each has characteristics that make it uniquely advantageous for particular measurement needs. The question is not "Which is better?" but "When is it better?" (p. 13)

Although the vast majority of published tests in physical education are norm-referenced, the use of criterion-referenced testing in the public schools has steadily increased in recent years. As shown by the findings of Hensley et al. (1987), 58% of the teachers surveyed reported using a criterion-referenced approach to evaluation, while only 37% reported using a norm-referenced approach. Given the variety of testing needs in physical education, the need for good tests of all types is becoming more important. Clearly the exclusive use of either the norm-referenced or criterion-referenced approach is neither necessary nor desired at this time.

Grading on improvement. Many physical education teachers contend that grading on level of achievement is unfair and penalizes those students who enter a class with a lower initial level of skill. They endorse the concept of grading on the amount of improvement a student has shown as opposed to achievement level. Such an approach is appealing to many physical education teachers, particularly if they equate improvement with learning. Usually scores on a pretest are used to provide a basis for initial status. The difference between the pretest scores and the scores on a subsequent test, or posttest, provide what many call *improvement* or *growth scores*. Conceptually this approach may sound appropriate, but there are several limitations to such a procedure:

- Improvement scores have been shown to be unreliable. Since each test score consists of a certain amount of measurement error, the process of subtracting the pretest score from the posttest score actually results in compounding the measurement error in the improvement score.

- The potential for improvement depends on the initial level of skill. Consequently, a student who performs well on the pretest has less opportunity for improvement than the student who performs poorly.
- Capable, test-wise students may purposely perform poorly on the pretest in order to increase the likelihood of attaining a large improvement score, a problem commonly called *sandbagging*.
- Considering that some of the skills or behaviors that may typically be taught in a physical education class have certain inherent dangers associated with them (archery, for example), the administration of a pretest is unconscionable and may be seen as negligence on the part of the teacher.

Apart from the limitations presented above, some teachers still consider improvement scores to be fairer than merely grading on achievement level. A few measurement specialists have attempted mathematical transformations of improvement scores in an attempt to increase reliability and to offset the inherent advantage of a low score on the initial test or pretest. For those individuals persisting in their use of improvement scores for grading purposes, the use of score transformations similar to the procedures described by Hale and Hale (1972) and modified by East (1979) might be considered. Refer to chapter 10 for an extensive analysis of procedures used to measure change.

Attributes used for determining a grade. A basic premise underlying the evaluation process is that grades should reflect the instructional objectives of the course. Every effort should be made to ensure that this basic tenet is not violated. The problem arises, however, in identifying the attributes on which to base a grade and in determining their relative importance. If stated properly, instructional objectives should refer to the specific behavior of a student in either the cognitive, affective, or psychomotor domain. Conceptually, then, attributes on which to base a grade may fall within any of these three domains, as long as they are identified in the instructional objectives. In practice those attributes often used for determining grades appear to have little in common with the instructional objectives of the class.

Philosophically, most physical educators would agree that one of the most important attributes to be used in determining a student's grade is achievement in some aspect of the psychomotor domain. This may include such factors as physical fitness, sport skills, or motor abilities. As noted previously, a student's improvement in performance is a variation of absolute achievement that may be used for determining a grade, although few measurement specialists would recommend it. Cognitive abilities and knowledge of movement principles, rules of games, safety standards, training theory, and so forth are also generally accepted as appropriate outcomes of the physical education class, and thus acceptable for use in determining grades. The problem arises when trivial knowledge becomes a significant part of the grading scheme. Perhaps the most controversial issue associated with determining a student's grade is the appropriateness of using affective factors such as sportsmanship, effort, attitude, attendance, and dressing out (see chapter 13). According to Baumgartner and Jackson (1987), first and foremost the attribute should be identified as an instructional objective of the physical education class. Although it is not uncommon for grades to be based on dressing out, showering, and attendance, it is unlikely that these can be legitimately thought of as instructional objectives of the class. Grading on these factors is often a punitive action, taken against students whose behavior is considered unsatisfactory. Whereas affective factors such as sportsmanship, attitude, and effort can be considered desirable outcomes of a physical education class, the ability to measure these attributes reliably and validly is highly questionable.

Typically, subjective observation is the basis for determining the degree to which a student demonstrates each of these traits. Such assessments are particularly susceptible to the **halo effect**, and few physical education teachers have received the proper training needed to use the observational analysis required here. Since effort and participation are used widely as factors in determining a student's grade in physical education and have been identified as the most important grading factors by nearly 50% of the respondents to the recent survey by Hensley et al. (1987), additional comments seem warranted. First is the lack of a standard definition for these terms. Is *effort* the same as *participation*? Are they related? Despite the difficulty of defining these attributes, they are perceived intuitively by many teachers as desirable outcomes for a physical education class. But these affective factors are extremely difficult to evaluate. How can a teacher determine if a student is putting forth a satisfactory amount of effort? Does the achievement level indicate how hard a student works or how actively he or she participates in the class? As previously mentioned, subjective observation is normally the means to judge these attributes. If physical educators insist on grading on effort and participation, such decisions must be made as objectively as possible. Furthermore, prospective physical education teachers should receive formal training in the use of observational analysis as a means of collecting information and measuring student outcomes.

The decision as to which attributes are appropriate bases for grades in physical education is somewhat philosophical. We recommend that those attributes that contribute to the uniqueness of physical education in the school curriculum (i.e., psychomotor attributes) receive the greatest emphasis in a grading scheme.

Marking and reporting systems. If instructional objectives have been defined properly and evaluation procedures have been applied correctly, the task of recording and reporting the grade would be a simple matter. Unfortunately this is not always the case. In fact, the issue of assigning marks (grades) and reporting student achievement has been controversial at all levels of education for the last 50–60 years. The problem is that no one has developed the ideal system of grading; nor is anyone likely to.

Marks are abstract symbols used by teachers to summarize their evaluation of educational achievement by the student. Such marks serve a variety of purposes for the students, parents, school personnel, prospective employers, and others. According to Gronlund (1981), an effective system of marking and reporting will (a) provide the type of information needed by the users of the report and (b) present it in a clearly understandable form. Traditionally, the accepted method of reporting student achievement is to assign a single symbol to the educational efforts of the student. The five-letter A-B-C-D-F system is the method most frequently used in the United States.

Hensley et al. (1987) reported this system to be the overwhelming choice among physical education teachers in their four-state survey, although elementary school teachers were more likely to use alternative reporting systems. Probably the most popular alternative to the five-letter system is the two-category pass-fail system. Such a system may be particularly appropriate when classes are taught under the mastery-learning concept. The pass-fail method of grading has been used at the elementary school level for many years and more recently at the high school and college level. A major shortcoming of the two-category system, however, is the loss of information and of the ability to discriminate among achievement levels. In addition, since most schools regularly require a composite grade index for each student, a system must be devised to combine five-letter and pass-fail marks. In the absence of clearly defined definitions of what each mark means, both of these systems are somewhat arbitrary. According to Ebel (1979), there are two major shortcomings of the marking systems commonly used: (a) the lack of clearly defined, generally accepted definitions of what the various marks should mean; and (b) the lack of sufficient relevant, objective evidence to use as a basis for assigning marks.

In order to provide a degree of uniformity in grading practices, most school systems dictate the marking system to be used. Unfortunately the type of system is often the only thing mandated, with no internal guidance on what each mark should mean. The result is that the meaning of marks varies from instructor to instructor and from department to department. A related issue, of particular importance to physical education teachers, concerns the use of a common marking system across all classes. Some classroom teachers and school administrators view physical education as a nonacademic class in which the students are merely provided with appropriate experiences. This type of class is more suitable for a pass-fail marking system or even for a system without grades.

Most physical education teachers contend that students in physical education class should be provided the same type of evaluative information that is provided students in other curricular areas. Philosophically this argument would probably be widely supported among physical educators. However, the inclusion of physical education in the school curriculum should not be justified on the basis that the grading system is similar to that used in other classes. Physical education is unique in the school curriculum, and alternative marking systems may be more appropriate for reporting student outcomes for these classes.

One alternative utilizes a multiple marking system in which evaluative information may be reported for a variety of instructional objectives for a single class. A classic example is one in which grades are assigned for both achievement-related objectives and behavioral objectives. Figure 14.3 illustrates such a multiple marking system adapted for use in a physical education class. Such a reporting form makes it possible to assign a grade based solely on achievement, because effort and other behavioral characteristics are reported elsewhere; or it is possible to combine all the factors into a composite grade. A marking and reporting system similar to this may be more appropriate for physical education. The fact remains, however, that there is no foolproof grading system. There are many questions that must be examined in detail and on which some

PHYSICAL EDUCATION PROGRESS REPORT

Name _____

Grade Level _____   Age _____   Date _____

Section _____   Teacher _____

Instructional Unit _____

I Achievement. *The category marked below is an indication of how well the instructional objectives for this particular unit were met.*

____ Excellent   ____ Fair
____ Very Good   ____ Poor
____ Good   ____ Very Poor

II Effort. *The category marked below is an indication of the amount of effort the teacher believes the student exerted to attain his/her achievement level.*

____ Maximal   ____ Moderate
____ Substantial   ____ Minimal

III Improvement. *The category marked below is an indication of how much the student improved during the instructional unit.*

____ Substantial   ____ Slight
____ Moderate   ____ None

IV Personal and Social Characteristics

+ Highly Desirable   √ Desirable   — Undesirable

____ Cooperation   ____ Perseverance
____ Responsible   ____ Attitude
____ Follows instructions   ____ Sportsmanship
____ Courteous and respectful

V Attendance

____ Good   ____ Acceptable   ____ Poor

COMPOSITE GRADE INDEX   _____

Figure 14.3   Example of a Multiple Marking System

consensus must be reached. Only then can measurement specialists provide the technical expertise needed to improve grading practices in physical education.

Conclusion

Research findings in physical education and exercise science have had a significant impact on the daily practices of many physical educators. Furthermore, research focusing on the theoretical foundations of measurement and evaluation, as well as the application and implementation of measurement principles to the world of movement, has led to modifications in testing practices, thus enabling physical educators to have a firm foundation on which to build assessment programs. Throughout this chapter we have attempted to present selected examples of research and illustrate how these research findings have affected or may affect measurement and evaluation theory and practice. The importance of clearly defining the attribute being measured was examined through a discussion of general motor ability and the impact specificity theory has had on testing is this area. Similarly, physical fitness has evolved from a rather broad term that combined a variety of attributes in a single test battery to a more definitive concept that differentiates between health-related fitness and performance-related fitness. Assessment of sports skills has traditionally received significant attention from physical educators. The development of sport skill tests, including examples of various methods of estimating reliability and validity as well as sport profiling and the application of item response theory, was discussed. For many physical educators, the opportunity to implement measurement principles culminates with the grading process and the evaluation of student achievement in the classroom. A review of evaluation practices in the public schools paints a poor picture of existing efforts, although there is evidence of improvement in some areas. The need exists to facilitate the translation of research findings into measurement practices.

References

American Alliance for Health, Physical Education, Recreation and Dance. (1976). *Youth fitness test manual*. Washington, DC: Author.

American Alliance for Health, Physical Education, Recreation and Dance. (1980). *Health-related physical fitness test manual*. Reston, VA: Author.

American Alliance for Health, Physical Education, Recreation and Dance. (1988). *Physical best*. Reston, VA: Author.

Barrow, H.M. (1954). Test of motor ability for college men. *Research Quarterly, 25,* 253–260.

Barrow, H.M., & McGee, R. (1964). *A practical approach to measurement in physical education*. Philadelphia: Lea & Febiger.

Battinelli, T. (1984). From motor ability to motor learning: The generality/specificity connection. *The Physical Educator, 41,* 108–113.

Baumgartner, T.A., & Jackson, A.S. (1987). *Measurement for evaluation in physical education* (3rd ed.). Dubuque, IA: Wm. C. Brown.

Clarke, H.H. (1971). Basic understanding of physical fitness. In H.H. Clarke (Ed.), *Physical Fitness Research Digest* (pp. 1–24). Washington, DC: President's Council on Physical Fitness and Sport.

Clarke, H.H., & Clarke, D.H. (1987). *Application of measurement to physical education* (6th ed.). Englewood Cliffs, NJ: Prentice-Hall.

Coker, G.E. (1972). *A survey of senior high school physical education programs for boys in selected Louisiana public schools.* Unpublished doctoral dissertation, Louisiana State University, Baton Rouge.

Davis, M.W. (1983). Let's Talk About Johnny's 'C' in P.E. In L.D. Hensley & W.B. East (Eds.), *Measurement and Evaluation Symposium Proceedings* (pp. 17–23). Cedar Falls, IA: University of Northern Iowa Press.

Disch, J. (1986). Status of research in sports skills testing. *Research Consortium Newsletter, 9,* 2.

Disch, J. (1987). Recent developments in measurement and possible applications to the measurement of psychomotor behavior: A response. *Research Quarterly for Exercise and Sport, 58,* 210–212.

East, W.B. (1979). *Mathematical techniques for estimating motor performance improvement.* Unpublished doctoral dissertation, University of Georgia, Athens.

Ebel, R.L. (1979). *Essentials of educational measurement* (3rd ed.). Englewood Cliffs, NJ: Prentice-Hall.

Falls, H.B. (1980). Modern concepts of physical fitness. *Journal of Physical Education and Recreation, 51,* 25–28.

Fleishman, E.A. (1964). *The structure and measurement of physical fitness.* Englewood Cliffs, NJ: Prentice-Hall.

Fox, J.W. (1959). *Practices and trends in physical education programs for boys in selected Oregon schools.* Unpublished doctoral dissertation, University of Oregon, Eugene.

Gallahue, D. (1976). *Motor development and movement experiences for young children.* New York: Wiley.

Green, K.N., East, W.B., & Hensley, L.D. (1987). A golf skills test battery for college males and females. *Research Quarterly for Exercise and Sport, 58,* 72–76.

Gronlund, N.E. (1981). *Measurement and evaluation in teaching* (4th ed.). New York: Macmillan.

Hale, P.W., & Hale, R.M. (1972). Comparison of student improvement by exponential modification of test-retest scores. *Research Quarterly, 43,* 113–120.

Henry, F.M. (1958). Specificity and generality in learning motor skills. *61st Annual Proceedings of the College Physical Education Association,* 126–128.

Hensley, L.D. (1987). Grading practices in Iowa. *Iowa Journal for Health, Physical Education, Recreation and Dance, 19*(2), 4–5.

Hensley, L.D., East, W.B., & Stillwell, J.L. (1979). A racquetball skills test. *Research Quarterly, 50,* 114–118.

Hensley, L.D., Lambert, L.T., Baumgartner, T.A., & Stillwell, J.L. (1987). Is evaluation worth the effort? *Journal of Physical Education, Recreation, and Dance, 58,* 59–62.

Hopkins, D.R., Shick, J., & Plack, J.J. (1984). *Basketball for boys and girls: Skills test manual.* Reston, VA: AAHPERD.

Imwold, C.H., Rider, R.A., & Johnson, D.J. (1982). The use of evaluation in public school physical education programs. *Journal of Physical Education and Recreation, 2,* 13–18.

Johnson, B.L., & Nelson, J.K. (1986). *Practical measurements for evaluation in physical education* (4th ed.). Edina, MN: Burgess.

Larson, L.A. (1941). A factor analysis of motor ability variables and tests, with tests for college men. *Research Quarterly, 12,* 499–517.

Morrow, J.R. (1978). Measurement techniques—who uses them? *Journal of Physical Education and Recreation, 49,* 66–67.

Patterson, P. (1986, April). *Validity generalization as a type of meta-analysis.* Paper presented at the national convention of the American Alliance for Health, Physical Education, Recreation and Dance, Cincinnati, OH.

Safrit, M.J. (1987). The applicability of item response theory to tests of motor behavior. *Research Quarterly for Exercise and Sport, 58,* 213–215.

Safrit, M.J., Costa, M.G., & Hooper, L.M. (1986). The validity generalization model: An approach to the analysis of validity studies in physical education. *Research Quarterly for Exercise and Sport, 57,* 288–297.

Safrit, M.J., & Wood, T.M. (1986). The health-related physical fitness test: A tri-state survey of users and non-users. *Research Quarterly for Exercise and Sport, 57,* 27–32.

Scott, M.G. (1939). The assessment of motor abilities of college women through objective tests. *Research Quarterly, 10,* 63–83.

Scott, M.G. (1943). Motor ability tests for college women. *Research Quarterly, 14,* 402–405.

Shifflett, B.S. (1985). Reliability estimation for trials-to-criterion testing. *Research Quarterly for Exercise and Sport, 56,* 266–274.

Singer, R.N. (1966). Interlimb skill ability in motor skill performance. *Research Quarterly, 3,* 406–410.

Smith, L.E. (1969). Specificity of individual differences of relationships between forearm strengths and speed of forearm flexion. *Research Quarterly, 40,* 191–197.

Spray, J.A. (1983, April). *Sequential testing in physical education: An overview.* Paper presented at the national convention of the American Alliance for Health, Physical Education, Recreation and Dance, Minneapolis.

Spray, J.A. (1987). Recent developments in measurement and possible applications to the measurement of psychomotor behavior. *Research Quarterly for Exercise and Sport, 58,* 203–209.

Spray, J.A., Sorenson, C., & Hooper, L.M. (1985). Inverse sampling procedures for criterion-referenced testing of motor or sport skills in the elementary school. *Motor Skills: Theory into Practice, 8,* 103–112.

Texas Governor's Commission on Physical Fitness. (1973). *Physical fitness-motor ability test.* Austin: Author.

Wood, T.M. (1987). Putting item response theory into perspective. *Research Quarterly for Exercise and Sport, 58,* 216–220.

Supplementary Readings

Safrit, M.J. (1981). *Evaluation in physical education.* Englewood Cliffs, NJ: Prentice-Hall.

Program Evaluation

Rosemary McGee
University of North Carolina at Greensboro

The assumption of program quality is no longer acceptable. The fact that well-meaning, qualified professionals are delivering a particular program is no guarantee that adequacy, much less effectiveness, is present. In business, the balance sheet attests to effectiveness. In such areas as medicine, law, social work, and education, however, the impact on the quality of human life is the telling point. The former deals with *things*, the latter with *people*. The focus of this discussion is on assessing the value of programs that concern people. More specifically, the emphasis is on people participating in programs of physical education and exercise science and such related fields as athletics, intramurals, youth sports, corporate fitness, and sports medicine.

Initial discussion focuses on some of the reasons for conducting program evaluations and the possible outcomes. Several of the theoretical models for program evaluation are presented, along with their advantages, disadvantages, and most appropriate applications. Various measurement considerations are addressed, such as internal validity, the role of the evaluator(s), sources of data, and standards. Finally, the process of program evaluation itself is outlined for the benefit of those who plan to conduct an evaluation.

The philosophy behind program evaluation centers around wanting to improve programs for the people they serve. If there is no desire or motivation to ask the tough questions about what can be done to make programs better, then no program evaluation needs to occur. The process of program evaluation not only has the potential for ultimately improving of the programs but keeps professionals on their toes by causing them to continually ask questions about ways of doings things differently and better. There may be various reasons for evaluating programs, but the ultimate reason is to better serve the people the programs serve.

Reasons for Conducting Program Evaluation

There are several reasons for conducting program evaluation, some forced and others optional. It is true, however, that required program evaluation is what has caused the field of program evaluation to be studied, refined, expanded, and given some scientific credence. The whole process is no longer a superficial look at sparse data but a carefully conceived, detailed process resulting in a well-prepared document that presents information upon which decisons can be based.

Accreditation

Accreditation is a licensing procedure attesting that a program meets specified standards. It is customary for state departments of public instruction to accredit public schools, and for regional and national accrediting bodies to authorize the quality of programs offered in colleges and universities. There are even specialized accrediting agencies that look at particular subject matter areas, such as chemistry and education. Graduates of accredited high schools are recognized as having received a quality education and being better prepared to proceed to college and other endeavors. Accredited schools are, likewise, eligible to receive state funds to supplement local tax money. Accreditation is thus a type of quality control, which the various states and agencies have undertaken to ensure that programs meet standards.

Standards for accreditation differ from state to state and from agency to agency. They usually, however, cover such areas of concern as philosophy and objectives of the program, organization and structure, personnel, budget, facilities, curriculum, and evaluation. Reference to state accreditation guidelines will illustrate the detail of standards stated under each section. The National Study of School Evaluation (1987) has presented *Evaluative Criteria for the Evaluation of Secondary Schools*. This school improvement model includes the self-evaluation phase, the visiting committee phase, and the follow-up phase. Table 15.1 outlines the broad headings covered in the criteria for evaluating secondary physical education programs; each subsection contains detailed criteria. Although geared to a school program, the subsections and criteria can be adapted to the evaluation of other human services programs, such as fitness centers and youth sport leagues.

Program evaluation for accrediting purposes occurs by law in designated cycles, usually every 5 or 10 years. Following a year of self-study by the school community and a review of materials and observations conducted by a visiting team of expert consultants, a final report is submitted; it can recommend accreditation, provisional

Table 15.1   Subsections of Criteria for Evaluating Secondary Physical Education Programs

---

    I. Major Expectations
   II. Follow-up to Previous Evaluations
  III. Organization for Instruction
  IV. Description of Offerings
   V. Components of the Instructional Program
        A. Faculty
        B. Instructional Activities
        C. Materials and Media
        D. Student Assessment and Program Evaluation
  VI. Facilities and Equipment
 VII. Learning Climate
VIII. Evaluations
  IX. Judgments and Recommendations

---

accreditation, or no accreditation. Because accreditation is required by law, it is by far the most prevalent reason for conducting program reviews.

Typically, the measurement field has reacted to measurement needs. For example, skills tests were developed only after sports were offered in school programs and there was a need to assess achievement. Likewise, program evaluation documents were developed as a result of required accreditation procedures. And now, primarily for accrediting purposes, numerous program evaluation instruments have been developed by the various states and accrediting agencies (National Study of School Evaluation, 1987; Educational Testing Service, 1983; Illinois Association for Health, Physical Education and Recreation, 1984a, b).

Program Development and Faculty/Staff Development

Many departments of physical education, athletics, and intramurals conduct program evaluations annually to reexamine their progress toward objectives and to decide on any refocusing needed in the future. This in-house evaluation carries no threat of revelation to the outside world or of lack of accreditation. Annual, ongoing program evaluation is consistent with good evaluation practices. It serves to keep (a) the faculty and staff up to date and growing and (b) the program responsive to the needs of the students and athletes and to current philosophy about what programs should include. Penman and Adams (1980) and the Secondary School Physical Education Council (1977) are two sources of guidelines and materials developed for assessing athletic and physical education programs.

The evaluation process is an excellent activity for faculty/staff development, because professionals conducting the evaluations interact about philosophy, content, scheduling, budget, and so forth. In addition, an outcome of the evaluation may be a decision to include new content areas in the curriculum that no present faculty member or coach is prepared to teach. Staff development is then indicated, an opportunity for re-tooling so that the faculty and staff can deliver the program considered best in a particular setting. The incidence of teacher burnout can be reduced if faculty are involved in the planning of future programs.

Program Justification

Periodically, physical educators have had to fight for the place of physical education in school programs. This is true at both the K-12 and collegiate levels. Sometimes the question of appropriateness of physical education has been a philosophical one; at other times the question has been a financial consideration. Regardless of the reason, professional physical educators need to conduct program evaluations in order to have the evidence to present their case for inclusion—or even survival.

Funding

In this day of government, corporate, and foundation support, many special programs have been designed to tap into these funds. These sources of funding are outside the funds usually designated by tax dollars for educational purposes. Learning resources programs, remedial programs, reading programs, health-related programs, and staff development programs are examples of the many and varied projects that have been designed. Such requests require the writing of grant proposals that describe the special project and attest to the ability of the requesting agency to carry out the proposed project. Consequently, some program evaluation has occurred in preparation for the funding request, and subsequent program evaluation has occurred at the end of the project. One unique difference in this type of program evaluation, as opposed to that used for accrediting purposes, is its focus on a limited part of the total program, i.e., the funded project. Another difference usually attributed to this type of program evaluation is its necessity for good grant writing skills and able lobbying efforts to actually acquire the money.

Another reason for conducting a program evaluation is to justify current funding. In these days of tight funding for education, accountability for budget expenditures is essential, and requests for additional funds must be persuasive. Program evaluation can help make the case.

Decision Making

An underlying reason for conducting program evaluation is to assist with decision making. Little progress will be made in program development if no decisions are made about such topics as staffing, content, budget, and scheduling. *Indecision* and *no decision* result in *no progress*. Decisions can be made more confidently if information is available on which judgments can be based. Physical educators need to be able to make sound decisions, and they need to be accountable for those decisions. Other leaders in responsible positions (e.g., the military, the corporate sphere, and human services agencies) likewise need to make decisions about the continuation of programs of various kinds. Program evaluation is the process that makes wise decision making possible.

Accountability

Accountability is a term discussed a great deal in current educational parlance. Accountability means that you are accomplishing what you said you would, and that you have the evidence to support that claim. Are you teaching what your curriculum guide says you should? Are the students/performers achieving at the level designated? Is their fitness attainment meeting predetermined standards? Does your program reflect the espoused philosophy of physical education/fitness? Is your faculty qualified to teach the activities offered? Are your students and participants aware of the benefits of physical education, physical fitness, and athletic training? Are the objectives of your program being met? Not only are answers needed to these and many other related questions but the evidence must be present to support the answers. Accountability is related to each of the purposes presented for conducting program evaluations. Whether it is undertaken for reasons of accreditation, program development, program justification, funding, or decision making, the program evaluation must be trustworthy. Accountability, therefore, is an integral part of program evaluation.

Models of Program Evaluation

When anticipating program evaluation, it is good to be familiar with the various theoretical models that are available to guide and focus the process. The purpose of the evaluation and the types of questions to be answered will dictate the theoretical model(s) selected. The literature on program evaluation models is replete with schema and ambiguous terminology. Anywhere from five to 49 types of models or studies have been identified. The taxonomy proposed by House (1978), however, seems the most clear and most informative. House identified eight basic models from which there are many mutations; a brief description of each is given here.

Current thinking in the field indicates that a multiple approach to program evaluation is desirable (Worthen, 1987). The design can be enhanced by using many of the beneficial aspects of various models and perhaps minimizing the less attractive features. In addition, a cross-proofing or triangulation effect can be achieved which gives greater authenticity to the results.

Since the models use both quantitative and qualitative approaches to data collection, some clarification may be helpful. Reichardt and Cook (1979) stated that

> by quantitative methods researchers have come to mean techniques of randomized experiments, quasi-experiments, paper and pencil "objective" tests, multivariate

statistical analyses, sample surveys, and the like. In contrast, qualitative methods include ethnography, case studies, in-depth interviews, and participant observation. (p. 7)

Jacobs (1988) summarized several important themes characteristic of qualitative research: conducting research in the natural setting, understanding participants' perspectives, researchers knowing subjectively and empathetically the perspectives of the participants, and having questions and theories emerge from data collection rather than being posed before the study begins. Jacobs further stated that qualitative research has been interpreted too narrowly. She used such traditions as ecological psychology, holistic ethnography, cognitive anthropology, and symbolic interactionism from the disciplines of psychology, anthropology, and sociology to make the point of different and broader interpretations of qualitative research espoused by different people.

Each method-type, qualitative and quantitative, has its advocates. Unfortunately many of them often feel that only one approach is suitable. Ianni and Orr (1979) stated that it is essential to develop theoretical and practical qualitative measures that can be integrated with quantitative approaches. The diversity of qualitative research makes it even more appropriate for inclusion in various models of program evaluation, especially if the multiple approach to program evaluation is adopted.

Quantitative Models

Two models seem to be essentially quantitative in nature: Behavioral Objectives and Systems Analysis.

Behavioral Objectives Model The **Behavioral Objectives Model**, also known as the *Desired Outcomes Model*, made famous by Tyler (1942, 1983), is based on investigating objectives attained on the basis of predetermined standards. Student performance is compared with behaviorally stated objectives. This is a highly quantitative model because of the extensive use of test scores. Worthen and Sanders (1973) stated that the advantages of this type of model are (a) the ease of assessing whether behavioral objectives are being met, (b) the ease with which a practitioner can design this type of study, and (c) a focus on the clarity of objectives. They also stated that this model oversimplifies the program and focuses on summative rather than formative information. In addition, it focuses on objectives with little consideration of their worth. The myriad of behavioral requirements written to cover each detailed objective makes the model tedious to carry out.

The Behavioral Objectives Model seems similar to the *Discrepancy Model* devised by Provus (Popham, 1975) which involves a comparison between performance and standards. With results available, decisions are made to change the performance or to change the standards. As in the Tyler model, however, there is some difficulty in setting the standards to be attained.

The Behavioral Objectives Model has not been used widely in physical education and exercise science, because the curricula have not been sufficiently detailed in behavioral objectives. The concept of mastery learning is consistent with this model if the attainment of desired objectives means mastery sufficient to progress to further objectives.

Systems Analysis Model The **Systems Analysis Model** (Madaus, Scriven, & Stufflebeam, 1983; Patton, 1980; Rivlin, 1971) addresses efficiency and productivity. Considerable statistical sophistication and design control are needed. This model is used extensively by the government to study separate components of its programs. Systems analysis seems inconsistent with the educational setting, partly because it does not provide information on the whole picture of the program.

Professional Judgment Models

Three models are characterized by the use of professional judgment: accreditation, artistic, and adversary.

Accreditation Model The **Accreditation Model** is used widely because of the legal requirements for programs to prove they are qualified to grant certificates in such fields as teaching, accounting, and nursing. The accrediting agency, usually a state department of public instruction, a commission of higher education, or a professional association, establishes guidelines that need to be met. A faculty evaluates its program on the basis of the set of guidelines and then invites a team of outside consultants to review the materials and judge the strengths and weaknesses of the program. Quantitative student data such as grading profiles, fitness tests, and skill and knowledge test performance are made available. Data about the size of the facilities and the budget are provided. Qualitative information (e.g., questionnaires and/or interviews with parents and students) may be used. An examination of curricular materials (e.g., unit plans, learning resources, knowledge tests) is possible. Collectively the visiting team makes a professional judgment about the quality of the program and whether or not it meets accreditation guidelines.

Worthen and Sanders (1973) identified some strengths and weaknesses of this model. It is easy to implement, a large number of variables can be studied, it can become an annual activity reflecting self-study as a habit for program improvement, and it is economical in time requirements. Some of the possible weaknesses are the quality and number of personnel on the roster for the visiting team, the lack of potential for replication because each setting is unique, and that the process may be overlooked by the results of the accreditation study.

Dumke (1986) acknowledged that accreditation is the weak link in education reform but encouraged more responsible use of the model, so that the government will not take over the role of professional educators in the accreditation process. The Accreditation Model often is flawed and often not rigorous enough, but it can be improved and remains more desirable than governmental control of education.

The use of the Accreditation Model is widespread in physical education, because this subject area is included whenever the total school is evaluated. Unfortunately the legislated time for evaluation is often the only time the physical education program is studied. The model, however, is amenable to use for program improvement, with faculty or neighboring colleagues serving as the evaluation team. Such a procedure may be repeated every year, or at least every two or three years, providing a mechanism for ongoing program evaluation.

Evaluative criteria in physical education designed by the National Study of School Evaluation (1987), an accrediting agency, were revised by representatives from the National Association for Sport and Physical Education (AAHPERD, 1985). Stronger criteria for fitness acquisition were included with suggestions about the learning climate, staff, and facilities.

Artistic Model   The **Artistic Model** is also known as the *art criticism model* and the *connoisseur model*. Eisner (1976) is credited with developing this model, which relies on the expertise of one person whose experience and knowledge is so widely respected that he or she can be counted on to critique a program wisely. Eisner distinguished between *connoisseur* and *critic* by crediting the first with appreciation, such as a wine connoisseur, and the latter with disclosure to the public in words. The critic is hoping to reveal what has not been seen previously. Such a revelation comes through a process of description, interpretation, and evaluation. It is not sufficient for the critic to merely describe and interpret; the critic must, on the basis of these two, *evaluate* the program. Because of the critic's focus, the critique may highlight only certain aspects of the program and may not be as comprehensive as other types of program evaluation. For example, the critic might comment on the quality of the educational environment but not on the credentials of the faculty.

The Artistic Model requires a substantial time commitment and money for the critic. It is also frightening because so much rests in the hands of one person who is his or her "own evaluative instrument" (Jewett & Bain, 1985, p. 238). The model is innovative, however, and might be appropriate to use in such areas of the physical education curriculum as adventure education, dance, and new games. The resulting information for decision making may be less helpful, because the connoisseur-critic has not necessarily been presented with a set of questions to address. Rather than using this procedure alone, the Artistic Model might be used in conjunction with other models.

Adversary Model   The **Adversary Model** (Levine, 1974) is the most legalistic of the models, because it utilizes two teams to investigate and debate. One team is the advocate team, the other is the adversary voice for the curriculum evaluation. A jury is selected to adjudicate the debate and declare the winner. Topics that clearly can be decided on a go/no-go vote are the most appropriate for this format. For example, should: the program change from a required to an elective offering; physical education be dropped from the college curriculum; the school upgrade its athletic program; the philosophy of the high school physical education curriculum be based on fitness attainment and maintenance; or a sport management program be added to the curriculum. By draw, the teams are decided and charged with preparing their cases and presenting them to an impartial panel. Jewett and Bain (1985) highlighted some pros and cons of this model. Among other points, they commented on the apparent fairness of the model and its potential for covering all points pertinent to the debate. There may be some question about the competence of the team members and the objectivity of the jury in this type of evaluation. Popham and Carlson (1977) suggested one remedy for possible team bias by advising that each team be required to debate both sides of the issue. This model is expensive in the use of time, money, and personnel. It may also cause a split in the faculty over a controversial issue, although it presents an in-service challenge for the faculty to respond in a professional manner and on a professional, not personal, level. The Adversary Model has not been used in physical education and exercise science but provides an innovative approach to program evaluation if everyone involved understands and accepts the ground rules.

Qualitative Models

The three models just described use a combination of quantitative and qualitative data; three other models are essentially qualitative in their orientation: Transactional, Decision-Making, and Goal-Free.

Transactional Model The **Transactional Model** centers on the process of the program. The evaluator studies the process and becomes a part of it. This model is also known as a *responsive evaluation* (Stake, 1967, 1975); it espouses a naturalistic approach. The curriculum is studied in its natural environment without manipulation (Patton, 1980). The evaluator (specialist) is committed to considering descriptive and judgmental data.

The Transactional Model seems quite similar to the Artistic Model but differs in its emphasis on process and the use of case study as the primary method. The model has not been used in physical education and exercise science but has potential for those wishing to approach program evaluation from a naturalistic viewpoint.

Decision-Making Model The **Decision-Making Model** focuses on supplying information to decision makers and is essentially formative. Stufflebeam (1968, 1983) developed this model using the acronym CIPP to represent evaluation in the areas of context, input, process, and product. The information is used to make four kinds of decisions respective to the CIPP: planning, structuring, implementing, and recycling. Stufflebeam's model makes a commitment to *improvement* of educational programs and not just proof that objectives have been met. Patton (1980) commented that the Decision-Making Model is "the most open of all models to a full variety of methodological strategies" (p. 58), depending on the types of future decisions to be made and the information needed to make them. The CIPP approach has been used extensively and was the central topic of the International Conference on the Evaluation of Physical Education in Jyvaskyla, Finland, in 1976.

Worthen and Sanders (1973) summarized some of the favorable features of this model, including its service dimension to administrators, sensitivity to feedback, facility to provide for evaluation to take place at any stage in the program, and holistic orientation. They also pointed out that, among other limitations, there seems to be little emphasis on value concerns, and that use of the model may be costly and complex.

The Decision-Making Model has promise for use in physical education and athletic evaluation procedures. It has a future-oriented approach and is especially helpful to administrators. It is less helpful to teachers and coaches, except as an in-service staff-development activity, unless, of course, they are the decision makers.

Goal-Free Model The **Goal-Free Model**, developed by Scriven (1967, 1974), is designed deliberately to reduce bias in program evaluation by looking at outcomes of programs without knowing what the goals are. In this way many outcomes can be identified, some not expected or planned, and many types of instruments can be used to collect data. The focus is on the consumer, and the role of the evaluator is to judge the merit of the program for producers and consumers (Worthen & Sanders, 1973). The model is complex because many measurement instruments can be used. The outcome provides a sort of *reverse validity* of a program. Purposely avoiding any notion of what the program goals are, the evaluator identifies the goals that have been attained. The program provider can then see whether the intended goals are the attained goals identified by the evaluator. If indicated, program revisions can be made. Many more goals probably will be identified by the evaluator than were stated in the program plan; this scope and thoroughness is an advantage of the model. Operating blindly in relation to program goals is Scriven's answer to ensuring greater objectivity in program reviews. The Goal-Free Model is appropriate to program evaluation in physical education, athletics, and related areas. It is comprehensive and nonthreatening, and provides a means of enhancing program development.

Multiple Method Approach

Each of these eight models probably could be used appropriately in selected situations. Each has its idiosyncrasies. Worthen (1987) suggests that the best approach is to use combinations of models. Then, depending on the purpose of the evaluation study and the situation, a model unique to each setting can be developed. This approach would increase the credibility of the evaluation and probably would reduce bias and enlarge the focus of the evaluation project. It requires, however, the added task by the curriculum evaluation specialists and evaluators of tailoring each model to each situation.

Measurement Considerations

The measurement considerations for program evaluation are different from those usually considered when evaluating students. Measurement of process may be a somewhat softer, less precise method than assessment of the performer. Formerly, a program was assumed to be creditable if participants were showing good achievement. Now it is considered sound measurement practice to assess both the process and the product of the program.

Threats to Internal Validity

Early writing on threats to internal validity is attributed to Campbell and Stanley (1963). Subsequently, Popham (1975), Wolf (1984), and Posavac and Carey (1985) discussed the topic in relation to program evaluation. Internal validity addresses factors that cause results to be meaningful. Usually the concept of internal validity is used in the context of experimental or quasi-experimental designs. Even though not all program evaluation models use experimental design, many of the concepts related to internal validity are applicable to qualitative and judgmental models as well. Most of the threats to internal validity can be controlled—if not statistically, then by careful planning. But they are so serious that if they are not accounted for, the interpretation of the program evaluation results may be hampered. These factors are not associated directly with the program but do influence it. Pretest and posttest scores often are used to measure improvement toward program goals. It is essential that the improvement can be attributed to the program and not to extraneous factors. (See chapter 10 for a discussion of analyzing change.)

Two factors that create threats to internal validity are maturation and history. Due to the *maturation* of students, some progress is expected as a natural occurrence. If progress toward program goals is the result of the growth and development of the students, it cannot be credited to the impact of the program. *History* relates to events in the world, nation, community, or even in the school or program that occur between pretests and posttests and that might influence changes in performance scores. A labor strike in the local community and a fire in the school building are examples of historical events that might prejudice achievement.

Three more threats to internal validity concern the participants themselves: selection, mortality, and regression. *Selection* is critical in comparing groups if the groups are not identified in the same way. For example, one group may consist of volunteers for a certain program while the other group has no volunteers. One group may be motivated and the other may be uninterested. Selection deals with the characteristics of people as they enter a program. *Mortality* refers to the differences in people who leave a program. Mortality refers to the dropouts from a program regardless of the reasons. *Regression* to the mean is a statistical concept. Students who score at the extremes of a test scale probably will be closer to the mean on the next testing, regardless of any educational treatment. This threat is more likely to come into play if a program is designed specifically for especially talented students or if a program is remedial in nature.

In addition to the threats mentioned by other authors, Wolf (1984) expressed concern about *communication* among group members who are receiving different treatments and about resentfulness of learners who think they are receiving less desirable experiences. These are equally important concerns when thinking about the threats to internal validity related to participants in a program.

Instrumentation and testing, the responsibility of the evaluators, are two additional threats to internal validity. *Instrumentation*, as a threat, is related to using different standards for grading, using different tests, and using observers (instruments) of different proficiency. There is also concern about the stability of the instruments being used (Popham, 1975). *Testing*, as a factor of internal validity, concerns the ability of students to take tests—especially posttests—because of their previous experience with the tests. Another concern of testing is the psychological condition of students when they are taking tests or are being observed. Posavac and Carey (1985) referred to this condition as *reactivity*. In addition to the influence of the evaluator on testing and instrumentation, evaluators also can be faulted for looking for specific findings by manipulating the data and by trying to make sense out of almost any finding once the data are examined (Posavac & Carey, 1985). When information is presented, most researchers can come up with an explanation for it; in doing so, they often make erroneous conclusions. The last of the threats to internal validity is any of the interactions that may occur among the factors previously listed.

Obviously threats to internal validity are a serious concern for the program evaluator, because they identify reasons why changes in human performance may not be caused by the program being offered. Many of these threats can be minimized by planning carefully, being alert to possible delusions, and by selecting an appropriate research design. The program evaluator who is not aware of threats to internal validity and who does not study them carefully will often report an incorrect conclusion about program effectiveness.

A curriculum based on the goal of fitness achievement and maintenance for eighth-grade students will be used to illustrate this concept of internal validity. The students are growing; the Olympic fever is prevalent. All of the students are in the fitness program. Only 80% complete the program. The fitness test selected for use is one designed for elementary school age children. It is administered in the fall without training and is repeated in the spring following the spring recess. Some students like the fitness emphasis, and some would prefer a program with a lifetime sports orientation. The evaluators analyze the data by age, gender, race, test item, and by test battery using both pretest and posttest scores. They conclude that the program being offered is effective for the fitness achievement and maintenance of the eighth-grade students. Do you believe that conclusion, and what would you do differently to control for some of the threats to internal validity?

The Evaluator

The *role* of the program evaluator is as a member of an evaluation team, the chair of the team, or the solo evaluator. An in-house evaluator probably knows the program well, usually can be trusted, and is especially helpful when viewing formative information. An outside evaluator, generally termed a *consultant*, is better able to assess summative information and can be credited with more objectivity than the in-house evaluator. Feedback is important to either type of evaluator and is usually better for the in-house evaluator because of personal contacts and trust factors. The consultant can, however, create an atmosphere of trust and sensitivity that can enhance the effectiveness of the consultant's role.

The evaluator also controls the *ethics* of the evaluation process. Personal decisions about who benefits and who suffers from evaluator decisions must be tempered with utmost objectivity. This difficult role is especially demanding of an evaluator but is essential to credible program evaluation. In addition to personal ethics, the evaluator must be sensitive to the way data are collected and to whether students, parents, faculty, and administrators have given consent, whether their privacy is protected, whether they have been manipulated, and whether they are protected from harm. In summary, as Popham (1975) stated:

> . . . not only should the educational evaluator be responsible for appraising the worth of particular instructional programs as they affect learners involved, but the evaluator should also be attentive to the ultimate impact of the program on the society at large. (p. 305)

The role of a program evaluator is considerable in its responsibility, and the *qualifications* of the evaluator(s) are important. Academic qualifications should include courses in measurement and evaluation, research design, statistics, program evaluation, and curriculum. In addition to formal coursework, the evaluator should have experience observing and conducting program evaluations in the field. Michael Wargo, director of the Program Evaluation Staff in the Food and Nutrition Service of the U.S. Department of Agriculture, stated that "most people coming out of school usually lack the social, political, and communication skills required to be an effective evaluator immediately" (Hendricks, 1986, p. 26).

In addition to professional qualifications, personal qualifications often make the difference in the effectiveness of the evaluator. Even with considerable technical competence, an evaluator who is not sensitive, objective, compassionate, honest, and approachable will be unsuccessful in completing an effective program evaluation.

Worthen (1987) listed several factors that should be considered when selecting an evaluator. They are summarized in Table 15.2. Needless to say, the selection and performance of the evaluator is crucial. A good selection combats many of the weaknesses that can occur in program evaluation.

Types and Sources of Data

Comprehensiveness of data is essential. Considering both formative and summative information in both quantitative and qualitative formats is congruent with the multiple method approach to program evaluation. The amount and type of data will be governed somewhat by the evaluation model being employed and the questions being addressed. It is essential that information specific to the purpose of the evaluation is gathered from various publics.

The publics include parents, teachers, administrators, patrons, students, program recipients, and the general public. Interviews, questionnaires, observations, test scores, grade profiles, and attitude surveys are examples of vehicles for obtaining information. Moreover, other types of information will be essential, such as philosophy and goal statements, curriculum materials, media resources, promotional materials, credentials of faculty/staff, program description, facility and equipment inventory, budget, support services, and evaluative procedures.

Depending on the evaluation model in use, not all types of information will be appropriate or needed. In addition, the evaluator should be alert to unexpected sources

Table 15.2   Factors to Consider When Selecting an Evaluator

Specifications	Components
Formal Training	Degree specialization Courses in evaluation methodology Qualifications of major professors
Previous Evaluation Experience	Amount Similarity References
Professional Orientation	Philosophical position Evaluation models Congruence with plan
Personal Style and Characteristics	Honesty Communication skills

of information. An alert evaluator will take note of information that surfaces in unexpected places and formats. Then the evaluator(s) is responsible for synthesizing, interpreting, and, finally, judging, based on the information available and the areas identified for scrutiny by the evaluation team.

Criteria for Judging Evaluation Studies

The Joint Committee on Standards for Educational Evaluation developed *Standards for Evaluations of Educational Programs, Projects, and Materials* (1981). The compilation has become the recognized document in the field of educational evaluation standards. The 30 standards are grouped according to four primary factors that influence educational evaluation: (a) utility, (b) feasibility, (c) propriety, and (d) accuracy.

The standards listed under the utility heading require that the evaluation be informative, timely, and influential. The feasibility standards relate to the realistic, prudent, diplomatic, and frugal conduct of the evaluation in its natural setting, while ". . . the propriety standards require that the evaluations be conducted legally, ethically, and with due regard for the welfare of those involved in the evaluation, as well as those affected by the results" (p. 14). Finally, the accuracy standards relate to the correctness of the data and to their connection to the conclusions. This category of standards reflects the overall validity of the evaluation. The Joint Committee realized that not all standards can be met and that standards should not detract from the creativity of the evaluation effort. The standards, however, do present a comprehensive picture of requirements that, if met, can raise educational evaluation to new levels of excellence. The checklist in Figure 15.1 shows all 30 standards. The Joint Committee admonishes the user to refer to the full text of the standards for complete understanding.

The *Standards for Evaluations Programs, Project, and Materials guided the development of this (check one):*

request for evaluation plan/design/proposal   evaluation report
evaluation plan/design/proposal   other
evaluation contract

To interpret the information provided on this form, the reader needs to refer to the full text of the standards as they appear in Joint Committee on Standards for Educational Evaluation, Standards for Evaluations of Educational Programs, Project, and Material. New York: McGraw-Hill, 1980

The *Standards* were consulted and used as indicated in the table below (check as appropriate):

Descriptor		The Standard was deemed applicable and to the extent feasible was taken into account	The Standard was deemed applicable but could not be taken into account	The Standard was not deemed applicable	Exception was taken to the Standard
A1	Audience Identification				
A2	Evaluator Credibility				
A3	Information Scope and Selection				
A4	Valuational Interpretation				
A5	Report Clarity				
A6	Report Dissemination				
A7	Report Timeliness				
A8	Evaluation Impact				
B1	Practical Procedures				
B2	Political Viability				
B3	Cost Effectiveness				
C1	Formal Obligation				
C2	Conflict of Interest				
C3	Full and Frank Disclosure				
C4	Public's Right to Know				
C5	Rights of Human Subjects				
C6	Human Interactions				
C7	Balanced Reporting				
C8	Fiscal Responsibility				
D1	Object Identification				
D2	Context Analysis				
D3	Described Purposes and Procedures				
D4	Defensible Information Sources				
D5	Valid Measurement				
D6	Reliable Measurement				
D7	Systematic Data Control				
D8	Analysis of Quantitative Information				
D9	Analysis of Qualitative Information				
D10	Justified Conclusions				
D11	Objective Reporting				

Name: _____   Date: _____
     (typed)

     _____
     (signature)

Position or Title: _____

Agency: _____

Address: _____

Relation to Document: _____
                    (e.g., author of document, evaluation team leader, external auditor, internal auditor)
Used with permission of the Joint Committee on Standards for Educational Evaluation.

Figure 15.1   Checklist of Evaluation Standards

The increase in the number of evaluation studies, in the number of people conducting them, and in the amount of money involved in conducting the studies and assigned to the programs being evaluated makes adherence to standards imperative. Whether mandatory or self-imposed, program evaluations must be trustworthy if recommendations for decision making are to be taken seriously.

Steps in the Process of Program Evaluation

The significant decisions that may result from program evaluation and the expenditure in personnel and money make it imperative that the process be planned carefully and implemented efficiently. A poorly conducted program evaluation is a waste of valuable resources, and the validity of the final report will be in question. Stufflebeam and Madaus (1983) showed a matrix of the 30 evaluation standards with 10 evaluation tasks developed by the Joint Committee on Standards for Educational Evaluation (1981). These 10 crucial steps in educational evaluation will be elaborated, because of their close tie to the 30 standards endorsed in this chapter.

Decide Whether to Do A Study

Some program evaluations are mandated by law. For self-initiated evaluations, however, such topics as the people who sponsor the program, the people who deliver it, the people who receive it, and the people who may resist the evaluation should be considered by the evaluators before proceeding (Posavac & Carey, 1985). The time frame also should be examined, and resources for conducting the evaluation should be assessed.

Often an effective evaluation cannot be conducted because of support restraints, design flaws, or the political climate. Posavac and Carey (1985) enumerated several potential sources of resistance to program evaluations. Among the fears they identified are program termination, abuse of the information gathered, insensitive methods of evaluation, expense, and futility. These fears and others are important to consider at the early stages of the process and again when recommendations are being implemented.

Clarify and Assess Purpose

Once all of the significant people in the program have been considered, along with the technical points of money and time, it is imperative to determine the real purpose for conducting the evaluation. Several reasons were discussed earlier in this chapter. Some of those reasons, and others, may be pertinent. Whether the evaluation is undertaken for funding, accreditation, public relations, or other reasons, it would be futile to proceed without a full and detailed definition of the purpose of the program evaluation. The purpose also has a significant impact on the theoretical model selected for use and the research design needed to implement the model.

Ensure Political Viability

The term *stakeholders* is used in program evaluation to identify people who have a vested interest in the program. They are the sponsors, producers, and consumers of the program. Jobs, salaries, reputations, and program benefits are at stake. Open and full discussion will help promote political viability. When the appropriate political climate is set early, the chances of the evaluation results being implemented are improved greatly.

Prepare Contract

Formal contracts usually are not considered necessary for internal evaluations, even though their use can minimize many problems along the way. External evaluations, however, should make use of formal contracts for both professional and legal reasons. Contracts clarify the exact task; detail by whom, how, and when the task is to be accomplished; and stipulate the financial arrangements. Worthen and White (1987) gave a detailed discussion of eight issues to be considered in contracts; they are summarized in Table 15.3.

This listing in Table 15.3 assumes a sophisticated, large-scale program evaluated by an external evaluator(s). Many of the issues identified, however, should be considered for project evaluations on a smaller scale.

Budget preparation is another aspect of program evaluation agreements. Costs related to such budget items as personnel, supplies, support services, communications, indirect costs, and unanticipated expenses should be allocated and agreed upon. Nearly all the information on cost analysis written in the context of program evaluation concerns the program and not the process of evaluation. Budget formulation is a fairly common procedure. The need to prepare a program evaluation budget should not be overlooked.

Staff the Study

The administrative structure of the evaluation personnel should be outlined, showing the line of command and the actual names of persons filling each role. It seems rather obvious that the prime evaluator must be identified, as well as team members for a site visit, if such a design strategy is being used. In addition, technical assistance for handling statistical, graphic, and editorial assignments should be accommodated in the plan. Secretaries, drivers, hosts and hostesses, guides, and so forth are also important and necessary personnel for efficient evaluation projects.

In addition to identifying all personnel needed for such a study, the qualifications of each should be considered. The characteristics of evaluators were addressed in the earlier section on measurement considerations. To reemphasize, lack of bias, consideration of stakeholders, and impunity are some of the critical factors that should be checked if the results are to be treated with confidence.

Manage the Study

At this stage the evaluator becomes the manager of the project who consults with and informs various publics as the process unfolds. In addition, the collection, analysis,

Table 15.3 Contract Issues and Topics

Issues	Topics
General descriptive information	Client description Program description Purpose Authorization
Information to be produced	Clarification of questions asked
Work and resource specifications	Scope of study Design of study Sources of information Instruments for data collection Reporting of results
Responsibilities of client and evaluator	Scope of inquiry Access to data and records Management of disruptions
Control and use of evaluation information	Editorial authority Misuse and nonuse of information Dissemination rights Uses of evaluation information
Ethical issues	Conflict of interest Confidentiality Anonymity Professional autonomy
Legal issues	Tort Statutory rights Constitutional rights
Other contractual issues	Arbitration Adjudication plans Payment agreement

and reporting of information must be given direction and leadership. Delegation of responsibility and a participatory management style will help to keep the program evaluation open, thereby minimizing suspicions of hidden agendas. The administrative skills of the evaluation project director will be put into play to guarantee the efficient and honest conduct of the study.

Collect the Data

Sources of data have been suggested earlier. It is prudent to comment that the evaluator should not be obsessed with amassing data. A careful review of the purpose of the evaluation should help identify the important data to collect. Comprehensiveness is important, but sampling is suggested. Protection of participants and collection procedures should be monitored carefully. Comprehensiveness means *type* as well as *amount*. Qualitative, quantitative, formative, and summative data all are needed if the multiple method approach to program evaluation is used.

Analyze the Data

Much more data will be available than can be analyzed and reported. Consequently, it behooves the director of the evaluation to return to the framing questions of the evaluation. Only those questions should be addressed in the analysis. Statistical accuracy and the use of tables and graphics to summarize the data are essential.

Report Findings

A program evaluation nearly always results in a written report that summarizes the project, procedures, and findings and then concludes with recommendations. Much has been written about the final report (Lynch, 1986; Popham, 1975; Posavac & Carey, 1985; Wolf, 1984; Worthen, 1987). Worthen (1987) even suggested that an outside critique of the report might be beneficial to help weigh its evaluative procedures and trustworthiness.

An executive summary of 3–5 pages is helpful. A news release prepared by the evaluator is usually more accurate than one prepared by the press. The report should be well-organized, succinct, enhanced by tables and charts, and accompanied by an appendix. The report language should be straightforward and geared to the publics affected by the study. The use of educational and statistical jargon is a good way to relegate the report to the unread and unimplemented stack.

The political climate is important to consider again at the reporting stage. Preliminary reports and oral reports can be helpful in alerting the client to unfavorable findings. The report findings, particularly any negative conclusions, should not come as a surprise with the reading of the final document. The report should not be viewed as a document to be fought and dreaded but rather as a document to be addressed positively for the benefit of the people served by the program under study.

The report, or at least its executive summary, should be widely distributed in a timely manner to as many stakeholders as possible. It should have a press release and be presented in open forums.

Apply Results

The role of an evaluator (evaluation team), whether internal or external, sometimes extends to offering suggestions for implementing recommendations. Considering the political climate, the extent of dissemination of findings, and the importance of the conclusions, the implementation process is crucial and is the ultimate responsibility of the administration. Much of the negative feeling about program evaluation centers around loss of time and money and conducting studies that will not be implemented. It behooves the administration to take definite steps toward expediting the recommendations considered viable. Even if some recommendations must be delayed temporarily, that strategy should be communicated widely, just as the immediate steps taken toward action should be announced.

Conclusion

Program evaluation in such fields as physical education and exercise science, athletics, intramurals, youth sports, corporate fitness, and athletic training needs to receive much more attention than it has in the past. Accountability by word of mouth is unacceptable. Evaluation designs should measure up to the best in practice. They should be founded on well-conceived theoretical models. They should be implemented with utmost care to achieve measurement integrity. They should be acted on forthrightly. Physical educators and exercise scientists need to be attentive to evaluating their own program evaluation procedures and to training evaluators who can serve our fields. This discussion has highlighted some of the points to be considered when an evaluation is anticipated, under way, and completed.

References

American Alliance for Health, Physical Education, Recreation and Dance. (1985, October). NASPE sets criteria for national study of school evaluation. *Update*, 5.

Campbell, D.T., & Stanley, J.C. (1963). *Experimental and quasi-experimental designs for research*. Chicago: Rand McNally.

Dumke, G. (1986, January 15). Accrediting: The weak link in education reform. *Chronicle of Higher Education*, 31 (2), 18, 104.

Educational Testing Service. (1983). *Graduate program self assessment*. Princeton, NJ: Author.

Eisner, E.W. (1976). Educational connoisseurship and criticism: Their form and functions in educational evaluation. *Journal of Aesthetic Education*, 10, 135–150.

Hendricks, M. (1986). A conversation with Michael Wargo. *Evaluation Practice*, 7(4), 24–34.

House, E.R. (1978). Assumptions underlying evaluation models. *Education Researcher*, 7, 4–12.

Ianni, F.A.J., & Orr, M.T. (1979). Toward a rapprochement of quantitative and qualitative methodologies. In T.D. Cook & C.S. Reichardt (Eds.), *Qualitative and quantitative methods in evaluation research* (pp. 87–97). Beverly Hills, CA: Sage.

Illinois Association for Health, Physical Education and Recreation. (1984a). Criteria for evaluating secondary physical education in Illinois schools (7–12). *Illinois Journal of Health, Physical Education and Recreation*, 19(Fall), 34–38.

Illinois Association for Health, Physical Education and Recreation. (1984b). Criteria for evaluating elementary physical education in Illinois schools (K-6). *Illinois Journal of Health, Physical Education and Recreation, 19*(Fall), 39–43.

Jacobs, E. (1988). Clarifying qualitative research: A focus on traditions. *Educational Researcher, 17*(1), 16–24.

Jewett, A.E., & Bain, L.L. (1985). *The curriculum process in physical education.* Dubuque, IA: Wm. C. Brown.

Joint Committee on Standards for Educational Evaluation. (1981). *Standards for evaluations of educational programs, projects, and materials.* New York: McGraw-Hill.

Levine, M. (1974). Scientific method and the adversary model. *American Psychologist, 29*, 661–677.

Lynch, K.B. (1986). Style versus substance in evaluation reports. *Evaluation Practice, 7*(4), 75–76.

Madaus, G.F., Scriven, M.S., & Stufflebeam, D.L. (Eds.) (1983). *Evaluation models— viewpoints on educational and human services evaluation.* Boston: Kluwer-Nijhoff.

National Study of School Evaluation. (1987). *Evaluative criteria for the evaluation of secondary schools* (6th ed.). Washington, DC: Author.

Patton, M.Q. (1980). *Qualitative evaluation methods.* Beverly Hills, CA: Sage.

Penman, K.A., & Adams, S.H. (1980). *Assessing athletics and physical education programs.* Boston: Allyn & Bacon.

Popham, W.J. (1975). *Educational evaluation.* Englewood Cliffs, NJ: Prentice-Hall.

Popham, W.J., & Carlson, D. (1977). Deep dark deficits in the adversary evaluation model. *Educational Researcher, 6*(June), 3–6.

Posavac, E.J., & Carey, R.G. (1985). *Program evaluation—methods and case studies* (2nd ed.). Englewood Cliffs, NJ: Prentice-Hall.

Reichardt, C.S., & Cook, T.D. (1979). Beyond qualitative versus quantitative methods. In T.D. Cook & C.S. Reichardt (Eds.), *Qualitative and quantitative methods in evaluation research* (pp. 7–32). Beverly Hills, CA: Sage.

Rivlin, A.M. (1971). *Systematic thinking for social action.* Washington, DC: Brookings Institution.

Scriven, M. (1967). The methodology of evaluation. In R.W. Tyler (Ed.), *Perspectives of curriculum evaluation* (pp. 39–83). Chicago: Rand McNally.

Scriven, M. (1974). Pros and cons about goal-free evaluation. *Evaluation Comment, 3*, 1–4.

Secondary School Physical Education Council. (1977). *Assessment guide for secondary school physical education programs.* Washington, DC: National Association for Sport and Physical Education; American Alliance for Health, Physical Education and Recreation.

Stake, R.E. (1967). The countenance of educational evaluation. *Teachers College Record, 68*, 523–540.

Stake, R.E. (1975). *Evaluating the arts in education: A responsive approach.* Columbus, OH: Charles E. Merrill.

Stufflebeam, D.L. (1968). *Evaluation as enlightenment for decision-making.* Columbus, OH: Ohio State University, Evaluation Center.

Stufflebeam. D.L. (1983). The CIPP model for program evaluation. In G.F. Madaus, M. Scriven, & D.L. Stufflebeam (Eds.), *Evaluation models* (pp. 117–141). Boston: Kluwer-Nijhoff.

Stufflebeam, D.L., & Madaus, G.F. (1983). The standards for evaluation of educational programs, projects, and materials: A description and summary. In G.F. Madaus, M. Scriven, & D.L. Stufflebeam (Eds.), *Evaluation models* (pp. 395–404). Boston: Kluwer-Nijhoff.

Tyler, R.W. (1942). General statement on evaluation. *Journal of Educational Research*, *35*, 492–501.

Tyler, R.W. (1983). A rationale for program evaluation. In G.F. Madaus, M. Scriven, and D.L. Stufflebeam (Eds.), *Evaluation models* (pp. 67–78). Boston: Kluwer-Nijhoff.

Wolf, R.M. (1984). *Evaluation in education—foundations of competency assessment and program review* (2nd ed.). New York: Praeger.

Worthen, B.R. (1987). *Curriculum evaluation* (National Curriculum Study Institute). Alexandria, VA: Association for Supervision and Curriculum Development.

Worthen, B.R., & Sanders, J.R. (1973). *Educational evaluation: Theory and practice*. Belmont, CA: Wadsworth.

Worthen, B.R., & White, K.R. (1987). *Evaluating educational and social programs: Guidelines for proposal review, onsite evaluation, evaluation contracts, and technical assistance*. Boston: Kluwer-Nijhoff.

Supplementary Readings

Chelimsky, E. (1987). What have we learned about the politics of program evaluation? *Evaluation Practice*, *8*(1), 5–21.

Dobbert, M.L. (1982). *Ethnographic research: Theory and application for modern schools and societies*. New York: Praeger.

House, E.R. (Ed.). (1986). *New directions in educational evaluation*. Philadelphia: Falmer Press.

Palumbo, D. (Ed.). (1987). *The politics of program evaluation*. Newbury Park, CA: Sage.

Patton, M.Q. (1986). *Utilization-focused evaluation* (2nd ed.). Newbury Park, CA: Sage.

Pitz, G.F., & McKillip, J. (1984). *Design analysis for program evaluators*. Newbury Park, CA: Sage.

Simons, H. (1987). *Getting to know schools in a democracy: The politics and process of evaluation*. Philadelphia: Taylor and Frances.

Stufflebeam, D.L., & Shinkfield, A.J. (1985). *Systematic evaluation*. Boston: Kluwer-Nijhoff.

Computers in Measurement and Testing

Harry A. King
San Diego State University

Computers—micro, mini, and mainframe—are being used for a great many purposes in physical education, exercise science, and sport. A recent, unpublished compilation by this author has identified more than 400 journal articles concerned with such applications. This chapter examines a restricted scope. Specific concern is given to examining those uses of the computer that provide facility in dealing with problems of measurement.

The restricted scope requires rather careful definition of what problems of measurement *are*. It will be necessary to think of measurement in more restrictive terms than common usage implies. This restriction will enable discussion of how the use of a computer can aid in planning strategies for taking measurements and analyzing them in studies dealing with quantitative data. Measurement being thus defined, some concepts about computers will be reviewed, particularly in light of the rapidly changing developments in hardware and software. The capabilities of modern-day computers that give them particular advantages in dealing with measurement problems commonly encountered in practical and research settings will be explained. The way in which each of these capabilities affects the kinds of problems that can be undertaken will be described. In doing this, a number of different studies that exemplify the capabilities will be explained.

What Are Measurement Uses?

The modern world seems to accept, almost without question, that a quantitative approach to problems is generally preferable to a nonquantitative one. It is assumed that by quantifying the characteristics of the physical world and its people, problems are more readily and efficiently solved. The view has become essentially implicit in our lives and seems to only rarely be questioned (e.g., Walberg, 1984). The process of measurement, in its all-inclusive sense, can be conceptualized as involving three discernible steps:

1. Collect quantitative information, preferably within the constraints of a prearranged, formalized plan. The investigator must carefully decide what to collect and how to collect it. Both decisions require many subdecisions.
2. Analyze this quantitative information, using the formal methods of statistics and/ or mathematics. This step results in a summary description of the entire set of measurement information.
3. Use the collected information to make an informed decision about the matter of interest.

The settings in which these processes of measurement occur may differ widely. The setting may be a scientific-research one, in which an investigator may be studying some hypothetical research proposition about how variables relate; or the setting may be a more practical one, in which an investigator has particular questions and needs that seem as though they can be better satisfied by using some form of testing and measurement.

In the research setting, many of the crucial parts of an investigation lie in considering how the decisions made about measurement are likely to affect success in providing a truthful answer to the posed problem. Questions such as the following come to mind:

- Can empirical measurement indeed be used to aid in the solution of the problem identified?
- Do the variables whose measures are being (or are being proposed to be) taken have validity (i.e., relevance and reliability) as indicators of the behavior of interest? Can they be defended as being more than merely convenient?
- To what extent does the way in which the measurements were taken (or are being proposed to be taken) affect the likelihood of our being able to reach a clear answer? Did (does) the study design permit sensitive detection of the effects studied?

- Do the collected measurements (or proposed ones) satisfy the assumptions inherent in the statistical analysis by which they were (or are proposed to be) reduced? If there is some doubt on this point, what can be done?
- Can the problem be investigated through examination of a mathematical or statistical model rather than through empirical data collection, simplifying it and perhaps giving different insights into it?

The consideration and application of measurement ideas within practical settings (including both instructional ones and the quasi-medical ones of the fitness club or exercise clinic) is more meaningfully embraced under the rather broader term **testing**. *Testing* is a more cohesive term in the practical setting than *measurement*, for it has a more ready relation to the kinds of standardized instruments that tend to be used in these settings. Testing, within these settings, evokes such concerns as:

- Can testing contribute to the success of instruction?
- Can tests of competency serve a useful purpose?
- Does the educational setting have differing conceptual needs for its uses of measurement than settings that do not have instructional outcomes as their focus?

Of essence for both the research and practical settings is the collection of measurement data, its reduction to a summary for the purpose of making inferences, and the use of this summary to make decisions about beliefs and/or subsequent practices. In this chapter both practical and research perspectives are kept in view when discussing the application of computers to measurement and testing.

The Generic Computer

The rapid technological developments of the past 10 years have blurred meaningful distinctions between the capabilities of the microcomputer, the minicomputer, and the mainframe computer. At the beginning of the microcomputer era, in the late 1970s, there were definite and obvious distinctions between the three types of machine: the microcomputer sat on one's desk and was operated interactively; it had limited memory capability; its speed of operation was relatively slow; its high-level languages were primitive; its graphic capability was meager; it was relatively friendly; and it often had color capability. Mainframe and minicomputer characteristics were generally opposite to these. The low cost of the microcomputers, their friendliness, and their ability to play fanciful games established them as tools to be used and enjoyed by educators and the general public alike.

In a mere eight years, these distinctions have become so blurred that the separate consideration of different types of computers is generally unimportant and irrelevant for the great majority of purposes. Mainframes and minicomputers no longer have a meaningful separateness and can be considered conceptually equivalent. The term **mainframe** will therefore here be used to signify any kind of centralized computer system, accessible simultaneously and interactively by a number of users, and making available for their use a wide variety of software facilities. Obviously the minicomputers commonly available on university campuses fall within this definition.

While a microcomputer still sits comfortably on one's desk or lap, so does the interactive terminal linked directly to the time-shared mainframe/minicomputer. The microcomputer can also now access memory, both short-term RAM and long-term hard-disk or floppy, in quantities perfectly comparable to what one can effectively access on a mainframe.

Microcomputers now have sophisticated versions of the high-level languages, lacking nothing required by any but the most advanced user. As acceptance of computer technology has become more common, more and more people have become computer literate; software developers for both microcomputer and mainframe environments have been forced to make their products friendly, easy to use, and more compatible with one another. This latter consideration has led to extensive development of hardware and communications software that enable the two environments—microcomputer and mainframe—to communicate readily with one another. Programs, raw data, and reduced data can be transferred back and forth in summary form, textual form, or graphical form, and the nature of the underlying environment is basically irrelevant.

For these reasons, for the majority of this discussion there seems little advantage, conceptual or practical, in distinguishing among the different types of computer environments. The word *computer* will therefore be generally used in its generic sense. For certain types of large-scale problems that are sometimes encountered, larger computers are faster and may be necessary for purposes of accuracy. Thus where the two environments do differ, and where a particular point needs to be made about this difference, note will be made.

The Use of Computers in the Investigation of Measurement and Testing Issues

The ready availability of the computer has greatly enhanced capabilities for investigating the kinds of measurement and testing issues that are likely to attend the investigation of substantive problems. This enhancement can be summarized as the computer's capability to:

- easily reconfigure and summarize collected information in a form that makes it much simpler to understand (statistical analysis capability);
- derive all the consequences of *what-if* models by virtue of its great speed of calculation (simulation capability);
- quickly acquire large quantities of measurement information on-line (acquisition capability);
- store large sets of data in a form that is readily accessible to many people (storage and retrieval capability); and
- aid in more efficient means of providing instruction and assessing its outcomes (instructional capability).

Some of these capabilities directly affect a user's ability to cope with the measurement and testing aspects of a problem, for example in making for much quicker reduction of data than would otherwise be possible. Other capabilities affect the user's abilities indirectly by altering the problem itself, enabling the use of approaches to a solution that would not be feasible without the computer's aid. Whether the effect is direct or indirect, the computer will certainly affect the level of sophistication that can be adopted in dealing with the measurement and testing aspects of the problem under investigation. The remainder of this paper explains some particulars of each capability, and, where appropriate, describes illustrative studies.

Statistical Analysis Capability

The end result of many investigations—research or practical—is a large collection of numerical data. The investigator needs to analyze this data set using the common methods of statistical analysis (e.g., comparison of group means, assessment of correlational relationship, or graphical summary). This statistical analysis might also include computation of derived variables from the measured ones, for example the calculation of percent body fat from collected skinfold measurements.

A few small data sets can be tackled by hand calculation, if with a little tedium. When rather more computational complexity is involved—in doing the computations for a two-factor ANOVA, for example—computer assistance is appreciated if not essential. Interactive input to a packaged computer program would probably cut analysis time by a factor of 50 or more compared with hand or calculator methods. For still larger problems, say a factor analysis of the scores taken on 150 subjects on each of ten variables, computer use would generally be deemed compulsory. In each of these cases, the computer serves the user's convenience, freeing him or her from the chore of calculation.

Traditionally, the mainframe computer and one of its common statistical software packages (such as SPSS^X, BMDP, and SAS) have been used for the statistical analysis of medium and large sets of data. These and similar major statistical packages are generally unparalleled in their capability to analyze a body of data in innumerable ways and with great accuracy. Nevertheless, the complexity of the programs (and the large number of assumptions that are necessarily built into the analyses) often create a complicated output that is difficult to fully interpret by all but the most sophisticated user. Gondek (1981) illustrates this kind of deviation of the results from what might be expected in some of the discriminant analysis programs of major packages.

In very recent years, with the availability of 16-bit chips and cheap memory for microcomputers, it has become feasible to undertake larger-scale statistical analyses on the microcomputer (rather than the small-scale analyses that were available before). All three packages commonly available on mainframes (SPSS^X, BMDP, and SAS) are now also available on IBM-compatible microcomputers. The microcomputer version of SPSS^X costs around $1,000, requires at least about 5 megabytes of hard-disk storage for the programs and at least 512K of RAM storage (and preferably 640K), and essentially demands the Intel 8087 math coprocessor. BMDP requires considerably less hard-disk space, because individual programs can be accessed from floppy disks, and generally costs about half the SPSS^X price. It still, however, needs the math coprocessor and about as much RAM as SPSS^X. SAS demands about 8 megabytes of hard-disk storage and otherwise has similar requirements to the other two packages. All three packages operate with almost exactly the same kind of user interaction as their mainframe versions.

Many statistical package programs are available for use in the microcomputer environment. Carpenter, Deloria, and Morganstein (1984) review 24 of these. The capabilities and specifications of these packages change with great rapidity as new and updated versions are marketed. Sporting such names as Statpro, Stat80, and Crisp, they are usually available for a few hundred dollars. The reader is advised to check current issues of computer magazines, or (more efficiently) to check major index reviews to magazines such as *Computer and Control Abstracts* (monthly) or *Microcomputer Index* (bimonthly) to find out what is currently favored in the market, and what capabilities the latest versions have.

Although the expanding hardware capabilities are continually changing the picture of the suitability of the microcomputer for larger-scale statistical analyses, the cautions noted by Swaine (1983) are still worth bearing in mind. In particular, larger-scale analyses on the microcomputer: (a) will often take too long (and certainly so unless they have special chips, such as the Intel 8087 math coprocessor, to speed numeric computations) and (b) sometimes run the risk of potential inaccuracies of calculation that occur because microcomputers are based on chips that process numbers in far fewer bits than do their mainframe cousins. Amateur programmers, programming their own solutions, are generally unaware of how weak programming algorithms combine with the limited bit representation to cause serious problems, even in rather small-scale analyses.

Though the various package programs are exceedingly comprehensive, some particular types of analysis cannot be made directly. For example, generalizability analyses cannot be computed directly by the package programs, but must be pieced together from portions of the output of relevant programs in the package. Godbout and Schutz (1983) describe the use of BMDP-8V for this purpose. Though this piecemeal strategy of analysis is often feasible, there are occasions when a still more tailor-made approach is necessary.

In such cases, two options are open to the investigator. The first option is to try to find a computer program that does what is wanted. Sometimes a program is available from commercial or noncommercial sources; for example, for generalizability analysis the program GENOVA is available from Crick and Brennan (1983). At other times, programs can be found by perusing measurement-related research journals. The journals *Educational and Psychological Measurement*, *Applied Psychological Measurement*, and *Behavior Research Methods, Instruments and Computers* all frequently contain a wide variety of task-specific computer programs for many different measurement-related purposes. Yet another source for programs is in published textbooks in measurement, statistics, and research methods. The textbooks by Baumgartner and Jackson (1987),

Safrit (1986), and Thomas and Nelson (1985) each offer programs useful to effect different types of simple data analyses. These include such common needs as the calculation of percent body fat from skinfold measurements, the calculation of max $\dot{V}o_2$, the calculation of standardized scores from raw scores, and the analysis of data collected from simple experimental designs.

The second option that can be used to carry out a quantitative analysis by computer is to write a program in one of the common programming languages. This approach is fairly time-consuming and prone to the kinds of numerical analysis errors noted above: it should therefore generally be undertaken only by someone fairly skilled in programming and cognizant of numerical analysis methods. If such programming is undertaken, the more comprehensive forms of the BASIC language will generally be found sufficient. In programs requiring more complexity, FORTRAN is preferable, particularly because of its ease of articulation to sophisticated preprogrammed packages, such as the IMSL (International Mathematical and Statistical Library) subroutines. The Pascal and C languages also offer great advantages for more comprehensive purposes.

Simulation Capability

There are a number of types of measurement problems that make the use of a computer compulsory. These are problems that use the *simulation* (or *Monte Carlo*) method. The method of simulation is applied to the investigation of problems where it is difficult to empirically collect the quantitative data necessary for a solution (Bronson, 1984). The difficulty usually stems from the need to understand the effect of a number of conditions (or factors) that affect the data—conditions that cannot easily be selectively and independently controlled. It is the number of combinations of relevant conditions that need to be considered in order to weigh all the different possibilities that makes empirical methods impractical.

Simulation methodology rests on defining the process to be simulated in terms of a mathematical (or statistical) model. The model can be either stochastic or deterministic. In *stochastic* models, the event-sequences studied depend on probabilistic (or varying) precursor-to-consequence relations; in *deterministic* models, the event sequences studied depend on invariant precursor-to-consequence relations. The model is then coded as a computer program that can be run many times under each of the conditions of interest that are built into the model. If the model was accurately constructed to mimic the problem under consideration, then results of the simulation can be assumed to represent how the process would behave in the real world.

Computer simulation methods have been applied to many pure measurement problems concerned with the validity of the assumptions underlying different statistical analysis techniques. Investigations of physical educators have included, for example: study of the reliability of criterion-referenced test scores as affected by sample size, score distribution characteristics, and the chosen cutoff score (Patterson, 1985); study of the effect of non-normality on tests of significance of differences between independent correlation coefficients (Chang, 1976); and study of the effect of disproportionality in subject numbers per cell on errors of inference in analyzing a two-way ANOVA (Looney, 1980).

A sweeping proposal for a general method of attack on practical statistical analysis problems by using a simulation-related methodology, *bootstrapping*, has been made by Diaconis and Efron (1983). They suggest the use of methods of analysis that are tailored directly to the data at hand, and that allow "freedom from two limiting factors that have dominated statistical theory from its beginnings: the assumption that the data conform to a bell-shaped curve and the need to focus on statistical measures whose theoretical properties can be analyzed mathematically" (p. 379). This methodology generates great numbers of simulated samples from the actual observed data (and not from a presupposed theoretical model) and examines inferential conclusions tailored to the data at hand rather than to a presupposed model. Such a method relies entirely on the enormous computational speed of the modern supercomputers—the kinds of computers (such as the Cray X-MP) in which a single machine can have the computing capability of 40,000 IBM PCs.

Another kind of simulation study that illustrates how computers can be used to investigate measurement problems was completed by King (1979). The basic question investigated was how accurately the relative abilities of a set of players engaging in a round-robin tournament (in tennis or table tennis, for example) could be estimated from *restricted* tournaments. Tournaments could be restricted by playing shorter matches or by completing less than the whole set of matches. The further question was posed of whether such restricted tournaments differed in their ranking accuracy as a result of the number and homogeneity of the players in the tournament, and also as a result of different methods of reducing the results matrix.

This is just the sort of problem that computer simulation methods are ideally suited for—the problem is just impossible to investigate by actual empirical observation. After a theoretical scoring model is set up (based on probabilities of players winning points against one another), the computer "plays" game after game, tournament after tournament. In the King study, 12,000 tournaments, some having as many as 171 matches (a 19-player round-robin tournament), were simulated, and the results were used to study how accurate different restricted-tournament types were in measuring the relative ranking of the hypothetical players. Thus a particular type of measurement problem, infeasible to investigate by any empirical means, could be studied.

Acquisition Capability

The actual physical collection of data is a time-consuming task. Because of this, we often need to restrict the number and variety of measurements we take. From a measurement standpoint, information is effectively lost when what is observed (or quantified) is too severely restricted. In many data collection situations, the loss of data and restriction of scope are now no longer necessary, because a computer can be used both as a device controller and as a data collector in a completely automated fashion. As a device controller it can initiate prompts to the experimentee with precise timing and

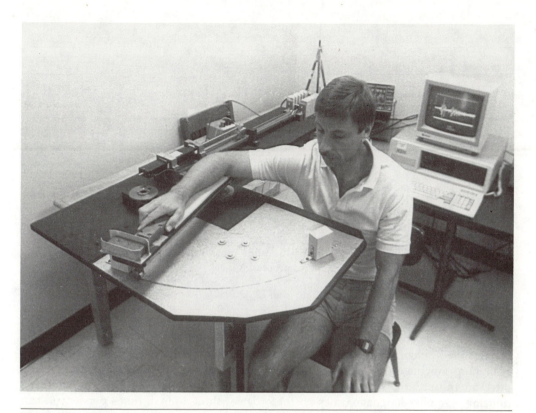

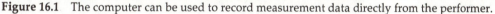

Figure 16.1 The computer can be used to record measurement data directly from the performer.

sequence. As a data collector, it actually acquires and records the experimentee's responses (Richards, 1987). The latter of these two functions is more directly concerned with the computer's role in affecting measurement capability, and will therefore be discussed here.

The computer can be used to record measurement data directly from the performer (or relevant equipment). Via suitable electrical gadgetry, the computer can record the occurrence and/or amplitude of motor responses (Figure 16.1). Instantaneous characteristics of the motor responses (for example, the distance of a marked point on the body from a reference point, or the sensing of a physiological event, such as a heart beat) are transduced into electrical voltages. These instantaneous voltages are then

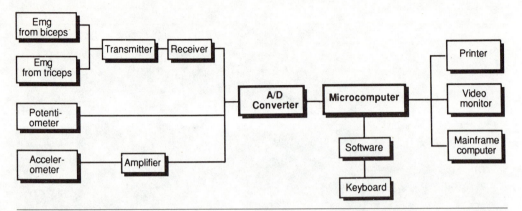

Figure 16.2   Four channels of data from an on-line motor control experiment are handled by an A-D converter for immediate computer processing.

converted, by an analog-digital (A-D) converter, into integer numbers (Belcher & Gale, 1980). Recordings of the motion can occur as frequently as the A-D converter is able convert the voltage to an integer and store it. This is in turn dependent on the programming language (and algorithm) used to control the A-D acquisition. Sampling rates on the order of several hundred times per second are fairly easily achieved; utilizing assembly language, rates on the order of thousands of times per second can be achieved.

It is commonly of interest to be sampling several motions of interest at the same time. A-D converters have several channels that allow this. Figure 16.2 shows an experimental arrangement in which four channels of data from an on-line motor-control experiment (two from EMG sources via telemetry, one from a potentiometer measuring distance, and one from an accelerometer measuring acceleration) are handled by an A-D converter for immediate computer processing. Of course a 4-channel converter that is recording four separate motions will sample one particular motion four times less frequently than if it were devoting its recording to one channel alone. For the recording of time-derived measures, the computer must have a built-in hardware clock.

This mode of on-line data collection can be used to great effect in all areas of sports and exercise science. There are a great many examples in the literature—for example, for collecting physiological (Riblett, Gallagher, & Dyer, 1985), sports medicine (Richards & Cooper, 1982), biomechanical (Olney & Winter, 1985), kinesiological (Kamen, 1983), motor learning (Crocker & Dickinson, 1984), and general motor-performance (McClenaghan & Williams, 1986) data in a laboratory setting.

Another way the computer can acquire performance data is indirectly, through the input of an observer of the movement performance. An observer records perceived events at a portable computer keyboard (or, perhaps, graphic tablet) as the actions are seen to occur in one or more performers' actions.

A common setting for this kind of behavioral observation recording is the instructional one, perhaps in public schools or public health instruction situations (McKenzie & Carlson, 1984). Behavioral recordings may be made, for example, for the purpose of finding out how well students are attending to instruction or how well teachers (or coaches) are following sound instructional principles in teaching. Such variables as the type, quality, and frequency of feedback being given to the learner (positive vs. corrective, general vs. specific), or the allocation of instructional time to different purposes (e.g., management time vs. active learning time) are often of interest. Recording these types of data on a portable computer greatly enhances the amount of data that can be collected. If the data are then sent, via a modem, to a larger-scale computer, fast and sophisticated analysis becomes possible.

Another setting in which the computer has been profitably employed to facilitate indirect behavioral recording is in the technical analysis of tactics, strategies, and techniques being used in different sports (Franks & Goodman, 1986a, 1986b). Occurrences such as shots made, turnovers, time of possession, and time on attack—occurrences common to many individual and team sports—can be easily recorded for concurrent or later analysis. Franks and Goodman have illustrated the use of these kinds of data collection and discussed the measurement concepts involved for sports such as fencing, water polo, field hockey, and soccer.

This facility of data collection must lead to several changes in the way measurement problems are approached. In the laboratory type of investigation, the computer makes it a simple matter to record multiple dependent variables at great frequency. In a behavioral observation setting, the measurements taken are necessarily more limited by the recording capability of a human observer, but their number and type can still be markedly increased. In both settings, then, use of the computer makes the process of recording data much easier, and thus the number and type of measurements taken can be profitably extended. From a measurement standpoint, investigators are faced with new decisions about whether this new bounty of data can be employed to good scientific advantage.

More measurement is not at all necessarily better measurement. Only insofar as one is able to make clear and wise decisions about how to handle the plethora of measures that computer data-acquisition methods bring to hand will scientific process be concomitantly improved. The researcher becomes faced with such issues as:

- How can one select from the multiple measures at hand those that pertain most validly to our specific question of interest?
- How is one to interpret results when several seemingly plausible dependent-variable measures do not lead to the same conclusions?
- How is it best to transform measures that do not fit the standard assumptions needed for traditional statistical analysis?
- When multiple dependent variables are taken in time-serial fashion (and where distinct autocorrelation patterns are seen), how is it best to analyze them?

It can be seen that the use of a computer as a data-gathering tool will lead to new and complicated measurement issues. It is this author's assumption that methods of multivariate statistical analysis will be increasingly used to deal with reducing the collected data. It is assumed, too, that methods of exploratory data analysis (Tukey, 1977) and time-series analysis (Spray & Newell, 1986) will need to be applied more frequently.

Storage and Retrieval Capability

Computers are readily capable of storing large amounts of data. The data can be stored extremely quickly and in a form that is easily accessible. The large set of stored data, coded and structured in various ways to allow multiple means of processing and retrieval, is termed a **database** in modern parlance. The data that comprise the databases can be sorted, transposed, rearranged, and otherwise manipulated with great versatility with appropriate software. Both **spreadsheet** software and **database-management** software allow these versatile manipulations of databases.

A database can be of two kinds: It can be comprised of data collected directly by an investigator, or it can be a set of reference data, probably gathered by someone else, against which the newly collected data are to be compared. In both cases, the investigator's capability to handle the database easily should have clear consequences for the measurement and testing aspects of research studies or practical projects.

In the former case, the ease of database management permits great flexibility in exploring different ways to combine, subdivide, reorder, and transform the collected data. A spreadsheet package, such as Lotus 1-2-3, can be used to manipulate a numerical data set rather easily (Figure 16.3), including its graphic display (Figure 16.4). Such a facility must be expected to greatly extend how an investigator can explore meanings and interrelationships contained within subsets of a body of data. In the latter case, where the database could be a reference set of norms specifying performance levels that are to be expected (on different motor tasks, different physiological and anthropometric measures, different nutritional standards, or other characteristics of interest), the analytic possibilities are equally widened. The norms can be arranged by percentile ranking in the population, by age, by gender, or indeed by any kind of categorization that may be of interest to someone wanting to make a particular type of comparison with known performance standards. The computer allows, then, the means not only to analyze data readily but also to compare them at once to any reference set of data we might choose.

An example of a large computer database of the first kind was compiled and reported by Carter as part of the Montreal Olympic Games Anthropometric Project (Carter, 1982, pp. 158–166). The meticulous structure and definition of this database and its computer accessibility have made it a superb resource for the investigations of many sports science researchers. A good example of a computerized database of the second kind was given by Purdy in his work on developing a system for more easily (and more accurately) scoring decathlon meets (Purdy, 1975). Other examples of databases will be cited in the section on instructional capability.

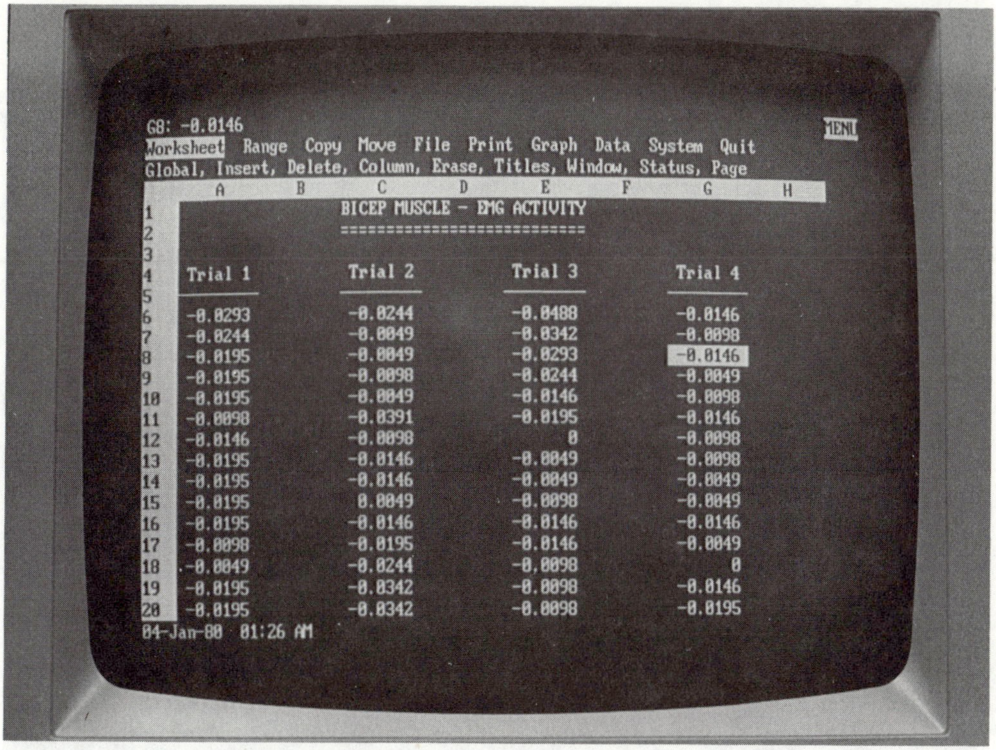

Figure 16.3   A spreadsheet package can be used to manipulate a numerical data set.

Instructional Capability

As noted earlier, issues concerning the way measurement and testing are (and can be) used in instructional settings in physical education have long been of interest to physical educators. It has been argued that present perspectives on the practical implementation of testing in these types of settings seem to have progressed little, conceptually or practically, from the ideas of thirty years past (King, 1984). The introduction of computer methodologies will be by no means a panacea for some of these deficiencies, but the new possibilities certainly offer potential for alterations of practice.

There are many ways in which computers can potentially assist in the teaching of physical education. King and Aufsesser (1986) and Baumgartner and Cicciarella (no date) both list computer programs that can be useful for different kinds of purposes in the instructional setting. Computer programs directly related to measurement and testing are evaluated according to three major criteria: (a) the easy storage and analysis of data collected via fitness performance tests; (b) the easy storage and analysis of test scores (and related data, such as attendance) for purposes of grading; and (c) the provision of means for improved cognitive testing. Each of these uses will be discussed separately.

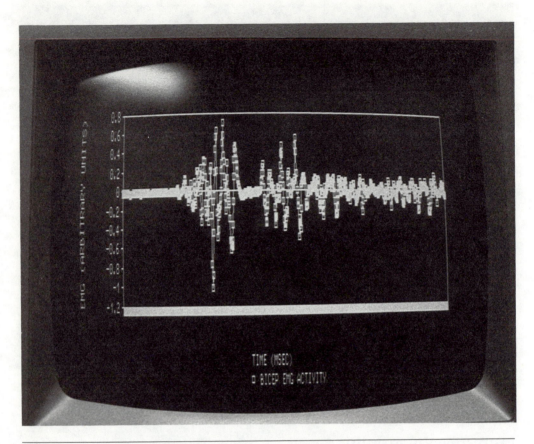

Figure 16.4   A graphic display of the numerical data set shown in Figure 16.3.

For several reasons, interest in fitness testing has increased in recent years. Computers are useful for assisting in the storage, analysis, and interpretation of group-collected fitness data for the reasons cited in the section on storage and retrieval capability. Many programs have been made available to assist educators in these data-handling tasks. King and Aufsesser (1986) reference 16 of these. These programs allow entry of data on a large number of measures by the teacher, and a variety of analytical capabilities that often include comparison with normative data, the printing of individual and group reports, and the compilation of improvement reports over a series of testing occasions.

Of particular note, because of the promotion that has been given to the AAHPERD's Health-Related Physical Fitness Test, are the programs that assist in gathering and analyzing its results. Though the test has not yet had widespread acceptance (Safrit & Wood, 1986), the improved means of analysis and data-handling using a computer might make the test more attractive. Of note, too, is the FITNESSGRAM program, described by Lacy and Marshall (1984). This program allows the recording of fitness data for school-age children, the comparison with different types of normative data, and the identification of children for different AAHPERD fitness awards.

In recent years, several physical educators have demonstrated the practical possibilities of using more individualized approaches to testing in school physical education—approaches stressing the importance of clear specification of performance objectives (or competencies) as the desired outcomes of each learner's interaction with the provided instruction (Reeve & Morrison, 1986; Viera & Ferguson, 1986). These kinds of approaches would seem to have great merit within the framework of the accountability movement that continues to have a significant impact on school instructional practices. A disadvantage of such systems of testing is the need for fairly copious recordkeeping. The computer undoubtedly has an important role in this process. Kelly (1987) has illustrated how the computer can play a central role in the management of test data within this kind of instructional setting.

The ability to maintain data files containing scores to be used in grading could potentially be a useful aid to physical educators. A large number and variety of programs are available (King & Aufsesser, 1986). These grading programs allow the entry of test data from tests of different types, allow scores to be combined in a variety of ways (often through conversion to standardized scores), and allow printouts of cumulative performance to be made at any time.

Even the relatively sophisticated grading programs (such as the PAR system available on IBM-compatibles) tend to have great flexibility in some aspects of the grading process but little flexibility in others. For example, though component scores can be combined in many ways, it is very difficult (and often impossible) to adapt the programs to the wide variety of nonstandard grading methods that many teachers use. Many real sets of grading data have *holes*, i.e., missing scores for different students on different combinations of tests. This fact makes standard reductions of data based on routine programs difficult and sometimes misleading.

Whether physical educators will use these types of programs is yet to be seen. Authors of textbooks on measurement and testing unfailingly explicate methods of formal grading, yet there seems little evidence that these formal prescriptions are followed by teachers (Morrow, 1978), or, indeed, that they use much formal testing as a basis for grading at all (Imwold, Rider, & Johnson, 1982). Whether computer capabilities will change these teacher practices remains to be seen.

Just as they are able to store large amounts of numerical and textual data of other kinds, computers are able to store large banks of cognitive test items. Test-item banks can be constructed to store questions thought to measure cognitive skills important for any particular courses of instruction in physical education—courses of either the theory type (e.g., anatomy or biomechanics) or of the activity type (e.g., tennis or aerobic dance). Computer programs that create and organize such test banks have been made available commercially (e.g., as listed by King and Aufsesser, 1986) and reported in the research literature (King, 1981).

The advantages of systems of cognitive testing based on computers are great. Large-scale banks of high-quality items would eliminate the need for instructors to invent their own on an *ad hoc* basis. The ease of handling computerized test banks affords the user the ability to update and improve questions easily, to create multiple different tests on the same material (and thus to implement instructional strategies based on mastery-learning concepts), and to generally use testing in a more direct way as an adjunct to the teaching/learning process. Such modern ideas as latent trait estimation and adaptive (or *tailored*) testing (Weiss, 1983) are dependent on computerized facilities for testing, and they, too, might find application to testing methods in our fields of study.

Once again, the question of whether such computer-based facilities will be used by teachers to improve their testing practices remains to be answered. But clearly the powerful computer capabilities now available can potentially change present-day practice.

Conclusion

Some of the various capabilities by which the computer aids researchers and teachers in applying methods of measurement and testing in new and powerful ways have been described, and illustrative studies have been cited. Yet any description of the status quo of computer methodology must be incomplete and quickly outdated. Within a rather short time, as the technology continues its relentless development, one must certainly expect to have to readjust perspectives on what is possible and what is wise practice. The computer is far more than a machine that aids industry and thinking. It alters and expands one's conception of the world. It radically alters the intellectual impress one can bring to bear on problems (Provenzo, 1986). Thus, it is to be expected that the computer will revolutionize the way that problems concerning measurement and testing in physical education and exercise and sports science can be conceptualized, and it will revolutionize the way in which methodologies can be applied to solve them. The computer will surely aid in the processes of measurement and testing, but it will also undoubtedly complicate the level of knowledge and insight that will be necessary to use these processes wisely.

References

Baumgartner, T.A., & Cicciarella, C.F. (Eds.) (no date). *Directory of computer software with application to sport science, health, and dance* (2nd ed.). Reston, VA: American Alliance for Health, Physical Education, Recreation and Dance.

Baumgartner, T.A., & Jackson, A.S. (1987). *Measurement and evaluation in physical education and exercise science*. Dubuque, IA: Wm. C. Brown.

Belcher, J.S., & Gale, A.S. (1980). The use of microcomputers for data acquisition and manipulation. *American Laboratory*, 12, 114–123.

Bronson, R. (1984). Computer simulation: What it is and how it's done. *Byte*, 8(3), 95–96;98;100;102.

Carpenter, J., Deloria, D., & Morganstein, D. (1984). Statistical software for microcomputers: A comparative analysis of 24 packages. *Byte, 8*(4), 234–256.

Carter, J.E.L. (Ed.) (1982). *Physical structure of Olympic athletes. Part 1. The Montreal Olympic Games Anthropological Project.* Basel, Switzerland: Karger.

Chang, C-O. (1976). Effects of non-normality and sample size on effectiveness of significance of differences between two independent correlation coefficients (Doctoral dissertation, University of Iowa). *Dissertation Abstracts International, 37,* 6217–6218B.

Crick, J.E., & Brennan, R.L. (1983). *Manual for GENOVA: A generalized analysis of variance system.* Iowa City: American College Testing Service.

Crocker, P.R.E., & Dickinson, J. (1984). Incidental psychomotor learning: The effects of number of movements, practice and rehearsal. *Journal of Motor Behavior, 16,* 61–75.

Diaconis, P., & Efron, B. (1983). Computer-intensive methods in statistics. *Scientific American, 248*(5), 116–130.

Franks, I.M., & Goodman, D. (1986a). A systematic approach to analysing sports performance. *Journal of Sports Sciences, 4,* 49–59.

Franks, I.M., & Goodman, D. (1986b). Computer-assisted technical analysis of sport. *Coaching Review, 8,* 58–64.

Godbout, P., & Schutz, R.W. (1983). Generalizability of ratings of motor performances with reference to various observational designs. *Research Quarterly for Exercise and Sport, 54,* 20–27.

Gondek, P.C. (1981). What you see may not be what you think you get: Discriminant analysis in statistical packages. *Educational and Psychological Measurement, 41,* 267–281.

Imwold, C.H., Rider, R.A., & Johnson, D.J. (1982). The use of evaluation in public school physical education programs. *Journal of Teaching in Physical Education, 2*(1), 13–18.

Kamen, G. (1983). The acquisition of maximal isometric plantar flexor strength: A force-time curve analysis. *Journal of Motor Behavior, 15,* 63–73.

Kelly, L. (1987). Computer management of student performance. *Journal of Physical Education, Recreation and Dance, 58*(8), 12–13, 82–85.

King, H.A. (1979). Effect of match length on accuracy of ranking in round robin tournaments: A computer simulation study. *Research Quarterly, 50,* 404–412.

King, H.A. (1981). Quiz: An interactive computer test generation program. *Educational and Psychological Measurement, 41,* 184–186.

King, H.A. (1984). Measurement and evaluation as an area of study: A plea for new perspectives. In C.M. Tipton & J.G. Hay (Eds.), *Specialization in physical education: The Alley legacy* (pp. 53–64). Iowa City: University of Iowa.

King, H.A., & Aufsesser, K.S. (1986). Microcomputer software to assist the school physical education teacher. *Physical Educator, 43,* 90–97.

Lacy, E., & Marshall, B. (1984). FITNESSGRAM: An answer to physical fitness improvement for school children. *Journal of Physical Education, Recreation, and Dance, 55*(1), 18–19.

Looney, M.A. (1980). Unweighted means and complete least-squares analyses of disproportionate cell data (Doctoral dissertation, Indiana University). *Dissertation Abstracts International, 42,* 1821B.

McClenaghan, B.A., & Williams, H.G. (1986). Design of an automated system to quantify dynamic stability. *Research Quarterly for Exercise and Sport, 57,* 78–81.

McKenzie, T.L., & Carlson, B.R. (1984). Computer technology for exercise and sport pedagogy: Recording, storing, and analyzing interval data. *Journal of Teaching in Physical Education, 3*(3), 17–27.

Morrow, J.R., Jr. (1978). Measurement techniques—Who uses them? *Journal of Physical Education and Recreation, 49*(9), 66–67.

Olney, S.J., & Winter, D.A. (1985). Predictions of knee and ankle moments of force in walking from emg and kinematic data. *Journal of Biomechanics, 18,* 9–20.

Patterson, P. (1985). An investigation of the dependability of criterion-referenced test scores using generalizability theory (Doctoral dissertation, University of Wisconsin). *Dissertation Abstracts International, 46,* 3286A.

Provenzo, E.F., Jr. (1986). *Beyond the Gutenberg galaxy.* New York: Teachers College Press.

Purdy, J.G. (1975). Computer generated track and field scoring tables: 2, theoretical foundation and development of a model. *Medicine and Science in Sports, 7,* 111–115.

Reeve, J., & Morrison, C. (1986). Teaching for learning: The application of systematic evaluation. *Journal of Physical Education, Recreation and Dance, 57*(6), 37–39.

Riblett, L.E., Jr., Gallagher, R.R., & Dyer, R.A. (1985). Computer-controlled instrumentation system for measurement of breath-by-breath responses from exercising humans. *Proceedings of the National Biomedical Sciences in Instrumentation Symposium, 21,* 63–71.

Richards, J.G. (1987). Interfacing peripherals for data acquisition and control. In J.E. Donnelly (Ed.), *Using microcomputers in physical education and the sport sciences* (pp. 13–32). Champaign, IL: Human Kinetics.

Richards, J.G., & Cooper, J. (1982). Implementation of an on-line isokinetic analysis system. *Journal of Orthopaedic and Sports Physical Therapy, 4,* 36–38.

Safrit, M.J. (1986). *Introduction to measurement in physical education and exercise science.* St. Louis: Times Mirror.

Safrit, M.J., & Wood, T.M. (1986). The Health-Related Physical Fitness Test: A tri-state survey of users and non-users. *Research Quarterly for Exercise and Sport, 57,* 27–32.

Spray, J., & Newell, K.M. (1986). Time series analysis of motor learning: KR versus No-KR. *Human Movement Science, 5,* 59–74.

Swaine, M. (1983). Can you do statistics on a microcomputer? *Infoworld* (November 14), 39;43–45.

Thomas, J.R., & Nelson, J.K. (1985). *Introduction to research in health, physical education, recreation, and dance.* Champaign, IL: Human Kinetics.

Tukey, J.W. (1977). *Exploratory data analysis.* Reading, MA: Addison-Wesley.

Viera, B.L., & Ferguson, B.J. (1986). Teaching volleyball: A competency based model. *Journal of Health, Physical Education, Recreation and Dance, 57*(7), 54–58.

Walberg, H.J. (1984). Quantification reconsidered. In H.W. Gordon (Ed.), *Review of research in education, Volume 11* (pp. 369–402). Washington, DC: American Educational Research Association.

Weiss, D.J. (Ed.). (1983). *New horizons in testing: Latent trait test theory and computerized adaptive testing.* New York: Academic Press.

Supplementary Readings

Brodie, D.A., & Thornhill, J.J. (1983). *Microcomputing in sport and physical education.* Wakefield, England: Lepus.

Cicciarella, C.F. (1986). *Microelectronics in the sport sciences.* Champaign, IL: Human Kinetics.

Donnelly, J.E. (1987). *Using microcomputers in physical education and the sport sciences.* Champaign, IL: Human Kinetics.

McKeown, P.G. (1988). *Living with computers* (2nd ed.). San Diego: Harcourt Brace Jovanovich.

Glossary

absolute reliability—an estimate of the amount of variability to expect in a person's score if the person was tested again within a short period of time.

accreditation model—method of program evaluation in which a team of outside consultants reviews qualitative and quantitative materials gathered by the faculty on the basis of guidelines set by an accrediting agency.

adaptive test—test that matches the difficulty of the test item to the ability of the examinee.

adversary model—method of program evaluation in which a jury determines the winner of a debate between an advocate team and an adversary team who have investigated the program.

affect—general class name for feelings, emotions, mood, and temperament.

affective behavior—manifestations of feelings, attitudes, interests, and values.

ANOVA—Analysis of Variance; a statistical procedure utilized to partition total variance in scores into contributing sources of variation.

artistic model—method of program evaluation in which an expert uses his or her knowledge to wisely describe, interpret, and evaluate a program.

attitude—a feeling about some *object*, such as a program, practice, group, person, or institution.

base-free score—*See* **true residualized gain score.**

Bayesian statistics—an approach that combines information from past research with current research to form a new distribution.

behavioral objectives model—method of program evaluation in which student performance is compared with behaviorally stated objectives.

BMDP8V—a series of computer programs for conducting statistical analyses.

body-image—the physical dimension of self-concept, i.e., one's perception of one's body.

canonical correlation analysis—CCA; multivariate product moment correlation between two sets of variables. Used primarily for construct validity.

canonical index—the relationship between a variable in one canonical space with a variate in the other canonical space. Similar to a factor loading in factor analysis.

canonical loading—the relationship between a variable in one canonical space with its corresponding variate in the same space. Similar to a factor loading in factor analysis.

ceiling effect—refers to the phenomenon of subjects who score high (on blood pressure, etc.) at the start of an intervention generally recording the smallest change in response to the imposed stressor, drug, or treatment. Leads to the negative correlation between initial status and gain.

Central Limit Theorem—if samples are drawn from a population at random, the means of the samples will tend to be normally distributed (Kerlinger, 1973, p. 207).

change score—*See* **gain score.**

classical test theory—a weak true-score measurement theory built around the concept of a true score and an error score.

closed item—an item that requires the examinee to respond in a specified way, such as selecting one or more alternative responses.

communality estimate—h^2; the sum of the square of factor loadings across the robust factors; represents the amount of variance of a variable accounted for by the factors.

concurrent validity—the extent to which a field test can be used in place of a criterion test.

concurrent validity design—validity studies that relate predictor test scores and criterion test scores at the same point in time, with the aim of substituting predictor scores for criterion scores.

confidence interval—an interval that is constructed to yield information about a statistical hypothesis.

confirmatory factor analysis—CFA; factor-analytic methodology whereby a given factor structure is tested against the data set or the data provided.

construct-related evidence—evidence that supports a proposed construct interpretation of scores on a test based on theoretical implications associated with the construct label (American Psychological Association, 1985, p. 90).

construct validity—a method of validation by which (a) common sources of variation are clustered to establish those measurement constructs provided or (b) predicted variables are related to preformed groups to establish the relationship.

content-related evidence—the degree to which samples of items, tasks, or questions on a test are representative of some defined universe or domain of content (American Psychological Association, 1985, p. 10).

content-related validity—subjective evidence gathered to demonstrate that the items comprising a particular test appropriately assess the abilities to be measured.

content relevance—assessing the appropriateness of the defined universe of test content and behaviors. Accompanies the assessment of content-related evidence for validity.

continuous variable—variable that can, in theory, be measured to finer and finer degrees.

convergent validity—evidence that indicates a strong relationship between different measures of the same construct.

correction for attenuation—correcting the validity coefficient by accounting for the unreliability in the predictor and/or criterion measures.

correlation—statistical procedure that quantifies the relationship between two variables.

criterion contamination—extraneous elements not directly related to the characteristic being measured that are introduced into a criterion measure during the construction of criterion measurement instruments.

criterion deficiency—failure to identify important components of a criterion measure.

criterion distortion—bias in criterion measures introduced as a result of combining criterion components to form a composite score.

criterion-predictor—the correlation between a criterion test and a predictor test. Used to assess validity. (A criterion test is the most valid measure of an attribute; a predictor test is one being considered as a substitute for a criterion test.)

criterion-referenced evaluation—an evaluation process in which a student's performance is judged against an explicitly defined criterion behavior.

criterion-referenced measurement—an approach to measurement emphasizing proportion of domain mastered. Can be either a domain-referenced test or a mastery test.

criterion-referenced test—an examination often having a predetermined performance standard required for passing.

criterion-related evidence—evidence that shows the extent to which scores on a test are related to a criterion measure (American Psychological Association, 1985, p. 90). *See also* **concurrent validity design; predictive validity design.**

criterion-related validity—*See* **criterion-related evidence.**

criterion scale unit bias—bias in criterion measures introduced via the scoring method employed.

criterion score—the recorded score on a test with repeated measures.

criterion test—the most valid measure of an attribute. For example, maximal oxygen uptake measured on a treadmill is an acceptable criterion test for cardiovascular endurance.

cross-validation—procedure that applies regression weights from one sample to a second sample in order to estimate the accuracy and stability of prediction equations in predictive validity designs.

database—an organized collection of data organized into rows (records) designating objects or people and columns (fields) designating information about the objects or people.

decision accuracy—the accuracy of classification of examinees as masters/nonmasters.

decision-making model—method of program evaluation in which information about context, input, process, and product (CIPP) are given to persons who make decisions regarding planning, structuring, implementing, and recycling.

decision rule—a rule used to determine if a statistical hypothesis has been confirmed or rejected.

dependent variable—the Y variable of a regression equation. Often called the *criterion variable*.

dichotomous scoring—a two-choice response, such as correct-incorrect.

difficulty index—the percentage of examinees who answer an item correctly.

dimensions—the common sources of variation in a factor structure identified by the factors.

discrete variable—variable that can assume values only at distinct or discrete points on a scale.

discriminant analysis—a procedure for estimating group membership by estimating the position of an individual on a line that best separates the groups.

discriminant validity—evidence that indicates a weak relationship between measures of different constructs.

discrimination index—a measure reflecting the degree to which examinees who are rated as good on some standard pass the item and those rated as poor by the same standard fail the item.

domain—the general area of study within a factor analysis. The dimensions of a study of a factor space describe the domain.

domain-referenced validity—the extent to which a test measures the objectives identified within a domain.

domain score estimation—the examinee's score (proportion correct or completed successfully) in the item domain.

D study—decision study; utilized following a G study (generalizability study) to make substantive decisions regarding appropriate measurement schedules.

effect size—a standardized contrast involving the difference between means divided by the standard deviation.

equivalent forms—two tests constructed from the same table of specifications and resulting in like means, variability, and reliability.

evaluation—process of making judgments about the results of measurement in terms of the purpose of measuring.

expected mean square—theoretical expectation of the sources of variation contributing to a calculated mean square value.

facet—a factor used in a generalizability theory analysis. For example, the *teacher* facet might be used in such a study where the researcher has four levels of teachers (i.e., four teachers are used).

factor analysis—FA; a multivariate correlational technique that attempts to reduce an N×N correlation matrix to an N×K factor matrix. The k factors represent common sources of variation represented by the original variables. FA is used to establish construct validity.

factor loading—an index of relationships between a factor and a variable.

factor structure—the matrix that is created by the factor-analysis methodology that relates the variables to the factors.

false negative classification—classifying examinee incorrectly as a nonmaster.

false positive classification—classifying examinee incorrectly as a master.

final score—last score obtained before change is measured; commonly abbreviated Y. Used in analysis of change.

floor effect—refers to the phenomenon of subjects who score low (on blood pressure, etc.) at the start of an intervention generally recording the largest change in response to the imposed stressor, drug, or treatment. Leads to the negative correlation between initial status and gain.

fully crossed random model—a generalizability (or ANOVA) model where the levels of all facets are considered randomly chosen from a universe of available levels and each level of each facet crosses all levels of all other facets.

gain score—score calculated by subtracting an initial score from a final score; measurement of change.

G coefficient—generalizability coefficient; numerical value between 0.00 and 1.0 that is interpreted like a reliability coefficient to indicate degree of generalizability (i.e., 0.00 is no generalizability; 1.00 is perfect generalizability).

generalizability theory—an extension of the intraclass reliability model that permits partitioning of observed score variation into various facets, which can be used to estimate the generalizability (reliability) of the data.

general motor ability—the present acquired and innate ability to perform motor skills of a general or fundamental nature (Barrow & McGee, 1964).

goal-free model—method of program evaluation in which an evaluator identifies the outcomes of a program without knowing the goals of the program.

G study—generalizability study; utilized to partition observed score variance and ascertain components and percentages of variation associated with the various facets analyzed.

halo effect—rater bias caused by previous knowledge about, or an impression of, an examinee.

health-related fitness—a specific type of physical fitness extending from birth to death that emphasizes a person's state of health and includes those physiological factors that afford some protection against coronary heart disease, obesity, and musculoskeletal dysfunction.

hierarchical linear models—HLM; procedures that are claimed to permit a more detailed examination of both the correlates of change and the identification of change (as well as its prediction). Somewhat similar to ANOVA methods.

homoscedasticity—equal spread; assumes that the variances of dependent variables for each value of the independent variable are the same.

independent variable—the X variable of a regression equation. Often called the *predictor variable*.

index of reliability—square root of the reliability (or generalizability) coefficient, which indicates the theoretical correlation between true and observed scores in classical test theory and between universe and observed scores in generalizability theory.

initial score—score obtained before change is expected to occur; commonly abbreviated X. Used in analysis of change.

interclass correlation coefficient—a correlation coefficient, based on the bivariate correlation coefficient, indicating the degree of relationship between measures on two test administrations.

internal consistency reliability—an estimate of the reliability of a set of repeated measures of a test that were all collected on the same day.

interval scale—scale that describes data with a meaningful order and equal distances between scores.

intraclass correlation coefficient—a correlation coefficient, based on ANOVA procedures, indicating the degree of relationship between two or more repeated measures of a test.

intrinsic rational validity—a method for assessing content-related evidence for written tests for which there is no clearly defined universe of content and behaviors (e.g., aptitude tests).

item bank—large pool of test items from which a subset can be drawn in order to create tests.

item calibration—estimation of item parameters from IRT models.

item information—a measure of how precisely abilities can be estimated.

item response—the answer to a test item as given by an examinee (e.g., the selected alternative in a multiple-choice item).

item response theory—IRT; a measurement theory treating the test item and the examinee's response to the item as a source of information about the underlying ability of the examiner and the characteristics of the item.

knowledge—a structure of ideas, concepts, and relationships known to an individual or humankind.

latent trait—ability of the examinee.

least-squares criterion—statistical criterion used to develop a regression equation. The sum of the residual scores equals zero.

Likert Scale—scale containing both favorable and unfavorable statements. The examinee selects one of several responses to indicate the degree of agreement or disagreement with each statement.

LISREL—a flexible computer program used to establish structural relationships within a set of data. Can be used either to examine a measurement model or to examine a structural-equations model.

logical validity—a method for assessing content-related evidence for motor skill tests. *See also* **intrinsic rational validity.**

logistic regression analysis—a regression model in which the dependent variable is categorical and the independent variable(s) may be continuous or categorical. The model provides a probability estimate of being in one category or another.

magnitude scaling—ratio scaling method of quantifying stimuli (physical, sensory, or social-psychological) on a continuum relative to a reference point.

mainframe—a centralized computer system, accessible simultaneously and interactively by a number of users; makes a wide variety of software facilities available. Typically requires a specialized support staff for maintenance and operation.

marker variables—the term for variables in a factor analysis that are selected to measure a specific dimension hypothetically.

mastery test—a type of criterion-referenced measure that uses a performance standard; designed to classify an examinee into two or more categories (e.g., pass-fail or master-nonmaster).

maximum likelihood—method of estimating parameters from observed data.

measurement—the process of assigning numbers to properties of objects, organisms, or events according to some rule.

memory drum theory—neurological theory of motor performance that suggests that motor ability is specific to individual tasks rather than general for many tasks.

meta-analysis—a method of quantifying the results of many studies of the same hypothesis.

microcomputer—a small computer that can be placed on a desktop and typically is used by individuals and organizations to handle small amounts of data.

Monte Carlo study—a computer simulation approach in which data are generated to test hypotheses. This is in contrast to an empirical study in which data are collected from subjects.

multiple attempt–single item tests—MASI tests (i.e., repeated attempts at a single task).

multiple discriminant analysis—MDA; multivariate correlation technique that establishes the relationship between a set of predictor variables and a categorical criterion measure. Used primarily in construct validity.

multiple regression—the regression method using one dependent variable and two or more independent variables.

nominal scale—classification of objects with attributes in common into categories.

nomological net—a hypothesized network of interrelationships between a construct and observables and other constructs. Validation of a construct is inferred from empirical analysis of the nomological net. *See also* **construct validity.**

norm-referenced evaluation—an evaluation process involving a hierarchical ordering of individuals in which a student's test score is compared with those of other students.

norm-referenced measurement—an approach to measurement based on individual differences; test score compared with other scores in the distribution.

norm-referenced standards—standards developed by comparing the performance of individuals against the performance of the group.

objectivity—the degree of agreement between two or more judges as to the scores of a group performing some task.

observed score—usually an examinee's number-correct score.

open item—item that asks examinees to respond in their own words, rather than select a response from a fixed set of possibilities.

ordinal scale—reflects the rank or order of scores, but not the amount of difference between scores.

parameter estimates—values of the parameters obtained from the item responses (i.e., a statistical "best guess" at the value of the true but unknown parameter).

parameter invariance—the idea that examinees' abilities should not change when examinees are administered a different set of test items and that item parameters should not change when the items are administered to a different population of examinees.

perceived exertion—subjective evaluation of the intensity of exercise.

physical fitness—the ability to carry out daily tasks with vigor and alertness, without undue fatigue, and with ample energy to enjoy leisure-time pursuits and to meet unforeseen emergencies (Clarke, 1971).

physicalism-subjectivism dilemma—deals with the issue of whether equal change scores at various points on the scale account for equal changes in the phenomenon being measured.

polynomial regression—method of developing a prediction model to define a nonlinear relationship between the dependent and independent variables.

posterior distribution—a combination of the prior distribution and new information that is used in a subsequent validity generalization study when the hypothesis has not been confirmed.

predictive validity design—validity studies that seek to assess the degree to which scores on a predictor test can accurately predict scores on a criterion test.

predictor test—a test being considered as a substitute for a criterion test.

primacy effect—tendency of an individual to select the first alternative in a set of responses, regardless of content.

prior distribution—information from past research used to test the validity generalization hypothesis.

proportion of agreement index—the proportion of decisions consistently made across test occasions.

randomly representative—the levels of a facet are said to be randomly representative when the levels were not selected but randomly chosen for inclusion; thus, they are said to be randomly representative of the possible levels available in the universe.

rating scale—a formalized subjective evaluation of a person with regard to specific traits, qualities, or behaviors.

ratio scale—scale that describes data with a meaningful order, equal distance between scores, and an absolute origin.

raw residualized gain score—score obtained by subtracting the predicted Y score (Yp) from the observed Y (final) score, where the Yp is the final score with X (initial score) partialled out; commonly abbreviated G_r. Measure of the degree to which an individual gained more or less than would be expected, given his or her initial status.

reactivity—influence of a prior test on a subsequent test due to a sensitizing or heightened awareness of the affective behavior being measured.

recency effect—tendency of an individual to select the last alternative in a set of responses, regardless of content.

redundancy coefficient—a coefficient created in a canonical-correlation analysis that relates the amount of variance of the original variables of one space to the variance of a set of variables in another space.

regression—statistical model used to predict performance on one variable, the dependent variable, from another, the independent variable.

regression intercept—the point at which the regression line crosses the Y-axis; represents the value of the dependent variable associated with zero on the independent variable.

regression line—often termed the *line of best fit*; the line defined by predicting the dependent variable from the independent variable.

regression slope—rate at which Y changes with change on X.

regression to the mean—the tendency of subjects who initially score at the extreme of the population distribution to score nearer to the mean on a second testing.

relative reliability—reliability estimated by utilizing a correlation coefficient.

reliability—consistency of scores or of an individual's performance on a test; absence of measurement error.

residual gain score—score in which that portion of Y (final score) that could be linearly predicted from X (initial score) was removed from Y, resulting in a G (gain) score uncorrelated with X.

residualized difference score—*See* **raw residualized gain score.**

residual score—difference between the actual dependent variable and the dependent variable estimated from the independent variable.

robust—in factor-analytic terminology, the result of a factor analysis that is consistent across a number of solutions.

SAS—Statistical Analysis System; a series of computer programs for conducting statistical analyses.

self-concept—feelings or cognitions about oneself. Dimensions of self-concept include personal, critical, and physical.

self-report—responses to a questionnaire, inventory, or interview made by an individual about his or her beliefs, opinions, or behaviors.

semantic-differential scale—scale consisting of bipolar adjectives pertaining to an attitude object. Addresses three dimensions of a concept: evaluation, activity, and potency.

sequential test—test which allows test length to vary as a function of examinee's ability.

single attempt-multiple item tests—SAMI tests (e.g., the usual written test that contains many different items, each attempted only once by each examinee).

Spearman-Brown prophecy formula—a formula for estimating the reliability of a test if its length is increased.

speed test—an examination having a time limit short enough to prevent many examinees from finishing it.

split-halves—a procedure whereby half the items on a test are used to establish one score for an examinee and the other half are used to establish another, independent score. The correlation between these two scores, corrected with the Spearman-Brown formula, is used to estimate test reliability.

spreadsheet—a matrix of columns and rows that can be used to manipulate numerical information. Typically used for financial planning, budgeting, and numerical analyses.

SPSS^x—Statistical Package for the Social Sciences; a series of computer programs for conducting statistical analyses.

squared-error loss agreement—the squared deviations of individual scores from the cutoff score.

stability reliability—an estimate of the reliability of a set of repeated measures of a test that were collected on two or more days.

standard error of estimate—SE$_{est}$; statistic used to quantify the accuracy of a regression equation.

standard error of measurement—an estimate of the absolute reliability of a test; the amount of error to expect in a person's criterion score.

state anxiety—temporary form of anxiety that reflects one's reaction to a perceived threatening situation.

statistics—a method of summarizing and analyzing data for purposes of interpretation.

systems analysis model—method of program evaluation which addresses efficiency and productivity but is inconsistent with the educational setting since it does not provide information on the whole picture of the program.

table of specifications—an outline of the content of a test specifying the percentage of items dealing with specific content areas and types of abilities.

tailored test—*See* **adaptive test.**

test reliability—a dimension of test validity that refers to the degree to which scores are free from measurement error.

test-retest—a procedure to estimate test reliability by correlating scores from two administrations of the test to the same examinees.

test-retest reliability—*See* **stability reliability.**

test validity—evidence supporting the accuracy of test score interpretation.

threshold loss agreement—the degree of misclassification error when *all* errors are assumed to be equally serious for a specified cutoff score.

trait anxiety—general, enduring form of anxiety that is part of one's personality; a predisposition to be anxious and to perceive certain situations as threatening.

transactional model—method of program evaluation in which the evaluator studies the curriculum in its natural environment without manipulation.

true change score—difference between the estimated true Y (final) and X (initial) score, that is, with both scores corrected for errors of measurement.

true residualized gain score—score uncorrelated with the true X (initial) score.

true score—expected number-correct score that an examinee should obtain if the test had perfect reliability or no error; also, the expected value of an examinee's observed score after an infinite number of (theoretical) administrations of the test.

Type I error—the probability of rejecting a null hypothesis when it is true.

Type II error—the probability of failing to reject a false null hypothesis.

validity—the extent to which a test measures what it is intended to measure.

validity generalization—a method of synthesizing evidence of validity from studies of the same predictor-criterion combination.

variance components—estimates of the variation associated with facets in a generalizability theory analysis.

INDEX

Discriminant validity, 39
Domain-referenced validity, 120–124

E

Evaluation
  definition, 11

F

Factor analysis, 158–165, 278

G

Generalizability theory, 9, 73–94
  applications, 92–93
  computer programs, 78–79
  D study, 76–77, 84–85, 90–92
  expected mean squares, 77–78
  facet, 74–75, 82, 86–87
  G coefficients, 84
  G study, 76, 82–83, 90
  multivariate generalizability, 93–94
  variance components, 79, 82, 87, 89–90

I

Improvement
  see change, measurement of
Interclass correlation coefficient, 47
Intraclass correlation coefficient, 47–60,
  303
Item analysis, 262–268
Item response theory, 9, 10, 230–239, 263,
  292–293, 360
  comparison with classical test theory,
  230–232
  goodness-of-fit, 238–239
  guessing parameter, 232
  item banking, 239–240
  item characteristic curve, 232
  latent trait, 231

local independence assumption, 235
mastery testing, 133
maximum likelihood estimation, 236–
  238
one-parameter model, 233
parameter estimation, 235–239
parameter invariance, 233
Poisson model, 243
three-parameter model, 235
two-parameter model, 234

K

Kappa coefficient, 141–146
Knowledge tests, 251–269
  item analysis, 262–268
    criterion-referenced tests, 267–268
    difficulty index, 263, 264–265
    discrimination index, 263, 265–267
  reliability, 252–260
    criterion-referenced test, 259–260
    examinee, 254
    factors affecting coefficient, 258–259
    scorer, 256–257
    standard error of measurement, 257–
    258
    test (internal consistency), 254–256
  validity, 260–262
    content, 260–261
    criterion-referenced, 261–262

L

Likert scale, 281–283

M

Mastery testing, 124, 241, 252
  see criterion-referenced measurement
Measurement
  advantages, 11
  applied, 5–8
  definition, 12